John :

2

(with thanks

On Madness

introduction to Gipps' work).

Also available from Bloomsbury

Great Philosophical Objections to Artificial Intelligence, by Eric Dietrich, Chris Fields and John P. Sullins
Knowledge and Reality in Nine Questions, by Matthew Davidson
Philosophers on Consciousness, edited by Jack Symes
The Evolution of Consciousness, by Paula Droege

On Madness

Understanding the Psychotic Mind

Richard G. T. Gipps

BLOOMSBURY ACADEMIC

LONDON • NEW YORK • OXFORD • NEW DELHI • SYDNEY

BLOOMSBURY ACADEMIC
Bloomsbury Publishing Plc
50 Bedford Square, London, WC1B 3DP, UK
1385 Broadway, New York, NY 10018, USA
29 Earlsfort Terrace, Dublin 2, Ireland

BLOOMSBURY, BLOOMSBURY ACADEMIC and the Diana logo are trademarks of
Bloomsbury Publishing Plc

First published in Great Britain 2022

Copyright © Richard G. T. Gipps, 2022

Richard G. T. Gipps has asserted his right under the Copyright, Designs and Patents Act,
1988, to be identified as Author of this work.

For legal purposes the Acknowledgements on p. vi constitute an
extension of this copyright page.

Cover Image: Josef Forster – Selbstporträt [Mann ohne Schwerkraft; 1916-1921],
Inv. No. 04494, © Prinzhorn Collection, University Hospital Heidelberg.

A catalogue record for this book is available from the British Library.

A catalog record for this book is available from the Library of Congress.

ISBN: HB: 978-1-3501-9253-9
       PB: 978-1-3501-9254-6
       ePDF: 978-1-3501-9255-3
       eBook: 978-1-3501-9257-7

Typeset by RefineCatch Limited, Bungay, Suffolk
Printed and bound in Great Britain

To find out more about our authors and books visit www.bloomsbury.com
and sign up for our newsletters.

Contents

Acknowledgements

For their good influence on my intellectual formation I owe a debt of gratitude to my excellent teachers Ron Pickering, Quassim Cassam, and Tim Thornton.

For her constant solicitude and also her intellectual companionship during the writing of this book I heartily thank my true friend Sanneke de Haan.

For his firm friendship, supportive challenging of my thought, and for reading and commenting on the entire manuscript, I'm ever grateful to Roger Teichmann.

Cover image

Josef Forster (1878–1949) – Selbstporträt [Mann ohne Schwerkraft; 1916–1921] – Self portrait [Man without gravity] – Inv. No. 04494, © Prinzhorn Collection, University Hospital Heidelberg.

Forster created this image whilst resident at a psychiatric hospital in Regensburg where he was an inpatient from 1916 to 1941. The man he depicts enjoys only a tenuous contact with the world (by means of stilts) and with other people (from behind a scarf). The text which Forster placed on the image tells of how it represents the fate of a body which has become weightless; it must therefore now be anchored using weighted stilts. His weightlessness does, however, also afford this man the ability to fly over the earth with great speed. Forster himself aspired to a condition both of utter self-sufficiency (nourishing himself with his own secretions) and of being able to float free of the world.

Introduction

The problem of delusion

The problem of delusion – *das Wahnproblem* – constitutes the central puzzle of descriptive psychopathology. The question 'what is it to suffer delusion?' is easy to ask, but surprisingly hard to answer. Hence the problem. Consider the following from Carlton Brown's *Brainstorm*:

> One day in July I discovered that the features of the Chinese lady [in the portrait on the kitchen wall] had become suffused with the absolute semblance of life. As soon as I had accustomed myself to the surprise of this discovery, I consulted her eyes for verification of each of my enraptured and increasingly convincing intimations of immortality, or for condemnation of the thoughts and actions that still marked me as a mortal, and found what I sought in their vibrant, eloquent depths. Our communion was wordless but complete. She was at once Judy's mother, my own, and Ann, the friend with whom my daughter was staying in the country, a warm, capable woman with two lovely children of her own. Her eyes mirrored the soul of the eternal Madonna whose son I was in the process of becoming, and from them I received implicit instructions in the filling of my new role.[1]

We find here no great problem of intelligibility if we read Carlton's words as poetic evocation, as expressive of metaphor. Perhaps we'd judge his prose and manner of thought overwrought or self-indulgent, but not unintelligible. And yet this would all be quite wrong: Carlton isn't here speaking in metaphor; his thought and experience instead evince delusion. Our recognition of this fact is of a piece with our failure to make sense of his words as expressing literal or metaphorical thought. But what is it to suffer delusion? And what could possibly legitimate taking our own failures in comprehension for a measure of his mind's derangement?

Delusion is sometimes thought of as just one amongst several symptoms of psychosis. In truth, however, it is its *sine qua non*, and so we may generalize our problem of delusion to include also such questions as 'what is it to be properly counted "psychotic" or "mad"?' And since certain psychoses (such as the schizophrenias, or mania-involving 'bipolar disorders' like Carlton's) constitute paradigms of psychiatry's central organizing concept (namely 'mental illness'), we may also fairly include within this problem's scope the question: 'what is it to suffer paradigmatic mental illness?'

Such questions are pressing for us because, whilst we know mental illness, psychosis, and delusion when we see them, we don't have a good reflective grasp of what it is we know; we can't readily articulate it. The following words penned in 1940 remain true today: 'no one has yet discovered a way of [accurately] defining ... delusion without invoking ... an underlying pathological process. Yet ... the word "pathological" pre-empts the very search for those criteria which make it pathological.'[2] The present text's central task, then, is to solve this problem of delusion by developing our understanding of what it is for our thought to become pathological in such a way as inspires description of its thinkers as 'delusional', 'mad', or 'mentally ill'. Along the way we shall see too why it need manifest no prejudice against our fellow man to use our own incomprehension as a measure of his rational disturbance.

What shall be our approach? It may help prepare the reader if at this point it's noted that what follows isn't a work of psychology – or, at least, it doesn't attempt to address the problem of delusion by making use of the methods of psychological science. Its form of enquiry is instead philosophical. Rather than aiming to increase our stock of empirical knowledge about psychosis, or offer new hypotheses, or help us better distinguish delusional from non-delusional thought in our practice, it instead tasks itself with developing our reflective understanding of what we mean when we talk of 'delusion', 'psychosis', and 'madness'. Readers of the scientific and clinical literature will often encounter there the tacit supposition that questions of what it is to be psychotic, or delusional, or mentally ill, can be quickly disposed of through definition, allowing the scientific work to then proceed apace. And yet – to now anticipate a theme of Chapter 2 – it's typical of such definitions to either misarticulate such phenomena (as when they conflate it with such false, non-standard, and ill-argued belief as is quite sane) or to be tacitly empty (as when they invoke an unexplicated concept of *pathological* belief). In truth, to think one could articulate the meaning of such fundamental concepts as 'delusion' or 'sane judgement' through mere definition is already to misunderstand just how tricky it is to bring such concepts into reflective view. The foundational concepts of our lives – concepts such as *space, time, life, value, meaning, sanity,* and *madness* – resist such easy capture. The sort of reflective articulation which is apt for the capture of the denizens of the higher floors of those conceptual buildings in which we live out our lives is scarcely adequate when we're considering these buildings' foundations. And so whilst the itch of the problem of delusion is immediately clear, the apt means to scratch it is not. We're called on, then, to stay with our questions rather than embark on empirical solutions, to more clearly articulate our puzzlement, to put aside pre-defined methods, and to simply think as hard and as clearly as we can about what it means to be in or out of contact with reality. To do all this is to practise what we call 'philosophy'. What follows, then, is a work not of empirical, but of philosophical, psychopathology.

An apophatic psychopathology

The central contribution of the present work is that which is herein styled an 'apophatic' psychopathology, and it will help situate the later discussion if something of this is spelled out in advance. The term is in fact owed to theology where we find talk of apophatic or negative, as opposed to cataphatic or positive, approaches to our understanding of God.[3] And yet the ambition in borrowing the term here is very far from one of importing theological concerns into psychopathology. It's instead to give clear shape to a certain form of understanding which is otherwise easy to overlook or misunderstand.

Consider first the term's theological use. Cataphatic theology is in the business of making intelligible and true claims about God's attributes – positively predicating of Him qualities such as beauty, love, truth, goodness, and mercy. Theology has however also developed the conviction that our language is essentially inadequate when it comes to articulating a transcendent God's being. Our terms are necessarily conditioned by their applications to this or that phenomenon within our sublunary lives. But turn not to another mere being, but to that 'ground of being' in which everything 'lives and moves and has its being', and their application falls apart. As the theologian has it, our very idea of God is essentially of that which exceeds what is thinkable for us. Yet rather than call it a theological day, an apophatic approach understands this collapse of predicative language as itself revelatory of God's being. It's precisely as we understand why and how God's transcendence is such as to prevent the cogent ascription of even those properties which we're most moved to so ascribe to Him that we approach closer to Him.

To turn now to psychopathology: the claim worked out in what follows is that we can best understand the depth and character of the psychotic subject's disturbance by understanding why some of the things we most want to say of her cannot strictly speaking be said. The fact is that various of our epistemic and psychological predicates presuppose, for their meaningful application, the sanity of their subject. They presuppose, that is, as conditions of their cogent application, that here we have to do with someone who may be found ordinarily intelligible because she has her feet sufficiently on the ground, and has expressions and acts and utterances which sufficiently hang together. To prescind from taking our ordinary meaning-reading, attitude-ascribing, stance when engaging she who's lost to delusion might look to some like a dehumanizing attitude to take towards the psychiatric subject. (And such an assessment may in some sense be correct whenever such prescinding is precipitate – although we should also note that to describe someone as delusional is already to characterize her as suffering a disturbance which only a human being could suffer.) But to insist on engaging in ordinary rational predication, when the object of predication is suffering from catastrophic degrees of inner and outer alienation and disintegration, is itself to radically falsify her – just as insisting on making positive predications of God is similarly to falsify Him. In the divine case, what's ignored is His transcendence; in the psychopathological case, what's overlooked is her brokenness – or to put it otherwise, what's overlooked is the particular form of her suffering.

Retrieval

Having sketched out something of the work's topic and approach it may help, before we turn to an outline of its contents, to share something of its rationale. Perhaps it could be said that a work of philosophy needs no motivation other than a desire to aptly characterize its subject matter. In truth, however, philosophy is most often called for in the face of pre-existing tacit tendencies to mischaracterize that subject – i.e. when we're not simply ignorant but latently confused. Especially when that subject is human life in its sane and insane aspect, the risk is that reflective self-mischaracterizations trickle down into and impoverish our psychological theory, our clinical sensibility and endeavours, and ultimately the very form of our self-enaction. (Iris Murdoch: 'Man is a creature who makes pictures of himself and then comes to resemble the picture.'[4]) Furthermore, whilst some mischaracterizations of human life are merely accidental, the product of the sheer difficulty of the self-reflective enterprise, others rather appear to result from a tacit motivated deflection. From deflection, that is, which takes us away from a topic that's too difficult or painful to stay with and towards one that's more rationally tractable and emotionally tolerable.[5] Our task, then, will be one of recovering or retrieving true understandings of psychotic life and thought from beneath the accretions of misunderstanding which have accumulated in the literature.[6]

Forms of psychopathological understanding, and our acknowledgement of aspects of psychopathological reality, rise and fall together. Should you be aiming to unfairly dismiss some or other description of psychopathological reality, the surest method you'll find will involve judging the method for disclosing that reality wanting according to criteria appropriate only to another method. By way of example, consider a clinical presentation I once attended at a psychiatric research institute. A psychologist presented a history and psychological formulation of a young woman who was sometimes psychotic. His patient and he had arrived at an idiographic (i.e. particular-to-her) psychological understanding of what triggered and maintained her relapses. But the dean of the institute asked rather pointedly if there was actually any published research evidence suggesting that events of such kinds really did typically cause psychotic episodes. The implication being that, if there was no such general evidence, then this particular psychological understanding was unsound. The dean's own psychiatric research, it should be said, was of a decidedly nomothetic form, which is to say that it aimed to provide evidence of the causation of mental illness through assessing correlations of putative causes and psychotic experiences in large population samples. Now there's nothing wrong with that, of course, but it hardly provides a useful model for assessing the validity of claims about the causes of an individual's relapses, since people differ in what they find disturbing. We have methods for distinguishing between valid causal explanations and just-so stories at the individual psychological level, but they typically don't reference population level findings. What seemed to have happened was that the dean's reflective grasp of what made for viable understanding of that form he himself was after had impaired his ability to recognize even quite ordinary other such forms. Hence the need for retrieval.

We just considered the importance of retrieving one form of causal understanding from under the shadow of another, but far more significant for what follows will be retrieving non-causal forms of understanding from under the shadow of the causal. Psychology as a discipline is notoriously bedevilled by forgetfulness concerning its own past insights into the inner life of psychosis, insights developed, in particular, within phenomenological and psychoanalytical psychology. (Nineteenth-century psychiatry developed the ability to paint the lot of the insane with tolerant and humanizing brushstrokes. Early twentieth-century psychopathological science, by incorporating the methods and understandings developed in the humanities, learned to also depict perspective and affectivity in its psychopathological portraiture. Later psychopathological science, now modelling itself more singularly on the natural sciences – i.e. to the exclusion of the humanities – sometimes degenerated into painting by numbers.) And all too often we find it scientistically misconstruing and dismissing such contributions as unscientific, unproven causal hypotheses – rather than recognizing them for the non-hypothesis-proffering attempts to richly describe or characterize psychological life that they are.[7] The problem is especially noticeable when a cognitive or experimental psychology takes an interest only in psychometrically assaying the objective performance of psychotic subjects. Such an assay may be quite proper in itself – but the difficulty which emerges is when those informed by such work, or the psychologists themselves, start to imagine that to be suffering from delusion and hallucination is nothing other than to perceive, reason, and speak in the ways they've discovered the psychotic person to do.[8] Much about the loss of reality contact, the substitute world of delusional and hallucinatory phantasm, the terror of self-dissolution, the chilling diminishment of vitality, the baffling negativism, and the dementing contradictions of schizophrenic ambivalence, now become quite lost from psychopathological view. With such a constraining vision in play, we may even lose sight of the fact that it was the goal of re-establishing some kind of meaningful empathic contact with the delusional person's interior that was our original psychopathological aspiration. (On Monday the art enthusiast enters the Sistine Chapel to learn to better appreciate its sublime artistry; she stays there until Friday when she emerges cheerfully sporting a mere pigment analysis, having somehow quite forgotten why she ever went in.)

Deflection

Philosophical retrieval is necessitated by forgetfulness, self-misunderstanding, and deflection. And we naturally deflect from what Cora Diamond has called 'difficulties of reality'. Working to retrieve psychotic experience, as this book does, requires standing up against that impulse. So what is a 'difficulty of reality'? Diamond introduces the concept with reference to a poem by Ted Hughes which concerns a photograph from 1914 of six smiling lively young country-dwelling men – who six months later were all killed in the war. She describes our experience of not being able to assimilate what we encounter when looking at this photograph, and how this:

> is capable of making one go mad to try, to bring together in thought what cannot be thought: the impossibility of anyone's being more alive than these smiling men, nothing's being more dead. . . . [W]e take something in reality to be resistant to our thinking it, or possibly to be painful in its inexplicability, difficult in that way, or perhaps awesome and astonishing in its inexplicability. We take things so. And the

things we take so may simply not, to others, present the kind of difficulty – of being hard or impossible or agonizing to get one's mind round.[9]

One place we find the urge to deflect from difficulties of reality is in such psychopathological research as wants to characterize psychotic thought as something to be 'decoded' so that a damaged surface may give way to an intact and hence assimilable interior. Thus: 'Some schizophrenic patients say things that are barely comprehensible, but very fascinating. It is easy to believe that, if we could understand what they are saying, we would also understand "schizophrenia".'[10] Or: 'the psychotic part of the mind … stores … ideographs … Our task in everyday psychiatry is to decipher the meaning of these ideographs. This is comparable to solving crossword puzzle clues.'[11] The philosopher Ludwig Wittgenstein offers much the same thought about Sigmund Freud's take on madness: 'Freud's idea: In madness the lock is not destroyed, only altered; the old key can no longer unlock it, but it could be opened by a differently constructed key.'[12] The desire runs strong to think that the intriguing and sometimes incomprehensible communications of the psychotic subject are ciphers awaiting decoding. And to be sure, delusional and disordered thought[13] truly are baffling and intriguing. Yet such approaches, especially ones that liken the desire to grasp delusion to a desire to solve crossword clues, can often be occlusive. What they occlude is, in part, the fact that psychotic thought is not simply puzzling but deeply disturbed – and deeply disturbing. Consider what the philosopher and psychopathologist Karl Jaspers says: 'The fact of the psychoses is a puzzle to us. They are the unsolved problem of human life as such.' So far so deflective, one might think – yet his thought redeems itself by how it continues: 'The fact that they exist is the concern of everyone. That they are there and that the world and human life is such as to make them possible and inevitable not only gives us pause but makes us shudder.'[14] Here we arrive at Jaspers' recognition of the fact that on encountering a psychotic person we meet on the one hand a human subject with her individual history and personality, someone who knowingly or unwittingly inexorably expresses to us something of her ownmost feelings, thoughts, and experiences – and yet, on the other, with someone whose human intelligibility can now, when she's in her psychosis, be so radically out of joint, her living meaning so deranged, her sensibility so jarred and jarring, that our sense of a common humanity can be jeopardized. None of this simply puzzles us. It instead inspires a deep disquiet, one connected in part to our fearful recognition of all of our sanity's contingency, but also one that's of a piece with our understanding that to encounter another in his psychosis is to visit a site of the tragic and the terrible. For psychotic experience is often terrifying for the sufferer, and even when it isn't explicitly that, what it constitutes an escape from – terror, brokenness, and overwhelm – often is.

A central claim of this work, then, is that psychopathology requires all the help it can get from philosophy to help it bear with, and offer acknowledgement to, the terrible facts of psychotic life, rather than deflect away from them into comfortable puzzle-solving pursuits such as armchair cognitive modelling. Three forms of this reassuring yet unhelpful deflective tendency appear as the object of critique in the pages to follow.

One such has it that what appear to be deep disturbances to mindedness itself are really only surface disturbances to the form taken by thought's articulation. If we could only find our way past these expressive distortions – so the thought goes – the underlying, and *ex hypothesi* intact, thought would be perfectly intelligible to us. This 'expressive' approach – sometimes met with in cognitive psychological explanations of psychotic experience – promises to draw the psychotic subject back within the fold of a common humanity; or rather asserts that they never really left in the first place. Its normalizing[15] agenda frequently presents itself as the rehumanization of psychiatry – as offering a humane recognition to the psychotic subject which has been lost by medicine's pathologizing disposition. But the clear risk is that it instead turns its face against the true dislocation of the psychotic subject and, in this way, fails to offer him any meaningful recognition in his mind-abrogating disintegration, reason-compromising uprootedness, and disintegrative terror.[16] (The perils of taking an 'expressive' tack are considered in relation to delusion in Chapter 2, formal thought disorder in Chapter 8, and diagnostic practice in Chapter 10.)

Another form of deflection, one that has been dubbed the 'lost tribe romantic' approach,[17] may be characterized with the suggestion that 'these words and deeds truly do make sense to her, if not to me; it's just that she lives in her own private world of meaning'. This proposal, which substitutes a mere incongruity of form of mindedness (between those dubbed psychotic and those dubbed sane) for any deep corruption of mindedness itself (within the psychotic), is surely a comforting one. (We find something of this romantic vision in some of our more radical philosophical expositors of psychotic thought.[18]) And yet we may rightly ask whether the notion of an essentially incommunicable private world of meaning on which it relies doesn't itself want for coherence. (This topic is pursued in Chapters 4 and 10.)

When encountering the psychotic subject in her delusion, we might find ourselves wishing we could, in Naomi Eilan's helpful formulation, 'solve simultaneously for understanding and utter strangeness'.[19] The two forms of deflection just mentioned ultimately sacrifice something of 'utter strangeness' in their attempt to redeem the psychotic subject from his dislocation. Both approaches typically pit themselves against a more traditional – third – strategy for managing the difficulty of psychotic reality. Such an approach, which sacrifices 'understanding' rather than 'strangeness', sometimes finds its practical expression in psychiatry's more biomedical strands. 'Medicate, watch, and sympathetically wait for the currently void human subject to return to the scene' becomes its ambition. The patient is now no longer engaged with in her psychosis; her body is, as it were, looked after until her mind returns. The approach is also met with in many a sufferer: 'the illness wasn't me; it didn't mean anything; now, however, *I* am back and we can forget about all of *that*'. Madness becomes but dysfunction. The temptations of this stance for both doctor and patient are clear: we don't now need to find a way to bear the difficulty of reality presented to us by psychosis since really, when the patient is in her psychosis, nobody is at home. The risks, however, are also clear: the intrinsically dignity-damaging psychotic process is compounded by an alienating clinical practice, and the opportunity is lost not only of offering recognition to the patient in her suffering, but also of grasping and working through her pains and predicaments, leaving her vulnerable to relapse.

Outline

The present work's focus is the question of what it is to suffer delusion, but Chapter 1 begins by stepping back a little from this to first ask: 'What is it for a mind to become ill?' The invocation of the 'illness' concept in the psychiatric context is often presumed, by psychiatry's critics, with little actual argument, to imply an ambition to medicalize madness or force a biological understanding of it upon us. That presumption is far from the tack taken in this first chapter, where the argument is rather that 'illness' here functions as something like a metaphor, one which serves to focus our attention on the suffering, the motivation, the internal (self-sustaining) causation, the diminished agency and especially the disturbed rational reality contact here met with.

Now disturbances of rationality make for disturbances of intelligibility, and it will be an essential theme of what follows that the delusional mind is essentially unamenable to a certain kind of (rational) understanding. The theme is famous from the work of Jaspers, and it has been frequently condemned by such psychologists as see it as dehumanizing or as invalidating of the psychotic subject. The book's second chapter, then, shall be concerned with understanding just what Jaspers had in mind with his claim of delusion's 'ununderstandability', with distinguishing the different forms that understanding can take, and with showing then the different ways in which delusion both may, and may not, be intelligible. The result is a retrieval of the central psychopathological claim that delusion is essentially opaque to rational understanding.

The claim that psychotic illness involves disturbed rationality requires considerable finessing, since reason's loss in the delusional mind is not primarily a matter of failures in reason*ing*. A disturbance to reason may propagate up to include aberrant inference, but (what in a purely formal sense would count as) valid reasoning may even be put in the service of a delusional system's elaboration. Rational impairment here rather has to do with a disturbance of the more fundamental matter of our reality contact, and the task of Chapter 3 is the elaboration of this central psychopathological notion. Of especial concern will be its differentiation from such far more trivial disturbances of mind as can be conceptualized as false representations of reality. At its hinges the mind is, we may say, itself of a piece with the world; it isn't here in the business of standing back from and representing it. And it's only by understanding that mind here takes an enactive form – one fully immanent within our active and interactive world-engagements, rather than one relegated to a hived-off, inner, domain of representation – that we can begin to understand what it is for us to become unhinged. Philosophers who take an interest in the nature of reason's most essential form, and who are suspicious of the relevance of deductive inference to their topic, sometimes reference 'madness' as an intuitive antonym for their topic.[20] The chapter's mission, then, is to render this more than intuitive, so that we may enjoy a true reflective understanding of what it is to be, as we say, 'in (or out of) one's right mind', to enjoy or suffer the loss of sane judgement.

Chapter 4 considers the related question of what it is to live, as we also say, in 'a world of one's own'. 'Reality testing', rather than 'reality contact', is the key concept here. And just as Chapter 3 deploys a notion of thought's faulty *mirroring of* the world as a foil for its own truer grasp of disturbed reality contact as a disturbance of thought's *footing in* the world, Chapter 4 deploys a concept of *mistaking imagination for reality* as a foil for its own truer characterization of lost reality testing. The analysis offered there consists not in any alternative positive psychological characterization of the phenomenon; it is instead 'negative' or – to now make use of that redeployed theological term of art, in the new sense spelled out above – 'apophatic'. To have reality testing fail is to suffer a state of mind which cannot now be properly characterized either in terms of imagination or in terms of world-directed cognition. Or, to put it otherwise, it is criterial of being in a world of your own that you no longer meet such conditions as are required before the question, 'is he indulging imagination or does he really believe what he's saying?' can sensibly be asked of you.

This 'apophatic' tack is continued in the next five chapters, which offer similarly 'negative' characterizations of various aspects of the psychopathology of psychotic illness. Thus Chapter 5 considers what it is to suffer such self-disturbances as are commonly styled 'passivity experiences' (as when I somehow seem to take my own thoughts, feelings, or movements for moments of another's agency or subjectivity). Positive psychological accounts aim to shed light on such disordered experience by showing how it could be possible to experience one's own thoughts as belonging properly to another. The apophatic account offered here, by contrast, sheds a truer light on the depth of disturbance met with in these phenomena by showing how their most apt evocation is instead necessarily in terms that articulate something quite impossible. Those positive accounts posit an inner sense of self ('pre-reflective self-consciousness', 'self-presence', 'ipseity') an intelligible breakdown in which is thought to result in the psychopathological experience. The claim of Chapter 5 is not merely the destructive one that such accounts are themselves incoherent – but also the constructive, if yet apophatic, one that it's precisely through understanding why and how such positive accounts fail that we can approach closer to the psychotic subject in her brokenness.

Chapter 6 considers that overlapping set of psychopathological experiences which are commonly theorized as manifesting a breakdown in 'ego boundaries'. These are confusional experiences in which I become unclear, for example, as to which of you and I is the author and which the reader of this book. Once again the claim will be that the 'ego boundary' concept, when put to explanatory rather than merely descriptive work, risks making too much sense, as it were, of pathological experience – chalking it up to an in-the-dismal-circumstances understandable mistake – whilst making a simultaneous nonsense of ordinary non-confusional experience. Thankfully, however, the critique once again has more than a destructive effect, for it's precisely through reflectively appreciating the difference between psychopathological confusion and representational mistake that we can approach more closely to the psychotic subject in the depths of his derangement.

The topic of hallucination is the concern of Chapter 7. The foil for the approach taken herein is again provided by such accounts of hallucination as attempt to provide a positive psychological understanding of what it is. Hallucination has, for example, been explicated as inadvertent imagining or self-talk, or as a matter of enjoying inner images variably projected into the world. Such explications, however, turn out to be either non-elucidating redescriptions or incoherent explanations. Yet we shall see that it's by staying with the paradoxical experience of seeing or hearing what isn't there to be perceived that we do a better justice to the phenomenology. And by setting hallucination in relation to the loss of reality testing and reality contact, it becomes clear why it should be the mentally ill who can be most prone to ongoing hallucinatory experience.

Chapter 8 concerns itself with the phenomenon of formal thought disorder – as when someone's reasoning becomes, unbeknownst to them, quite incoherent. Approaches which relegate the disturbance merely to discourse are shown both to trivialize the disturbance and to require an alienated conception of thought's relation to communication. They, too, are tempted to render the psychotic subject newly intelligible by imagining him as suffering a merely expressive disturbance – but the falsification they indulge ends up taking us further away from the psychotic subject in his brokenness. By recovering the immanence of thought in discourse, and of discourse in the emotionally alive interpersonal encounter, we can better appreciate the depths of the disturbance, and the relation of disturbed thought to emotional perturbation, to damaged reality contact, and to reality testing.

The final two chapters diverge from the symptom-based organization of the previous five in order to deepen and generalize some of the lessons of Chapters 3 and 4. Thus Chapter 9 asks what it is for delusions and hallucinations to be sometimes characterizable as 'symbolic'. One fairly popular suggestion has it that such experiences, or their discursive expressions, may be treated as metaphor, and their meaning thereby retrieved in the same way that the sense of otherwise opaque discourse may sometimes be retrieved – i.e. by grasping that we'd wrongly treated as literal what instead should have been read as metaphor. That suggestion provides an apt foil for the understanding of psychotic symbolization developed here. This understanding stresses instead that a disturbance to reality testing makes not for metaphor but rather for a form of thought which is characterized negatively by the inapplicability to it of the literal/metaphorical distinction.

The book's final chapter has to do with what it styles the 'politics of insanity ascription'. The question, in short, is: who gets to call who 'mad', and what is their justification? The demonstrable meeting of diagnostic criteria is one thing, but the question here in play aims deeper than this to instead ask with what right anyone gets to say of themselves that their judgements are sane and another's are mad. The figure herein called the Realist hopes to justify his judgement by appeal to natural facts; the Idealist tells us that someone is mad just so long as the Idealist and her tribe judge them to be so; and the Relativist tells us that we all belong to tribes the acts and utterances of which are intelligible only to their own members. The intelligibility of the 'with what right?' question inspiring these three answers may, however, be contested. The upshot is that the attempt to render psychiatric judgement accountable can, when taken beyond a certain point, be seen to amount more to a failure, than to a taking, of psychiatric responsibility.

Let's take stock. The work which follows offers an answer to the question, 'what is it to suffer delusion?' It offers critique of such approaches as aim to diminish the clinician's disquiet by making delusion rationally comprehensible. Instead, it takes an 'apophatic' tack which sheds light on what it is to be deluded precisely by showing the failures of such ambitions to achieve delusion's rational comprehension. The goal is to thereby make visible the suffering of the psychotic subject – including, especially, that suffering which delusion itself aims to evade. And the intent of that is to resource us to retrieve and sit with the patient in her brokenness, rather than to 'rescue' her by hallucinating an extant rational order lying behind it. Yet despite, or in fact sometimes because of, the brokenness of her rational intelligibility, other forms of understanding – symbolic, motivational, phenomenological – can be seen to be available. Available, that is, so long as they too have first been retrieved from the institutionalized forgetfulness of much contemporary psychopathology. Throughout the work the method shall be strictly philosophical: if what follows attempts at any point to substitute for the exercise of pure thought something which an empirical scientist would recognize as methodologically sound – to substitute, for the sheer reflective apprehension of a phenomenon, something like, say, psychology's qualitative or quantitative methods – it shall be failing at its self-appointed task.

The reader may also, and naturally enough, want to ask, 'so where's he coming from?' To this question I shall here only answer that, to those familiar with them, the voices of Martin Heidegger, Karl Jaspers, the early R. D. Laing, Maurice Merleau-Ponty, Eugène Minkowski, Gilbert Ryle, Louis Sass, and especially the later Ludwig Wittgenstein, will doubtless sometimes be audible in the background. However, I shall again be failing at my task if, and to the extent that, grasping what I have to say depends on a prior acceptance of the bent of their thought.

1

Mental Illness

Introduction

Madness – psychosis – comes in varieties. Thus we distinguish between that which is a passing effect of somatic disease or intoxication, and that which constitutes mental illness proper. And mental illnesses come in varieties too, not all of which involve psychosis. Even so, the psychotic forms are paradigmatic, and it's these which shall constitute this book's topic. The fundamental question we shall be considering is: what is it to suffer such madness as is sometimes met with in mental illness?

When thinking on what makes for mental illness we do well to keep the real human experience of it in mind. Not doing so readily results in various failures of reflective reason, not the least of which involve imagining we could grasp what it is to be mad without tracking the suffering intrinsic to it. So let's begin by considering a self-report. The seventeen-year-old Ilse has suffered a frightening psychotic break whilst taking her final school exams and after her first two brief and confusing sexual encounters with men. Here we find her largely recovered from active psychosis and looking back on her experience:

> My illness first showed itself in loss of appetite and disgust at food. My periods stopped; I became obdurate. I didn't speak freely anymore; I lost interest in life; I felt sad, distraught, humourless, and became startled when anyone spoke to me. I dressed badly despite spending hours in front of the mirror.
>
> My father, who owned a restaurant, said to me the cookery examination (which was to take place next day) was only a trifle; he laughed in such an odd tone that I felt he was laughing at me. The customers were looking oddly at me too as if they'd guessed something of my suicidal thoughts. I was sitting next to the cash desk; the customers were looking at me and I became haunted by the thought that I'd stolen something. For five weeks I had had the feeling that I'd done something wrong; my mother called me unseemly and sometimes looked at me in a strange, penetrating way.
>
> It was about 9.30 in the evening (she had 'seen' three white-robed ghostly figures who she feared would take her away). I got undressed and lay in bed rigidly still so they wouldn't hear me; I listened hard for the least noise; I believed the three figures would get together again and tie me up.
>
> In the morning I again feared that I'd stolen my father's money, and I ran away. As I went across the square the clock stopped and was suddenly upside down.

I thought it was working on the other side; just then I thought the world was going to end; on Judgement Day everything stops; then I saw a lot of soldiers on the street; when I came close, one always moved away; ah, I thought, they are going to make a report; they know when you're a 'wanted' person; they kept looking at me; I really felt that the world revolved around me.

Then came a strange afternoon in which the sun seemed to not be shining when my thoughts were bad but to come back when they were good. I thought the trucks and cars were all going the wrong way; when a car passed me I didn't hear it. I thought there must be rubber underneath; large lorries didn't rattle along anymore; as soon as a car approached, I seemed to emit something that brought it to a halt ... I referred everything to myself as if it were made for me ... people didn't look at me, as if they wanted to say I was altogether too awful to look at.

When at the police station I had the impression that I was really in the Afterlife. One official looked like Death himself. I thought he was already dead and had to write on his typewriter until he had expiated his sins. There was a small alarm clock next to the typewriter; every time the bell rang I thought they were fetching someone whose life had ended. (Later I realized the ringing came from the typewriter as it reached the end of the line.) I waited for them to fetch me also. A young policeman had a pistol in his hand; I was afraid he wanted to kill me. I refused to drink the tea they brought me as I thought it was poisoned. I was waiting and longing to die ... it was like being on a stage populated with puppets. I thought they were merely empty skin pods ... the typewriter seemed upside down; there were no letters on it, only signs which I thought came from the Other World.

At the clinic I found everything unnatural; I thought I was going to be used for something special; I felt like a guinea-pig; I thought the doctor was a murderer, because he had such black hair and a hook nose, big teeth, and a brown complexion. Another man outside pushing an apple-cart seemed like a jumping jack. He was walking so hurriedly, just like in the pictures ...

Later at home things were changed, partly they were smaller; it was not so homely as before, it had become cold and strange. My father had got me a book; I thought it had been written specially for me; I didn't think I'd lived through all the scenes it described, yet it nevertheless seemed that they applied to me. I was annoyed at how they knew how ridiculous I'd made myself.

Today I can see clearly how things really are; but then I always thought something unusual was up, even on the most trivial occasion. It was a real illness.[1]

'It was a real illness', Ilse says. Let's start there: what is that? For that matter, do *mental* illnesses even count as *real* illnesses?

Illness

Disease can afflict any living organism, yet only animals become ill or injured.[2] This is because illness and injury have to do with more than organismic impairment: they have to do with disturbance to activity and experience. Illness of its nature at some point involves the suffering of: discomfort, loss of concentration, and restrictions to agency such as sleepiness and lethargy, loss of drive to eat, groom, work, and socialize.[3]

In fact, it's not with animals in general but with human beings in particular that talk of 'illness' finds its most paradigmatic application. One reason for this is that illness typically involves not 'feeling or being oneself'.[4] A poorly dog may be lethargic and show no enthusiasm for food. Yet to say of her that 'she doesn't feel herself at the moment' would be peculiar; we reserve that attribution for such beings as enjoy self-understanding – for much of which understanding an expressive facility with language is required. A second reason is that certain features of illness such as increased pain sensitivity, depression, and irritability are concepts more readily applied to such beings as have the expressive, discursive, and purposive character of humans. A third is that illness attribution draws part of its purpose from the management of a moral status which non-human animals don't enjoy. Illness ascription, that is, both acknowledges a loss of dignity in the sick person who now struggles to perform her duties, whilst also providing moral exculpation for he who withdraws and suffers loss of drive. A secure illness ascription both validates rather than challenges 'I don't feel myself' pronouncements and defeats or reduces critical moral judgement of the sufferer's apparent sloth. Civilization itself partly depends on our use of such distinctions as that between the ill and the immoral.

It has been suggested that the specialty of psychiatry can be understood as belonging properly to medicine – that is, as belonging to that discipline which treats of, and treats, illness and injury – because 'mental illness' and 'physical illness' are sub-categories of a more general category of 'illness'. On one such understanding, illness involves not something done by or to us but rather a failure in action – a failure in 'just getting on and doing things' or in 'ordinary doing'. Such a failure is said to be found in both mental and physical illness, and to be that in virtue of which they're both illness.[5] In paradigmatic physical illness the failure consists in our not forming or effecting our usual intentions: we lose our drive. In paradigmatic mental illness, however, it consists in addition in our forming intentions that are quite aberrant or 'out of character'. Ilse's aberrant intentions include those underlying her suicidality, her lying stock still, her standing for hours in front of the mirror, her refusing what she took for poisoned food, her wish to strip and run naked into the street, and her attempts at setting the sun or stopping traffic by thinking and acting in certain ways.

The suggestion that mental and physical illness are two types of a more generally intelligible notion of illness is not without its difficulties. When trying to strip off and run outside, or control the sun or traffic with her thoughts and movements, Ilse shows no failure in 'just getting on and doing things'; it's just that what she's getting on with is 'crazy'. This isn't to say that such cases couldn't also be brought under some or other description of 'action failure'. However, the concept of 'action failure' now required will surely be disjunctive between mental and physical illness, and this in turn impugns its use in providing a unitary analysis of 'illness'. Furthermore, much of what in Ilse's experience and judgement is 'ill' is only incidentally related to her intentions.

The analysis of mental illness as a failure in ordinary doing itself fails, but it nevertheless puts us in touch with a significant feature of mental illness. That is, it reveals an aspect of how the concept of mental illness 'radicalizes' or 'sublimes' our

ɔncept.[6] In moving from failures within the domain of ordinary action
undertake projects, say) to failures of that very domain (failures to even
..,-oriented projects), it abstracts the concept of 'illness' from its normal
intelligibility-conferring context and deploys it of that very context. We might compare
this with walking into a shop to buy a drink, but finding you like the place so much that
you buy the shop itself. Were someone to describe this latter act as 'going shopping' we
should know what they meant, but we shall also be alive to the sense in which this
radicalizes the notion of 'shopping'. The shop owner is after all the one person who
cannot buy the drinks on the shelves. (To transfer money from one's left to one's right
hand is not to complete a financial transaction.) Similarly with mental illness: the sense
in which actions 'fail' in mental illness is a radicalization of the sense in which they fail
in ordinary illness. Notwithstanding this we still see the point of talking here of mental
illness.

Mental illness

So what then is it for Ilse to be mentally ill? We can't understand her as suffering from
an illness which has an *effect on the mind*, since many illnesses (fever, porphyria,
hyperthyroidism) affect the mind without thereby themselves counting as mental.[7] So
perhaps such illness is the effect of psychological factors? If by 'effect' we mean
something that is more than notionally separable from its cause, then the answer must
again be 'no': the common cold caught by a man who, lost to melancholic rumination,
locks himself out of his own home on a winter's night, does not become a mental illness
on that account. In mental illness we find the mind itself affected, rather than something
else – a brain disease, for example (neurosyphilis, Korsakoff syndrome, Alzheimer's
disease) – having an effect on the mind. Mental illness is in some sense *of the mind
itself*. But in what sense?

An oft-encountered criticism has it that the last-voiced question is itself but the
product of a misguided dualism: 'Now that we moderns no longer believe in immaterial
minds, now that we know the mind to be nothing other than the brain ..', goes the
objection, '... the psychiatrist's distinction between organic illness (e.g. neurosyphilis)
and mental illness (e.g. schizophrenia) can be revealed as outmoded.' At first glance the
argument perhaps seems valid, but in truth it fails to even begin to consider how the
concepts of 'mental illness' and 'organic illness' are actually deployed by psychiatry.
When we do consider that, what we find is that it's only the critic, and not the ordinary
user, of the distinction between mental and physical illness who locates in that
distinction the dualistic schematism which is then rightly diagnosed as confused.

The truth is that nobody here was talking about immaterial minds before our critic
showed up. The psychiatrists weren't even considering the metaphysics of the relation
of mind to brain, let alone basing a central psychopathological distinction upon it. To
be sure, a dualism of substances, such that the mind and the brain are taken to be
fundamentally different types of entity, truly does make for a peculiar and difficult
world. (What really is an 'immaterial entity' anyway? How on earth are they supposed
to causally interact with material entities?) But the concept of 'mind' we find at play in

psychiatry doesn't betoken an entity; instead, it signifies certain capacities and their loss, especially intellectual and volitional capacities for rational thought and action. It isn't misguidedly dualistic to distinguish between a car's engine and its acceleration, or between the law and the material paraphernalia (wigs, court rooms, legal documents) of its practice. 'Acceleration', 'law', and 'mind' no more pick out objects than does 'the nick of time' or 'the average Catholic with four and a half children'. 'Car' and 'person' pick out entities, but 'acceleration' and 'mental illness' designate properties of the aforementioned entities, rather than denoting further entities in the scene.

With this distinction in place, we can begin to sketch out what it is for a mental illness to be 'of the mind itself'. But before beginning with that it will pay dividends to first offer something more general about the kind of concept 'mental illness' is. Consider the following two forms of concept; the first we shall call 'classical', the second 'family resemblance'. A classical concept is demarcated by a neat set of necessary and/or sufficient conditions. Technical concepts provide the clearest examples of these, as they're typically introduced with a simple rule for their use or, to put it otherwise, there are a simple set of criteria for them that all instantiations of the concept must meet. On a family resemblance conception, by contrast, various criteria help define the concept, and so all are sometimes essential, yet not every instance of the concept requires the meeting of all the criteria.[8] (Examples: 'art', 'good', 'meaning', 'salad'.) Despite such a possible partial disjunction of criteria, the disjunction is not to such a degree that we're drawn to speak here of different concepts. The claim offered in what follows, then, is that our ordinary concept of 'mental illness' is a non-technical, family resemblance, concept. It grew up non-deliberatively over a long period of time and can be articulated by referencing a motley of criteria, all of which delineate what it is for certain conditions to be mental illnesses, but some of which may nevertheless not always be met.

Returning now to the question of what it is for mental illness to be illness 'of the mind itself': A key criterion for mental illness is that it implicates a particular aspect of a person's rational functioning. The aspect is called 'reality contact'; what that amounts to will be considered in Chapter 3. (Suffice it for now to say that it has little to do with inferential prowess or degree of intelligence; the distinction between mental illness ('lunacy') and learning disability ('idiocy') is an old one.[9]) Whilst ordinary ('physical') illnesses (such as porphyria or malaria) may have secondary effects on the mind, including the inducing of mental illness, unlike mental illnesses they aren't themselves individuated by reference to such effects.[10] Were a man diagnosed psychotically depressed found on autopsy to have nothing aberrant about his brain, the diagnosis would not on that account be challenged. Not so for one diagnosed with neurosyphilis. A study of the brain of he who has a mental illness may (or may not) be revealing in all sorts of ways.[11] Even so, it will no more tell us what it is to have such an illness than would an investigation of a combustion engine tell us what it is for a car to accelerate.

Consider now the question: how are we to meaningfully distinguish between such disturbances to human thought, feeling, motivation, and action as are caused by, say, spirochetes in the brain in neurosyphilis and those caused by schizophrenia? The answer now proposed proceeds by noting the two different senses of 'cause' here in play. The neurodegenerative process that eventually causes behavioural disturbance in untreated syphilis sufferers is intelligible separately from its behavioural effects, whilst the psychological processes which cause the characteristic behaviours of schizophrenic illnesses are themselves of a piece with such behaviour; reference to them instead offers a new description under which the behaviour may be brought. To borrow Aristotle's terminology, the disturbance of reality-contact and reason found in schizophrenic illness is its *formal* cause, whilst neurodegeneration is the *efficient* cause of the mental disturbance met with in neurosyphilis.[12] Or, now in Wittgenstein's terms: delusion is *criterial for* a schizophrenic illness, whilst the behavioural disturbance in neurosyphilis is merely *symptomatic of* the brain infection.[13] A final terminological variant: the spirochete infection *underlies* the symptoms of neurosyphilis in that it *precipitates* them; a disturbance of reality contact, however, *characterizes* or *shapes* various of the symptoms of a schizophrenic illness, thereby partly *constituting* the condition. Such distinctions help make clear what it is for a mental illness to be an illness of the mind, rather than being a disease of the brain or body manifesting in the mind.

Mental *illness*

Having considered something of what it is to suffer *mental* illness, let's return to the question of what it is to suffer mental *illness*. It was suggested above that mental illness isn't happily thought to relate to ordinary illness by way of both instancing a unitary illness category. Yet the concept of mental illness is surely used to marshal some of the same social consequences as are afforded to the ordinarily ill: the exculpatory sick note, the provision of care by those with a medical training, etc. Furthermore, the intuitiveness of the concept is rooted in certain similarities between losing one's mind and being ordinarily ill. (Particularly significant here are disturbances of agency, reduced openness to the world, inward preoccupation, often a depressed mood, and – as we shall discuss later – the presence of suffering.) The question remains, though, as to what kind of relation the concept of mental illness bears to that of ordinary illness, if it's not itself a sub-type of illness.

It's sometimes suggested that psychiatric talk of *mental illness* is itself metaphorical; this however is hard to understand since we have no clearer idea of a contrastive literal use of the phrase than that provided by psychiatry. The more plausible alternative has it that mental illnesses are *illnesses*, and the mentally ill are *ill*, in a metaphorical sense.[14] On such an understanding, when Ilse says she has 'a real illness' we should take her either to be in error or to mean that, whilst she's really suffering, this was yet not from literal, but rather from metaphorical, illness.

To evaluate this proposal with analogy's aid, consider some of the varying uses of 'attitude': in the seventeenth century as a technical term for the postures of painted figures; in the eighteenth century expanded to include ways of carrying oneself ('she walked with a graceful attitude'); in the nineteenth century used in conjunction with 'mental' to refer to dispositions or states of mind ('mental attitude'), then shortened to simply 'attitude'; in the twentieth century sometimes deployed as a shortened form of 'bad mental attitude' (i.e. being antagonistic and uncooperative). Is it evident that someone who today is said to have (a bad mental) attitude has but a metaphorical attitude? At least when compared with what all would admit are paradigmatic metaphors ('It is the East, and Juliet is the sun!'), 'metaphor' doesn't seem the happiest description for the new uses of 'attitude' and 'illness' in 'bad mental attitude' and 'mental illness'.[15] Even so it's surely plausible to suggest that, in a manner not dissimilar from the derivation of metaphors from their literal roots, the concepts of 'mental attitude' and 'mental illness' were formed by analogical extrapolation from extant uses of 'attitude' and 'illness' – from uses, that is, which post-extrapolation might, if the context did not take care of it, be helpfully disambiguated with the prefix 'physical'.

A happier description than 'metaphor' for the illness of mental illness is what philosophers have called 'secondary sense'.[16] Our ancestors, let's imagine, spoke of 'deep wells'; soon enough their descendants were intuitively extrapolating this to talk of 'deep sounds' and 'deep sorrow'.[17] We take a term which has a clear meaning in one semantic context, then spontaneously deploy it in another, it being only our disposition to use the word in the same way as one another that makes for ongoing mutual understanding. The concept of 'illness' was already in play to articulate both feeling unwell (ill) and suffering from this or that particular illness (flu, syphilis); the term and aspects of its conceptual structure could then be borrowed to articulate the predicament of those suffering 'nerves', 'melancholia', and 'insanity'.[18] No doubt such a use drew in part on similarities in the sickness behaviour of the physically poorly and some of the mentally unwell. But it also extrapolated from this: to include further aspects of suffering such as anguish, to cover the idea of a 'disordered' mind by analogy with the bodily 'disorder' underlying ordinary illness, to elicit the sympathies we feel for the ordinarily sick, and to license and cement the management of the mentally ill by physicians. The resources of these extant professions could now be mobilized to keep those judged 'lunatic' from the workhouse or the jail, and to develop theories of their 'pathology' and its corresponding apt 'treatment'.

We may defend our judgement that Ilse was truly and literally mentally ill by appealing to various of the things she believed (that the town clock was upside down, that the world was turning around her and about to end, etc.) and how she acted (trying to run out naked into the street). No similar appeal can, however, justify our conceiving of such human experiences as illness. Should questions of justification come up, those who disapprove of the concept may focus on its disanalogies from ordinary illness; those who approve of it may cite its similarities.[19] To take either tack, however, is to implausibly presuppose that the 'illness' in 'mental illness' isn't to be understood as either metaphor or secondary sense. Yet in the end it's only the concept's usefulness, and not its putative grounds, which provide it with its warrant.

Maintenance and motivation

In thinking on what it is for illness to be 'of the mind' we've so far encountered one negative and two positive defining criteria. The negative, exclusionary, criterion is that it's *not itself brain disease*. (It may involve altered brain function, it may even be triggered by brain disease, and someone may be unlucky enough to suffer both; even so mental illness is not itself such a disease.) The positive ones are that true mental illness involves some kind of radical *disturbance of agency*, and some kind of *disturbance to a person's rational relationship with reality.* Three further criteria of mental illness will be adumbrated below: the *self-maintaining* character of the disturbance, the *motivation* at play within it, and the *suffering* from which it emerges and which remains implicated within it.

The next of our criteria for mental illness – its *self-maintaining* character – has to do with it not being maintained by a purely environmental cause. Mental illness may be caused by disturbing experiences, whether these are one-off traumas or ongoingly disturbed relationships. Even so, what makes talk of illness, rather than simply of distress, apt is that genuine illness doesn't cease just when the source of distress is removed. Hot environments may provoke discomfort, yet we only talk of heatstroke once the body's thermoregulation is overwhelmed and an enduring malaise persists despite returning to the shade. Taking to one's bed doesn't immediately make one well. In this way is 'illness' distinguished from 'reaction'.

So too with mental illness. The dynamic systems theory notion of the personality as a self-regulating system that can get trapped in particular 'attractor basins' captures something of this.[20] Savanna, desert, and forest, for example, are alternative stable ecosystem states; intermediary states move towards one of these, and once formed are not easily destabilized. So too we may consider everyday mood states to be self-maintaining since they exercise a constraining force on the kinds of thoughts, memories, and action tendencies that are readily available, and in this way maintain themselves. When in a depressed mood, for example, we think dismal thoughts, become sedentary, lose interest in our lives, and can't access hope – and this all maintains the mood. So too when we're giddily happy or anxious: emotions come and go as we adapt to new situations, but moods are not ongoing flexible adaptations to our lives, but have their own inner dynamism. We can become trapped in them for a while, especially if we're somewhat emotionally blocked. Even so it's in the nature of ordinary mood to shift after a sleep or a significant sustained change in activity or environment. Mood becomes mental illness when it becomes a more deeply entrenched pattern.[21] Also relevant here is the notion of 'internalization'. A child may have occasional experience of an abusive relationship without internalizing it. If, however, the experience is protracted, the situation may become 'trapped' inside the child. Now she either comes to fearfully expect all others to be abusive, or tacitly casts the abuse as deserved and becomes unwarrantedly self-deprecating, or becomes abusive herself. The point of mentioning such possibilities here is not to lapse into a merely empirical psychology, but only to make clear what it is for mental illness to be self-maintaining.

The fifth criterion has it that essential to much true mental illness is that it's at least partly intelligible in *motivational* terms.[22] To borrow Aristotle's terminology again: essential to much mental illness is that somewhere on the scene are *final* causes. What distinguishes much mental illness as such is that in it the will turns against, rather than supports, contact with reality, at least in some limited domain of that contact.[23] Such a perversion of its own natural function informs key aspects of the analogical extrapolation from ordinary to mental illness, and in particular is what informs our intuition that in mental illness the mind has in some sense itself become ill. The significance of motivation is registered in different terms by different psychological systems – whether we're thinking of the behaviourist's 'avoidance' or the psychoanalyst's 'defence mechanisms' – but ultimately it belongs not to a contingent aspect of these systems' empirical science but rather to the essential nature of that which they here theorize. This motivation is, of course, not well described as 'to become mentally ill', or 'to become psychotically depressed'. Nor is it aptly thought of as conscious – i.e. as being readily avowable by the mentally ill subject.[24] Instead, it shows itself in a reflexive avoidance of anxiety, anguish, terror, and overwhelm in order to preserve inner equilibrium.[25] Contrast here such ('organic') disorders as merely affect the mind with those ('functional') disorders which are mental illnesses proper. In the latter cases the symptoms enjoy a form of intelligibility (i.e. perform a 'function') related to their sufferers' unconscious attempts to preserve selfhood, reduce overwhelm, and flee angst. That these attempts may sometimes eventuate in even worse psychotic terrors, or in cutting off not only what was terrifying but also what was nourishing in reality contact, does not itself speak against the idea of such reflexive avoidance being criterial of mental illness. (Compare: Fever may be our body's way of dealing with bacterial infection; this doesn't mean it won't damage you if it goes too far. Or: you take benzodiazepines to reduce your anxiety, but over time your chemical dependency makes your anxiety worse. . . . Welcome to the motivated yet hapless human world of temporary, compelling, and ultimately damaging fixes ascending over the far harder won delayed gratification of sustainable change.)

'Mental illness' is often taken as synonymous with 'mental disorder'. It is however in the former's allusions to a self-maintaining state, to suffering, and to the motivated avoidance of such suffering by psychotic or neurotic retreat, that it reveals itself as a more specific concept. (Consider too that the concept of 'mental disorder' includes not only mental illnesses but also developmental disabilities.) Yet despite the fact that motivation is an essential ingredient of our understanding of mental illness, it's not the case that it's always to be found. As suggested above, 'mental illness' is a family resemblance concept, and sometimes we may call 'mental illness' a condition which is unmarked by such motivation.

Suffering

Ordinary illness will, unless interrupted early, at some point result in suffering. The suffering will most usually be registered as pain, fatigue, or discomfort, although some illnesses damage dignity more than cause unpleasant sensation. Many mental illnesses such as melancholia and anxiety disorders present clear instances of distress and dysphoria: anxiety and angst, panic, inner torment, mental pain, etc. Yet when we think on certain paradigmatic mental illnesses (say a manic or schizophrenic psychosis) we may be struck by how their sufferers – sometimes even those who concurrently suffer such physical illness as would normally result in pain – don't always complain of such suffering.[26] Retrospectively, of course, a subject may – as Ilse did – acknowledge the deep mental distress that in some sense she was nevertheless in at the time. And whilst we can readily see the damage to her dignity – damage which the concept of illness will itself be called on to ameliorate – and how in this sense she suffers, she may well not be able to see this at the time, a fact which naturally compounds the injury.

At this point it may be tempting to appeal to the 'family resemblance' character of the suffering criterion and suggest that, whilst it's essential to some instances of mental illness, it need not always be present. Perhaps this is sometimes the case; even so, the appeal moves too quickly. Consider how, when discussing disturbances to agency above, it was suggested that whilst paradigmatic mental illnesses may seem to evince no 'failure in getting on and doing things', the criterion is met with if taken in a radicalized rather than ordinary form. The failure, that is, is not to ordinarly exercises of will, but is instead met with in that very will's derangement: it's not the absence of the fact of, but the continued possibility of speaking meaningfully about, 'ordinary doing' that's here negated. The parallel suggestion now is that whilst the psychotic subject may feel no conscious suffering, the very form of his thought now radically embodies suffering. The suffering which is here expressed in his thought and action is not that which he consciously feels, but instead that which has broken his ability to stay in touch with painful reality. Suffering's lostness to him here is, we might say, a symptom of his own greater lostness to suffering. If we clinicians and theorists deflect from the difficulty of reality that madness presents us, and take taxonomic refuge instead in terms like 'mental disorder' which carry no essential reference to suffering, we overlook how someone may be so broken by anguish that they're no longer alive to it.

None of this is to say that there's not also often a great deal of ordinary emotional suffering in mental illness. Instead, it's to urge that paradigm cases of it are those in which the greatest suffering now manifests in the collapse not only of agency but also of subjectivity – where by 'subjectivity' is meant, in part, the capacity to consciously suffer. Unfulfilled intention and unsoothed distress cannot now, as it were, be successfully suffered by the mind.[27] Now, when the mind buckles, its disappointment and emotional pain instead become inscribed in its very form, rather than being felt as such. Should this collapsed subject become able to tolerate emotional reality again, she will by that token once again become able to truly experience, rather than collapse into, her anguish. In the meantime, we might detect it simmering in the restless agitation underlying a manic patient's flight from anguish, or covered over by the insouciance accompanying the hebephrenic's delusion. We intuitively sense that the paranoiac's delusion provides, as Freud wrote, 'a patch over the place where originally a rent had appeared in the ego's relation to the external world', whilst the catatonic has frozen himself out of existence itself because of that anguish which temporal existence now engenders for him.[28] A patient called Joan described it thus:

> I had to die to keep from dying. I know that sounds crazy but one time a boy hurt my feelings very much and I wanted to jump in front of a subway. Instead I went a little catatonic so I wouldn't feel anything – I guess you had to die emotionally or your feelings would have killed you.[29]

Another schizophrenic subject talked of how he 'suppressed feeling as I suppressed all reality. I dug a moat around me.'[30] The philosopher Arthur Schopenhauer also put it well:

> if such a sorrow, such painful knowledge or reflection, is so harrowing that it becomes positively unbearable, and the individual would succumb to it, then

nature, alarmed in this way, seizes upon madness as the last means of saving life. The mind, tormented so greatly, destroys, as it were, the thread of memory, fills up the gaps with fictions, and thus seeks refuge in madness from the mental suffering that exceeds its strength.[31]

In such ways the 'mental illness' concept provides us with a reminder to maintain contact with the mentally ill patient's latent suffering. Ilse's psychosis developed when she was *utterly overwhelmed* by her first sexual encounters and her school examinations. Whether her delusions were a mere breakdown product of a mind overwhelmed by such suffering as 'exceeds its strength', or whether instead she 'seized upon madness' by way of motivated retreat from an anguish that was 'positively unbearable' to her, isn't something we can decide on from the information in the case report. But we anyway aren't forced to choose between these: the family resemblance concept of 'mental illness' includes both possibilities within it.

'Monstrosity'

The widespread shunning, disquiet, and fear encountered by the mentally ill – especially by schizophrenic people when psychotic – is often described as *stigma* and suggested to be due to widespread, erroneous, media-fed beliefs about their dangerousness or perversity. The suggestion is partly contradicted by the facts – which at the time of writing are (very roughly, and in the West) that, whilst most schizophrenic people are not dangerous to themselves or others, 10% of sufferers kill themselves within ten years of diagnosis, 10% of murders are committed by schizophrenics (whilst only 0.5% of the population have been psychotic in the last year), 10% of those having a first episode are seriously and repeatedly aggressive (weapon use, sexual assault, injury), and 0.15% kill.[32] Smoking skunkweed and not being tranquilized increase the risk of committing such offences, and given that most people known to have psychotic conditions are currently medicated with major tranquilizers, it's reasonable to conclude that the violence of those suffering psychotic illness would be considerably higher were it not for such treatments. Since the social disquiet primarily relates to the untreated condition, the widespread belief in dangerousness seems to not be entirely misplaced.

Approaches to tackling stigma often attempt to question the reasonableness of the beliefs held by those who shun the stigmatized person. Thus they ask the question, 'are the majority of psychotic people actually dangerous or perverse in the way you imagine?'; to which the right answer is, clearly, 'on the whole, no'. Yet extensive anti-stigma campaigns conducted along such lines have been largely ineffective.[33] Furthermore, reflection alone reveals that it's the psychotic individual in his psychosis who's feared, not simply such of his acts as would be fearful whoever commits them. We're disquieted by his acts under the description of 'psychotic', not simply under the descriptions 'violent' or 'sexually perverse'. We – and he too when he's sane – are disturbed by his delusional peculiarity, by his unpredictability, by his baffling admixture of comprehensible humanity and what may to some seem like an inhumanity which is in certain ways incomprehensible.

What such incomprehensibility amounts to will be discussed in the next chapter. To now take out a loan on that discussion's results: we may distinguish between the rationally (or humanly) and the psychologically (or motivationally) intelligible, or between the 'why' and the 'how' of belief. Thus we may understand the radical boost to self-esteem that is provided to a mentally unwell cobbler by his belief that he's a supreme commander. Even so, this speaks not at all to the rational intelligibility of his claim; we can't thereby really 'find our feet with' him, we can't 'get' how he could think what he does. And it's such foot-finding failures that are intrinsically jarring and deeply disconcerting.

It's worth recognizing that we're not inexorably disquieted by what we don't understand or relate to, or by what we find unpredictable. We're typically emotionally disturbed neither by quantum physics, nor by the birds of the air, nor by the quotidian vagaries of the weather. Instead, we blanch at that which is both close yet alien: we're phobic of phenomena which appear to us under the aspect of the *monstrous*. We fear what invites our efforts at understanding but then pulls apart our minds in the attempt. We tremble neither at the dead nor at the living but at the undead. We take fright at the psychopath all the more because of the extent to which he is, despite his sometime deathly inhumanity, on the whole largely human. We dread the beast that is half human, half animal. Throughout history our cultures have thrown up endless icons of the monstrous – from the minotaur to Frankenstein's monster – to help us articulate, and thereby gain some small degree of purchase on, such otherwise thought-stopping terror.

The layperson's conflation of the psychotic with the psychopathic may in part be due to the confusingly similar terms, or to misleading media reporting about the dangerousness of those with psychotic conditions. Yet it's also the case that people suffer an instinctive fear towards that which is, albeit in quite different ways, disassembling of the human and the humane. With respect to psychosis, what we fear is the unreason which is yet no disturbance of inference-making but rather a more primordial disturbance to thought's footing. We're made anxious by this jarring disconnection between us. We tremble at this unmooring within the psychotic individual – an unmooring which, when we attempt connection with him, threatens to unseat our own basic orientation in the world.[34] And we fear too this reminder that it's but a contingent fact that any one of us isn't also trapped in a waking dream, that the anchor chain of our mind doesn't break and the ship of reason be flung about on the dementing wave, and that insight can't be secured through reasoning or will.

To overcome stigmatizing reactions we do well to first articulate such concerns, so they may then be faced with understanding. This prevents our ignoring them by misarticulating them as, for example, being solely due to our overestimating the risks of the physical dangerousness of those with psychotic mental illness. This work of understanding inevitably involves work on oneself, and work on oneself is typically not a matter of learning further facts about the afflicted, but rather a matter of one's own gradual moral transformation, the careful deactivating of one's own defensive recoil, the growth in one's tolerance for the alien, the owning rather than the projecting of one's own monstrous aspect, and the growth in one's ability to hold onto that in the other to which, despite all that is awry, we can yet offer recognition. Especially when someone has suffered radical affliction and is deeply unwell, and when our tired glance detects nothing in them onto which ordinary sympathy and intersubjective resonance can find a purchase, it can take the radical disclosive power of the look of love to reveal that about them which makes it possible to still talk here of knowing someone and of having a sincere concern for them.[35]

Truly knowing – not simply being acquainted with – someone with mental illness is one of the best predictors of a greater tolerance for the mentally ill.[36] Yet we also do well to acknowledge the work already done by the concept of 'mental ill health' towards this end.[37] It offers a clear alternative to judgements of blameworthiness: the psychotic subject is unwell and not to be blamed or shamed for her acts; hence the value of the insanity defence. Furthermore, it offers an alternative to being judged monstrous, in part since it invites us to hold in mind that matters were not always thus: there was here once a sane person who fell ill, and a person who we hope will yet recover and who may require something of us (treatment, care, and understanding).[38] Our talk of 'mental illness' itself invites us to consider here a *person* who is *ill*, a person who – when in his illness – *is not himself*, a person who is grievously *suffering* and *incapacitated*. To urge that only those with the moral status of human beings can truly become mentally ill is to make no merely empirical point. In this way, to find someone ill is thus already at least an invitation to recognize their humanity. And in this way, too, does such talk of 'illness' itself help us manage the unthinkable shadow of the monstrous.

The term's use is, however, not without its risks, risks which arise when one forgets the categorical differences between mental illness and such ordinary illness as (after our analogical extrapolation of the former) is called 'physical illness'. 'Medicalization' is the term we give to this presumption: the assumption that mental illnesses will (like many physical illnesses) often be best explained by reference to somatic factors, that research funding will best be directed at discovering these, that it will not after all be psychologically explicable, that its apt treatment will be medicinal, and that the primary task for the patient and the doctor involves not the development of a more resilient self with a greater capacity for suffering and disappointment and relating but instead the recovery of premorbid functioning and the prevention of relapse. It might take a tin ear to not notice the conceptual slippage, yet such artificial organs are nowhere in short supply. The dangers are at their greatest when talk of 'mental illness' is taken to offer license for foregoing the ethical task of showing understanding, and offering recognition, to the psychotic subject – as if all by itself such talk of 'illness' somehow implied that there's nothing, and perhaps even nobody, here to understand, that we must just calmly await recovery before we once again take seriously the patient's inner experience and word.

Conclusions

Let's return to Ilse. Was her psychosis, as she suggests, a 'real illness'? If we mean by that a real mental illness or derangement of reason and will, and assuming no misdiagnosis, then the answer is 'yes, it's a paradigm of such an illness'. And if talk of 'illness' here helps preserve her dignity whilst acknowledging that it's yet in jeopardy; if it highlights her suffering; if it makes for the suspension of such moral judgement as her actions when she's 'not in her right mind' may otherwise attract; then this is a valuable outcome. However, if we'd hoped that such an answer as 'she's genuinely ill' would by itself entail a requirement of medical attention then we'll be disappointed. Whilst the concept of 'mental illness' relates to that of ordinary illness in its focus on moral exculpation, impaired agency, and suffering, such a focus doesn't itself necessitate a medical approach (it is, for example, but a contingent fact that only medics write sick notes for the mentally ill, and psychotherapy is often practised by non-medics). Furthermore, in the analogical extrapolation from the case of ordinary to mental illness, the significance of impairments of agency and of suffering is somewhat altered through what above was described as their 'radicalization'. The result of this is that any *a priori* rationale for medical treatment evaporates – unless one also analogically extrapolates the concepts of the 'medical' and of 'treatment' to maintain their synchrony with that of 'illness' in the psychiatric context. None of this is to say that medicinal treatment – such as the use of major tranquilizers – might not be supremely useful to someone in Ilse's predicament. It's only to say that the value here of medicinal treatment is to be underwritten by its effects and not by the fact that we're dealing with illness.

The above analysis brings to the fore of our reflective comprehension of what it is to be mentally ill: a collapse of mental functioning into an alternative equilibrium state which, whilst yet enjoying its own order, nevertheless no longer subtends that rational order which constitutes reality contact; mental suffering; that suffering's motivation by rationality-disabling avoidance; the deservedness of exculpation for what otherwise would be considered moral ills; a radical disturbance of agency; and a negative criterion: it's not merely the expression of brain disease. The analytical aim has been descriptive rather than revisionary. To disprove the analysis, all that's required is for those truly fluent in talk of 'mental illness' to find that it fails to accurately represent their discourse (bearing in mind, of course, that exceptions needn't prove troubling for a family resemblance concept in the same way that they would for a classical concept). Having said that, it's striking that much philosophy of psychiatry, at the time of writing, would take issue with some of the above-cited criteria. Thus it's typically only the suffering produced by the mental illness itself, rather than the unendurable pains of life which result in and are expressed by it, which are offered for consideration in philosophical analyses of mental illness. And it's typically only impairments to, rather than the positive presence of, motivation that are considered relevant to the analysis. The role offered it in this chapter may then be seen as an overreaching intrusion of an empirical hypothesis of psychodynamic psychology into the philosophical analysis. Exculpation is also seen as extrinsic to our understanding of what mental illness itself is – i.e. to represent a value judgement we independently bring to bear on those we deem mentally ill. What explanation can be offered for the disjunction of the perspective of this chapter and that of mainstream philosophy of psychiatry?

One explanation is that contemporary philosophy of psychiatry actually focuses not so much on *mental illness* but on *mental disorder*. Whilst sometimes treated as equivalent,[39] at other times the former is taken as the 'clinical manifestation' of the latter.[40] The result is that the allusions of 'illness of the mind' are rather lost, and an approach to 'mental disorder' is offered which stresses disturbances in 'mental functions' and 'underlying mechanisms'.[41] These analyses are, naturally enough, typically pursued in purely naturalistic terms, and so find little room in their understanding for the concepts more typically marshalled by the humanities. As a result they typically consider mental disorder in terms of mental dysfunction.[42] Concepts like 'human intelligibility', 'suffering' and its 'motivated avoidance', and 'moral status' are now inevitably seen as mere add-ons to a naturalistic core of disorder. Additional reasons for the neglect of illness-provoking suffering in the understanding of mental illness are the facts that it often finds expression there in a merely mute form, and that we're all anyway naturally motivated to deflect from, rather than bear with, it. Finally, but allied to all the above, is the widespread misunderstanding of the character, and fundamental significance for psychiatry, of the concepts of the 'understandable' (as opposed to the 'explainable'), of 'being in one's right mind' (as opposed to 'correct inference making'), and of 'lost reality contact' (as opposed to 'incorrect representation'). These final concerns constitute the topics of the following two chapters.

Delusion + me since I have not id ' "

2

Delusion's Rational Irretrievability

Introduction

Of the mental illnesses, the psychoses are our paradigm – and a sufficient condition of these is delusion. 'Since time immemorial, delusion has been taken as the basic characteristic of madness. To be mad was to be deluded.'[1] Perception, mood, thinking, and memory may all become delusional: 'A man in a brown jacket is seen a few steps away. He is the dead Archduke who has resurrected'; 'It suddenly occurred to me one night that Miss L. was probably the cause of all the terrible things I've suffered'; 'I feel certain that *something* is going on'; 'On reading about the waking of Lazarus from the dead I immediately felt myself to be Mary. Martha was my sister, Lazarus a sick cousin'; a 47-year-old clerical worker claims that '10 years earlier, I met an internationally famous orchestral conductor who proposed marriage to me whilst picking fruit alongside me on a farm in east Anglia.'[2] Despite this formal variety we often aptly call the articulations of diverse delusional phenomena the expressions of delusional beliefs. Such talk of 'belief' is not designed to align the delusion with, say, the consideration, the hypothesis, the conjecture – nor to suggest that perceptions, intentions, feelings, etc. cannot themselves be delusional. Instead, it registers both delusion's essential non-objectivity and the delusional subject's failure to acknowledge this non-objectivity.[3]

In the sense of 'thought' at play in this book – i.e. not the act of cogitation but the content of an intentional attitude – it is thought itself which is, and such thought's thinkers who are, delusional. Delusion implies disturbance of what we call 'reality contact', and disturbed reality contact makes for radical difficulties – in fact, for a particular kind of impossibility – in understanding such thought as proceeds from its basis. These difficulties arise both for the thinker and for the other who encounters him, yet it's a significant fact about delusion that only the latter is ongoingly aware of them.

The epistemological matter of delusion's intelligibility is this chapter's subject, whilst the following two treat of delusion's ontological roots in disturbed 'reality contact' and its manifestation in lost 'reality testing'. The reason for this topsy-turvy ordering is due to the fact that, despite the radical nature of the delusional mind's intrinsic disturbances, today we are everywhere invited – especially by the psychologists – to construe delusional thought as itself intelligible. To construe delusion, that is, as the sort of thought we could imagine ourselves arriving at were we to suffer various aberrant, yet not themselves intrinsically delusional, psychological predicaments such as failures or anomalies of memory, reasoning, perception, or sensation. If delusion could be handled

Bion 'agitation.'

in this way, then we should abandon, as the misguided stalking of an illusory prey, the subsequent chapters' ambition of limning that disturbed 'reality contact' and 'reality testing' which underlies and informs delusional breakdowns in meaning. It is, therefore, important to first tackle that objection which would otherwise vitiate the chapters to follow.

To help secure our bearings on the true phenomenon, let's consider an extract from Morag Coate's autobiographical *Beyond All Reason*:

In the short space between one half minute and the next I had lost my reason and become insane. . . . I forgot immediately and completely my normal, rational view of life.

I finished my lunch and walked out into town, ready for whatever adventure should befall. I was under direction. All I needed to do was to go wherever the impulse took me, and sometime during the day I would meet the special messenger who was being sent. . . .

I passed by my flat and glanced in through the window. A man was kneeling beside the armchair on which I had laid my head while deep in thought the previous night. . . .

There was a big football match on, and that was significant, for part of the plan for the future was that aggressive and competitive impulses should be channelled into sports and games as a substitute for war. I pressed on purposefully towards the cathedral which was my immediate destination, and I was soon joined by an unseen companion who walked beside me on my right. . . . I was surprised when he held back fifty yards from the cathedral and would not come any nearer to it. . . . a man of flesh and blood fell into step with me. We walked in silence; I felt no need to talk; I knew I had at last met my special messenger.

When we reached the quiet backwater where I lived he started, still in complete silence, to make love to me. . . . Eventually he spoke.

'Do you know who I am?'

'No.'

'I'm David.'

'David Stronsay?'

'Yes.'

This was the only conversation that we had. It was quite sufficient for me; it identified him as my grandfather's great-grandfather come back from the dead.

My contact was in fact a real and ordinary man. So much the worse for him, for he had been nervous from the start, and he got a serious fright when I told him suddenly that he was upside down. He ran away from me, after a short struggle in which I tried to stop him; and after that the solar system started to fall apart. I had certain, but purely abstract, knowledge of the danger that now threatened . . . The running man, as he went out of sight, could be seen now as four different men all present in one body at the same time. There was the stranger of my own time and district; there was the eighteenth-century ancestor; there was another contemporary man living at that time in a different place; and there was a semi-divine personage as well. . . .

I retired to my flat.... The superhuman personage was in blind flight and racing round the planets widdershins.... I knew also, as the racing figure did not, that at one point one of them was missing and he would fall through and disrupt the equilibrium of the others in his fall.... The main risk was that the balance of the moving planets would be lost. If I could provide some kind of counterpoise, all might be well. I stood in a passage swinging my arms like pendulums until the danger point had passed and all was well....

I was found soon afterwards, dancing naked in front of a mirror.[4]

The questions on our conceptual table are these: What is it to think as Morag thinks? How could she have believed what she reports? For that matter, are such *outré* thoughts as hers genuine, or merely ersatz, thoughts? Can we make sense of her in her madness – and, if so, in what way?

It's the philosopher and psychopathologist Karl Jaspers who sets the scene for our philosophical understanding of delusion, and it's largely with his work that this chapter engages. A key claim of his *General Psychopathology* is that there's an important sense in which thoughts such as Morag's are 'ununderstandable'. With this many psychologists have since taken issue, and done so in the spirit of restoring that humane comprehending contact with delusional persons which Jaspers appears to them to rule out. What's rarely considered, though, is what exactly he was ruling in and out by way of delusion's comprehensibility.

We may agree with these psychologists – and in fact, as we'll see, with Jaspers – that there are various senses in which genuine delusions are indeed intelligible. Nevertheless, what follows turns the tables on the psychologists by elaborating a centrally important further sense in which delusion essentially exceeds our comprehension's ambition. To this there will be an ethical corollary: that it's in following not Jaspers but the psychologists that we risk withholding adequate recognition to Morag in the depths of her predicament.

Delusion's marks

One way the question 'what is delusion?' gets foreclosed is by deployment of a definition which assimilates it to such belief as is merely

1) stubbornly maintained, even
2) in the face of contradictory evidence,
3) contrary to reality, and
4) socially unconventional.

We find something like this in nearly all the textbooks,[5] and the first three criteria may also be found in Jaspers' *General Psychopathology*. Delusion, he tells us, is belief

1) held with an extraordinary conviction, with an incomparable, subjective certainty,

2)   where there is an imperviousness to other experiences and to compelling counter-argument,

3)   and the content of which is impossible.[6]

What's often ignored, however, is Jaspers' description of such criteria as being but 'vague', 'merely external', 'superficial and incorrect'.[7] Whilst (1)–(3) certainly are true of most delusions, they don't hold true of all, and they also characterize many non-delusions. Modern psychiatric textbooks attempt to remedy this by stressing (4) the socially atypical character of delusional content. Yet whilst this allows the psychiatrist to avoid the awkwardness of diagnosing as delusional our many culturally prevalent, strongly maintained, poorly reasoned, and possibly false beliefs (various widespread religious, would-be-scientific, and political convictions, for example), it can scarcely be said to convey insight into delusion itself. To speak with the philosophers: this psychiatric bodge might help us hone in on delusion's extension (i.e. the criteria now pick out more delusion and less non-delusion) but it fails to elucidate its intension (i.e. the actual meaning of 'delusion'). The natural suspicion remains that we'd do better to consider, say, the cultural scarcity of delusion to be a function not of its definition but of a merely empirical fact – of the thankful fact, that is, that most people are, because of circumstance or temperament, fairly invulnerable to psychosis. Something similar may be said of the first three criteria: they are merely accidental ('merely external') properties of most delusions that don't reach to the ('internal') psychotic core of delusion itself.

Let's unpack this argument a little. In what ways may taking the standard definition to provide a truly operational set of criteria result in false negatives – i.e. result in the error of taking something to be absent which in fact is not? By way of genuine delusions that may yet be true, Jaspers offers us world war and jealousy. Delusions of world war are not so uncommon in schizophrenia, and yet a diagnosis of such delusion in someone who in late 1939 hadn't heard of the war's development would not have to be retrospectively revoked. Similarly with delusional jealousy, which 'does not cease to be a delusion although the spouse of the patient is in fact unfaithful – sometimes only as the result of the delusion'.[8] To these we may add the paradoxical delusion of mental illness: someone who hypochondriacally believed he was suffering mental illness was still properly judged delusional; not, of course, because his belief was false – but because of the extraordinary manner and context of its arrival and the fashion of his cleaving to it.[9] Such delusions' truth is not, as it were, to be held against them. A final false negative springing from the standard summary definition concerns the widespread idea that delusions are necessarily 'fixed beliefs'.[10] The fact however is that delusion may wax and wane in response to changing circumstances, changing stress levels and therapeutic interventions; several of Morag's delusions were but short-lived.[11] And in any case the incorrigibility of her delusion cannot be allowed to characterize it for all time – for that would make recovery from it a logical impossibility. Once more our suspicion must surely be that the fixity of certain beliefs is a function of their delusionality (rather than vice versa), and that the textbook authors here again mistake an empirical cart for a conceptual horse.

And what of the false positives encouraged by the standard definition? Regarding these we may simply ask, with Jaspers: 'If incorrigible wrong judgments are termed "delusion", who will there be without delusion, since we are all capable of having convictions and it's a universal human characteristic to hold on to our own mistaken judgments?'[12] Whilst 'normal mistakes are also very largely incorrigible', and whilst it 'is astonishing how most people tend to maintain the realities they believe in during a discussion, although the mistakes they are making seem to the knowledgeable person little else but "sheer delusion"', we surely do not here actually meet with 'delusion in the psychopathological sense'.[13]

So much for the under- and over-inclusivity of the standard definitions. But we should recall that our true concern here is not with definition.[14] What we want is instead, and abstractly put, to answer *das Wahnproblem* – the problem of what it is to be deluded – that 'unsolved problem of human life as such' which 'not only gives us pause but makes us shudder'.[15] More concretely, what we want is to understand Morag in her delusion. It's not simply that delusions are false, unusual, and strongly maintained beliefs; rather they are, as psychopathology used to put it, 'pathologically falsified' beliefs, and we want to know just what is pathological about them.[16] Their atypicality is no mere matter of statistical rarity, but rather one of normative peculiarity. We're struck by how forcefully they're maintained – not because intransigence is scarce in human life, but because we can't readily grasp how anyone could stubbornly cleave to claims like those. In short, Morag has beliefs which, as we say, one 'would have to be mad' to entertain, and what we want to understand is just what it is to be mad in this way. We want to know what it could mean for Morag to think, seemingly out of the blue, that she was due to meet a special messenger, that the solar system was falling apart, and that she could remedy this with arm movements.

Jaspers vs. the psychologists

Definition hasn't helped us understand what it is to be deluded – but might psychology succeed where lexicography fails? Psychological approaches often lead with attempted rebuttals of Jaspers' pessimistic declarations that it 'is not possible to understand the genesis of delusion proper'; that much 'has been explained as meaningful which in fact was nothing of the kind'; that delusion is 'psychologically irreducible'; that 'we cannot really appreciate these quite alien modes of experience' which 'remain largely incomprehensible, unreal and beyond our understanding.'[17] For Jaspers – the great champion not only of a psychology of *Erklären* (causal explanation from without) but also and especially of *Verstehen* (empathic understanding from within)[18] – to have made so little headway with, and even pronounced the impossibility of, 'empathically understanding' the delusional person, has seemed to the psychologists a great and regrettable irony.

Psychologists of diverse schools have agreed on the charge that Jaspers' pessimism regarding the empathic intelligibility of delusion was ill-founded.[19] And one might think there's cause for their concern because, at least since Aristotle, the human has been understood as ζῷον λόγον ἔχον – as the animal whose rational capacity is integral to its being what it is. To find Morag more than passingly ununderstandable may, then, seem to amount to finding her, when she's in her delusion – when she is, as she herself puts it, 'beyond all reason' – to have a temporarily compromised humanity. Jaspers' tack, the psychologists quite naturally worry, encourages us to baulk at offering humane recognition to her. Which, in the context of psychiatry's sometime humanizing ambition and humanistic ethic, could hardly seem but a regressive step.

As will now be demonstrated, something has, however, gone seriously wrong in such psychologists' critique of Jaspers. Perhaps such matters of scholarship matter little per se. Nevertheless what follows argues that this same error, when propagated more widely outside the scholarly context, has significant implications: it impedes our understanding of Morag in her delusion. For this reason, then, let's survey some criticisms from the literature.

Consider first the quite typical claim, from a survey of *Cognitive Approaches to Delusion*, that the psychological suggestion that

> delusions are explanations of experience [that] represent the individual's attempt to make sense of events . . . contrasts very markedly with the conventional wisdom regarding delusions, dating from Jaspers (1913), that (primary) delusions are 'ununderstandable' and psychologically irreducible.[20]

Next, this, from a work entitled *Madness Explained*:

> Jaspers held all truly delusional beliefs to be ununderstandable, by which he meant that they are meaningless and unconnected to the individual's personality or experience. [Yet if we make] the effort . . . to understand them . . . it is apparent that the most common delusional themes observed in clinical practice . . . reflect patients' concerns about their position in the social universe.[21]

And this, from a prominent review of Jaspers' *General Psychopathology*:

> Jaspers . . . fails to understand the dialectic of the person's life before the supposed alien, meaningless intrusion occurs. It is because he has lost track long before, that the person's experience finally loses all meaning to Jaspers, and [merely causal, ununderstandable] process is then invented. I devoted a book (*The Divided Self*) largely to demonstrating that the way from apparent sanity to apparent madness could be understood well past the point where Jaspers tells us to give up.[22]

A text called *Making Sense of Madness* tells us that it's only

> if looked at from a narrow perspective which posits biological causes such as faulty neurotransmitters or deviant genes as sole or primary causes [that psychotic] experiences become incomprehensible.
>
> . . . Jaspers' (1963) influential contention [is] that a defining feature of psychosis is that it is fundamentally 'un-understandable' and therefore not amenable to psychological intervention. We believe that Jasper's [*sic*] position is untenable: psychosis may be complex and confusing, but . . . not only is it understandable, but also at least some of those who actually experience psychosis can, if given the opportunity, help contribute to making it so.[23]

Or see this from a work entitled *Understanding and Treating Schizophrenia*:

> Primary delusions, Jaspers assumed, result from biological causes that completely overwhelm the capacities of the individual and have no link to the subject's psychological history.... Jaspers argued that these experiences are not explainable in terms of life history, trauma, defences, or conflicts, and thus he referred to them as primary.... Psychodynamic and interpersonal theorists, in contrast, emphasize the relationship between delusions and life history. Their focus is on the role of current and past relationships, underlying conflicts, and defensive structures in understanding the origins and meaning of delusions.[24]

Finally, consider the claim that Jaspers' distinction between

> what is meaningful and allows empathy and what in its particular way is ununderstandable, 'mad' in the literal sense,

... such as manifests in

> the seeming nonsensicality, the *logical* impossibility, of the following passage from the diary of the dancer Vaslav Nijinsky, who suffered a schizophrenic breakdown in his late twenties: 'Once I went for a walk and it seemed to me that I saw some blood on the snow. I followed the traces of the blood and sensed that somebody *who was still alive* had been killed.'

... is of a piece with his having

> insisted so adamantly on the utter incomprehensibility of [schizophrenia].[25]

In short, the guiding thought appears to be that, so long as we can contextualize delusional utterance within a social, existential, narrative, or psychological frame, then delusion isn't ununderstandable in Jaspers' sense. Nevertheless, when we turn to Jaspers' *General Psychopathology* we find him actually maintaining all that the above-cited critics claim he denies.

Thus, contra the idea attributed to him that delusions aren't attempts to make sense of inner and outer experiences, we find him writing that

> Thinking accompanies the first step which brings delusion about. This may be no more than the unsystematic, blurred thinking of the acute psychoses ... yet even here patients look for some kind of connection. Or the thinking may be more systematic... Here the thought works over the delusion on the basis of the primary experiences, trying to link them harmoniously with real perceptions and the patient's actual knowledge.... In this way a *delusional system* is constructed which in its own context is comprehensible, sometimes extremely closely argued and unintelligible only in its ultimate origins, the primary experience. These delusional systems are objective meaningful structures ...[26]

Rather than claiming that delusions don't reflect their sufferers' personality we find him writing that

> ... every illness and every psychosis too is *elaborated* by the affected personality; the attitude of the personality to the illness is to be understood in terms of the personality-traits.
>
> [We can't equate psychosis with personality type but can ask] whether and to what extent the original personality-Anlage and the [psychotic] process reveal any relationship to each other.[27]

Far from claiming that delusions do not express recognizable concerns regarding, for example, one's position in the social universe, Jaspers in fact proclaims it to be

> self-evident that the *content* of every psychosis depends on the content of the earlier life experiences and that, for example, the delusional preoccupations of a shoemaker will differ from those of a publican.
>
> A sexual lapse is transformed by embarrassment and remorse into a fear of being discovered and into delusions of being watched and finally of being persecuted. Sexual inadequacy and poor contact with the environment are transformed into the delusion that sexually one is being influenced and that one is being persecuted. Sexual deprivation is transformed into delusions of being loved and being asked to marry. Yet however understandable the connections, the specific character of the relationship and of the transformation still remains ununderstandable.[28]

Rather than denying that delusion is motivationally intelligible, springing from personal and social, rather than merely biological, causes, Jaspers can be found voicing that

> We may well understand from the context how a delusional belief's content provides the delusional individual with relief from something unbearable, or seems to deliver him from reality and lends a peculiar satisfaction which may well be the ground for why it is so tenaciously held. But in this very moment when the understandability of delusion is taken to concern not simply this content but instead its development, this understandability vitiates the diagnosis of delusion, for in that case what we actually shall have grasped is ordinary human error, not delusion proper.[29]

As for the claim that Jaspers' take on delusion's ununderstandability rules out psychotherapy, it's worth noting that psychosis simply doesn't feature in the 'limits to psychotherapy' he describes. His caution regarding the psychotherapy of psychotic individuals instead concerns the need for psychotherapists to first have an adequate training in psychopathology:

> When there is no proper grounding in the reality of the psychoses and no passionately sought understanding of them, every individual or anthropological

presentation will . . . carry serious flaws. . . . Psychotherapy cannot live simply on its own resources.[30]

True ('primary') delusion, as Jaspers understands it, is then actually – contra what we're often told he thinks – at least sometimes: intelligible as an attempt at making sense of inner and outer experience; intelligible as an attempt reflecting the subject's personality and which may be motivationally intelligible; intelligible as an attempt with a content expressing recognizable concerns; and responsive to psychotherapeutic treatment. Yet even so, despite elaborating the ways in which delusion and psychosis may be understood psychologically, Jaspers still frequently proclaims their essential 'empathic unununderstandability'. Rather than assume, then, that 'empathic understandability' means 'psychological intelligibility', we will do better to suppose that, on Jaspers' lips, it means something different which we've yet to grasp.

What is Jaspers' 'empathic understanding'?

Jaspers' talk of 'empathy' (*Einfühlung*) and of 'empathic understanding' references both a pre-reflective and passive experience of 'seeing from within', and a more effortful, reflective analogue of this in the phenomenology of understanding (*Verstehen*), such empathy contrasting with that impersonal 'seeing from without' met with in explanation (*Erklären*). It's sometimes assumed that in such talk, or in his occasional mention of 'transposing oneself' or 'sinking into' others' mental lives, Jaspers is telling us *how* interpersonal understanding arises.[31] Yet we can fruitfully distinguish between (a) acknowledgement and (b) explanation – i.e. between (a) modest attempts to simply offer recognition to the distinctive character of such understanding and (b) more ambitious attempts to actually explain how it's achieved. And nothing in his text suggests that Jaspers even considers such 'how?' questions as answered by (b) to be so much as coherent. He doesn't, for example, construe our interpersonal understanding as involving us in the business of somehow finding our way (by inference perhaps, or by imaginative projection) from bare externals (movements, expressions, situations) to meaningful internals (thoughts and feelings). Nor does he spell out 'transposing oneself' in terms of imaginative projection (as when I'm supposed to grasp what you're feeling by first imagining what I'd be feeling were I you and then taking you to be feeling what I just imagined myself feeling). Instead, and along with other phenomenologically-oriented philosophers and psychiatrists, he offers us a conception of human expression-in-context as itself replete with perceptible meaning (I can, as long as I'm receptively open to you, simply see what you're feeling).[32] We therefore do well to construe his mentions of 'empathy' not as references to a method for, but as acknowledgements of a basic form of, interpersonal understanding.

This form of understanding – 'understanding from within', 'empathic understanding' – has to do with our grasp of speaker's meaning (or, to coin a phrase, 'agent's meaning') – i.e. with our comprehending grasp of *what* someone's saying (or doing, or expressing) and of *why* it's said (or done). This grasp of 'why' takes various forms; it includes both our grasp of reasons – i.e. of why saying or doing something makes rational sense – and of such matters as, say, the choice of a particular metaphor to describe a certain piece of music. When this kind of understanding eludes us we say, 'I didn't get what you meant', 'I didn't catch your drift'. Accordingly, when Jaspers says that delusional utterances are ununderstandable we may take him to mean that here we meet with a drift which simply cannot be caught or, more perspicuously put, with but an ersatz drift.

So, what are the essential characteristics of 'seeing what someone's getting at' or 'grasping the point of what someone's saying or doing'?

The first thing we might note is what it's directed at – which is not mere events but rather discourse, actions, expressions and their products (works of art, texts, smoke signals, etc.).

A second characteristic of 'empathic understanding' is that it's usually more helpfully described in terms of *what* someone's doing and *why* they're doing it – and not in terms of 'understanding X *as* Y'. Above we saw both Jaspers and his critics understanding delusional utterances *as* attempts at sense-making, *as* reflections of personality, *as* expressing social concerns, *as* motivationally intelligible, *as* material for therapeutic intervention, etc. These are not examples of 'empathic understanding' in the sense here under consideration.[33] I may understand what someone's doing as her making of a dismissive gesture; I may take what someone's saying as a request. Yet, whilst often interdependent with it, such understanding is not identical with my understanding of the dismissive gesture or with my understanding what's being requested. It's this latter understanding which delusion thwarts.

A third characteristic is that, in its essential form, empathic understanding is *without method*. Because of this it's typically rather meaningless to ask *how* we ordinarily understand one another. Whilst we do sometimes use methods – either to resolve perplexity (by newly contextualizing what initially was baffling), or to overcome ignorance (by asking for clarification, looking up unknown terms in a dictionary, etc.) – this itself depends on our enjoying a prior method-free understanding of the clarification. Furthermore, after we've used such a method it may be safely set aside without our thereby suffering a loss of understanding. Relatedly, empathic understanding isn't typically superposed upon an experience of an object which is first grasped independently of that understanding.[34] For example, if we empathically understand what someone's saying, we don't in the ordinary case first need to project ourselves into her shoes; we don't need, as it were, to simulate her predicament and preferences within ourselves and then add to our prior grasp of her the results of our simulation. Instead, we can simply relate to her, without first having to relate her to ourselves. It's in the midst of our experiential engagements with her, and not in some extra ratiocinative or imaginative overlay, that we catch her drift, grasp what she's doing, saying, feeling, or thinking.

The final marker offered here concerns explicability and apt response. If I'm properly to be said to understand what you're getting at, I should typically be able to paraphrase your words. If you ask me a question which I understand, my understanding is demonstrated in my response – either in an action (e.g. I fetch what you requested), or in discourse (I refuse to fetch it), or, if I don't know the answer, in a demonstration that I do at least know what general kind of response is here being invited. Or, if I understand the use of a metaphor, then I will sometimes be able to say something about its basis.

('I am the good shepherd; and I know My sheep, and am known by My own ... and I lay down My life for the sheep.'[35] Christians who understand this see themselves as members of Christ's flock, called into close relationship with him.) Yet it should be noted that at other times my appreciation of the aptness of a non-literal use will not be something that can be further cashed out: that I too find myself moved to use the same musical terms to describe just this sunset will be enough for talk of 'grasp of speaker's meaning' to be secure. Or I may find relatable particular 'secondary sense' uses of terms to express psychological states. For example, I will properly be said to understand what you mean by telling me 'I've got pins and needles' if I too am sometimes disposed to articulate a sensation thus. Finally, far from it being a requirement on empathic understanding that I'm always able to cash out all metaphors, our comprehension of poetry can involve us in appreciating precisely the non-paraphrasability of the poem when it comes to (what, borrowing from Jaspers, we may call) 'sinking ourselves into' it.

In sum, empathic understanding may be understood as what at root is a fundamentally method-less grasp of the meaning of what's said and done, which grasp has its life in our variously apt sense-registering attunement to these sayings and doings.[36] With this in mind, consider again the extract from Nijinsky's diaries quoted above: 'Once I went for a walk and it seemed to me that I saw some blood on the snow. I followed the traces of the blood and sensed that somebody *who was still alive* had been killed.' In his treatment of delusion Jaspers nowhere implies that we can't understand this as Nijinsky's attempt at sense-making, as reflecting Nijinsky's personality or preoccupations, as an utterance motivated by strong affect and profound ambivalence. What he might say, however, is that it expresses an attempt at sense-making which itself is marked by delusionality. Even though we may be able to see in his delusional remark much of his psychology, his history, and his social and political circumstances, there yet remains an important sense in which we can't understand what Nijinsky says. Again, understanding is not one thing: understanding a speaker's meaning is irreducible to understanding what emotional forces motivate his utterance. I may be motivated by loyalty to defend Jaspers; you may grasp this motivation underlying my writing; your grasp of that, however, is a different matter than your grasp of the meaning of my sentences. All being well I shall now be intelligible to you in at least two different ways, one of those ways being the matter of your grasping what I'm on about. Alas, all was not well with Nijinsky.

Delusion as epistemically primitive

Of particular interest to Jaspers is what he calls 'genetic understanding'. This refers to our immediate apprehension of a mental state as arising intelligibly out of a particular worldly or psychological context. Jaspers stamps on your foot; you cry out and are angry; I straightway understand your cry and your anger as intelligible responses to Jaspers' act. You suddenly realize that you've left it too late to catch the last train; I immediately understand your worry, your self-recriminations, your annoyance. Such phenomena themselves have an intelligible form, and our 'empathic' understanding of others' sayings and doings is informed by our appreciation of the intelligibility of such acts' genesis. Furthermore, that your crying out and anger constitute intelligible responses to Jaspers' foot stomping is not itself something for which evidence could reasonably be requested or provided. Instead, it's something we describe as 'self-evident' or (with Jaspers) as 'ultimate'.[37]

Jaspers' principal articulation of delusion's unununderstandability is in terms of it having no empathically intelligible genesis: delusion is not genetically intelligible. It's for this reason that he compares it with such phenomena as organic illness or those aspects of character which reflect inherited constitution.[38] If we wish to understand the genesis of organic illness and constitution we must look to matters such as environmental influences, physiology, genetics – i.e. to matters which are not rationally or empathically intelligible. Such phenomena are, from the point of view of *Verstehen*, simply there as 'basic and primary' givens that must be acknowledged rather than accounted for.[39]

This lack of genetic intelligibility also explains why Jaspers says of delusion that 'phenomenologically it is an experience', arrived at 'in a direct way, non-mediated by reflection or inference', coming 'before thought, although becoming clear to itself only in thought', manifest in delusional judgement whilst having 'none of the characteristics of a judgement in itself'.[40] Its experiential nature isn't a matter of it having, say, a perceptual origin (although perception may indeed become delusional); it's instead due only to it coming 'before thought'. And such priority is itself best understood not in temporal or psychological, but in logical, terms. Consider the difference between mistaken and confused thought: mistakes are made whereas confusions are suffered; mistakes are errant whilst confusions are aberrant. The ascription of confusion impugns descriptions of what's said or done as expressive of intelligible thought or intent. And since genuine thought is in principle intelligible, the thought met with in confusion is thought in name only. So too for that form of confusion we term 'delusion'.

This also explains why Jaspers describes delusion as 'an immediate, intrusive knowledge of meaning', such 'immediacy' referencing not the psychological phenomenon of rapidly arriving thought but rather the fact that this (false pretender for) knowledge cannot be conceived of as deriving from reflection.[41] The upshot is not that delusion can't be elaborated by reflection; it's rather that such delusion as does become thus elaborated is delusional because of the delusionality that's already there within the experience or the reflection. The upshot of this is that if we 'try to make the actual formation of the delusion, as well as its content, understandable, any diagnosis of delusion becomes impossible, for what we have grasped in this case is ordinary human error, not delusion proper'.[42]

Consider in this light Morag's psychotic episode. We might be able to understand how her underlying delusion – that a new cosmic plan is afoot in the world – organizes certain of her thoughts and experiences. Various of her beliefs – that a stranger is a secret accomplice, that sports are orchestrated to sublimate warmongering aggression, that her four great's grandfather has come back to life, that she can avert cosmic catastrophe by moving her arms – can be understood in the light of her organizing delusion. We may also be able to see how her delusional system provides relief from the anguish of her life, and how, in this sense, she's strongly motivated to form and cleave to it. Finally, we may even sometimes be able to imagine being drawn to speak as Morag speaks. Yet what we cannot do is comprehend her underlying delusion whilst treating it as a sincere, non-metaphorically meant, attempt at sense-making: our judgement that it isn't comprehensible in this way is instead of a piece with our judgement that here we truly do meet with delusion.

Psychological theories of delusion

In her narrative Morag tells us that she 'lost her reason', and with this Jaspers would agree. Yet at least since Jaspers' time, various psychologists have suggested that she and he are both at least partly wrong about this.[43] And perhaps a fair consideration of such psychological studies will force us to reopen the question of delusion's intelligibility. For what is often argued is that, contra Jaspers, we can achieve an empathic understanding of Morag's delusion if we see it either as an ordinary attempt to make ordinary sense of various non-delusional experiential abnormalities, and/or as the natural result of trying to make sense of ordinary experience whilst suffering certain impairments or biases in her reasoning that are not themselves intrinsically delusional in form. What follows presents a brief excursus into matters empirical, then returns to properly philosophical concerns regarding delusion's intelligibility.

It's an undisputed fact that sufferers from schizophrenic illnesses, the most prevalent of the psychoses, can experience deficits in cognitive abilities such as attention, memory, executive function, and understanding others' mental states.[44] That such psychological difficulties correlate with thought disorder and the so-called negative symptoms (demotivation, social withdrawal, diminished emotional and verbal expression) is also indisputable.[45] So too is the fact that delusions are often found in those who suffer schizophrenia, and that, compared with their coincidence in the general population, the coincidence of delusion and thought disorder in schizophrenic individuals is high.[46]

What, however, is not evident in any of this is a causal link between cognitive deficit and delusion. Taken as a whole the empirical evidence rather stands against the hypothesis that delusions primarily result from trying to use an impaired (but not intrinsically delusional) cognitive resource to reason about, or otherwise understand, the kinds of personal, social, romantic, religious, and metaphysical matters typically thematized in delusion. An alleged disposition of delusional schizophrenic subjects to jump to conclusions is, for example, not a good contender for explaining their delusionality, since their allegedly jumpy cognitive disposition is also associated with a tendency to quickly relinquish their beliefs, a tendency incompatible with the intransigence of many schizophrenic subjects regarding their delusions.[47] Furthermore, delusions are usually circumscribed: large stretches of the psychotic subject's thought, knowledge, and belief may remain quite unaffected by delusion. A quite general impaired reasoning capacity is not, then, an obvious contender for a causally sufficient condition of delusional difficulties. Such theories also fail to explain why some delusional individuals don't appear to suffer such general biases in judgement, and why non-psychotic individuals may suffer significant impairments in cognitive ability without becoming deluded.

An alternative hypothesis has delusion resulting from the use of unimpaired cognitive resources to discern the origin and significance of disturbed (but not intrinsically delusional) sensory experience.[48] Schizophrenic individuals do after all experience not only delusions but also perceptual and somatosensory hallucinations, and so – the thought goes – perhaps the former result from attempts to make sense of the latter. Such a theory, however, is empirically limited since it accounts neither for such delusion as develops without disturbed sensory experience, nor for the absence of delusion in those non-schizophrenic individuals who experience sensory disturbances (tinnitus, phantom limb, hypnagogic hallucinations, the hallucinations met with in Charles Bonnet syndrome, etc.).[49]

So much, perhaps, for matters empirical. From a philosophical point of view, however, the question still remains as to whether such psychological theories really are theories of delusion, or whether, as Jaspers suggested, they offer us 'no clear differentiation … of the specific phenomenon, the actual delusional experience' but only 'an understandable context for the emergence of certain stubborn misconceptions'. In other words, might the explanation and that which it's aimed at here risk passing one another by? For sure, delusions are paradigms of unreason. For sure, delusional subjects may reason poorly. Even so, superior reasoning abilities may yet be 'put into the service of the delusion', elaborating it and defending it against disconfirmation.[50] For this reason, the psychologists' restriction of their own interest to cognitive processes leaves us quite in the dark as to what it is to suffer delusion. Even if they correctly detect deficits in Morag's inference-making, and even if such deficits do somehow contribute to the formation and maintenance of her delusional beliefs, we're still left unclear as to how she's able to seriously maintain beliefs as strange as hers. How could a mere tendency to, say, jump to conclusions lead Morag to think that moving her arms in a pattern will help avoid a cosmic crisis? How could a tendency to make substandard inferences lead her to think that she's just met and made love to her deceased four great's grandfather? And how could perceptual or inferential difficulty lead her to think that four people inhabit the same body? What is it, in any case, to think such thoughts? Would not a more reasonable conclusion, regarding any perceptual anomaly, be that something is awry with the mind, brain, ear, or eye? Or, to return to Ilse from Chapter 1: how, really, is it that Ilse could think that everything now happens in reference to her, that others know her secret intentions, that the clock in the square has stopped upside down, that others shall make a report on her, that the police station was the Other World, that a police officer is dead and has to type on an upside-down typewriter until he has expiated his sins, that her tea is poisoned, that there are other people lying in her bed, that everyone is bewitched, and that the doctor's black hair and hook nose means he is a murderer?

These are the real puzzles which the delusion of Morag and Ilse presents to us. Far from making psychologically describable mistakes of reasoning, they instead appear to have lost touch with reality in such a way as makes it apt to describe them as no longer in their right mind. With their feet no longer on the ground, it matters little how inferentially impeccable or awry the cogitations in their heads are found to be – for the delusionality of what obtains there is rather a function of the underlying slippage in their reality contact. And saying what that actually amounts to surely requires a different kind of investigation altogether – one such being offered in the next two chapters.

For such reasons, Jaspers' scepticism about psychological attempts to understanding delusion ('should we ... try to make the actual formation of the delusion, as well as its content, understandable, any diagnosis of delusion becomes impossible, for what we have grasped in this case is ordinary human error, not delusion proper'[51]) would appear to remain as pertinent today as a century ago when he first declared it.

Contexts of enquiry and treatment

When we ask 'what's meant by "understanding someone's thought"?', we may have in mind any of the following:

i) Does someone have reasons for – wherein the rational intelligibility of her – thinking as she does? (Why does she think he's coming back late tonight? Because he left her a note to this effect.)

ii) Does an author's use of metaphor resonate with us? (I understand E. E. Cummings' 'nobody,not even the rain,has such small hands', from his poem 'somewhere i have never travelled,gladly beyond', if, resonating too with his talk of silence, frail gestures, slightest looks, intense fragility, etc., I'm thereby drawn to appreciate the tender gentleness of the form of love of which he writes.)

iii) What is it to think such thoughts? (What is it to be deluded?)

iv) What psychologically motivates – what function is served by – the development and maintenance of such thought? (What are delusion's typical psychodynamics?)

v) What sustains, and what are the material conditions of possibility of, such (valid or aberrant) thought? (Are there specific disturbances to attention, thought, brain activity, inner or outer experience, etc., to be met with here?)

vi) What developmental trajectory provides someone with the mental, neurological, personality, etc., structures in which such thought may take root? (Does an abusive upbringing make an individual psychosis-prone?)

vii) What if anything precipitates such thinking? (What are its typical efficient causes – environmental stressors, drug abuse, romantic breakdown, etc.?)

viii) Can we recover the (i) rational intelligibility of someone's thought by seeing her as making the best of a bad job – i.e. as labouring to make sense of the world whilst (v) suffering disturbances to inner experience, outer experience, or reasoning?

It was as a result of not distinguishing between such different senses of 'understand' that the above-mentioned critics talked past, rather than rebutted, Jaspers' claim that we cannot empathically understand delusion. That claim of his is best understood as emphasizing the impossibility, when what we have to do with is a delusional subject, of answering (i) and (ii), whereas the psychologists instead emphasize the availability of answers to (iii)–(viii).

The essential nature of delusion lays down a constraint on what may count as its satisfactory genetic explanation, since it's senseless to seek the rational elucidation of an essentially irrational thought. This, however, is not the only constraint in play. Others are provided by what Chapter 1 offered as criteria for mental illness: that it involve breakdown or motivated flight in the face of suffering. Not all the symptoms of mental illness need carry such traces; some may arise adventitiously once the state of reality-detachment supervenes. Nevertheless, flight from suffering, or pseudo-coherent compensation to breakdown, is essential to our understanding of such delusion as characterizes psychotic mental illness. When it comes to the delusions met with in mental illness, explanations of their arising that leave out reference to pathic and motivational factors will at best be partial and may well only pertain to their more incidental aspects.

To illuminate other constraints, consider first that permissive proposal known as 'interventionism'. This has it that causes – or at least, what interventionism calls 'causal factors' – are properly identified and individuated by interventions: 'A is a cause of B if intervening on A disrupts B.' If we intervene pharmacologically on Morag's amygdala activation, and as a result she no longer thinks planetary catastrophe may be averted by arm movements, then we would, says the interventionist, be right to offer her amygdala activation as a bona fide cause were we asked why she became deluded.[52]

If our interest in the causes of delusion happens to include not only their precipitating (efficient) but also their constituting (material) causes, it will be hard to fault the interventionist's proposal. Furthermore, there are good reasons to think the technical notion of 'causal factor' a useful addition to psychiatric discourse. So long as we expand it to also include such factors as are only jointly sufficient for producing and maintaining psychopathology, the notion usefully summarizes the procedures for ruling out invalid aetiologies and treatments, and enables ready articulation of the logical distinction between truly causal and merely coincidental correlations. Yet difficulties emerge once we turn from the technical notion of a 'causal factor' to our non-technical concept of a 'cause' as, roughly, 'that which may be properly cited in a causal explanation'. This is because what counts as valid explanation depends upon the context of enquiry, which context includes, in particular, the interests and concerns of the enquirer.

Consider Morag. One of her psychiatrically illiterate relatives visits and, shocked by her strange behaviour, asks an attendant psychiatrist why on earth Morag thinks she can mend a damaged cosmos with arm movements. His fruitful answer situates Morag's belief in the context of her mental illness: 'Morag is mentally ill and this is one of her delusions.' The answer helps the questioner get her bearings; it effectively tells her both that a certain other set of questions and answers is here to be ruled out (we aren't here to resolve the puzzlement by reference to Morag's reasoning) and that Morag has been overwhelmed, has lost contact with reality, is living in a world of her own.

Later on another relative visits, one who's more psychiatrically literate and who moreover has seen Morag in the throws of a previous episode. Knowing full well that she's once again psychotic, and that her cosmos-mending beliefs and activities are delusional, he nevertheless asks the psychiatrist the same question. What now might he mean by it? Well, perhaps he's after a further elaboration of the delusion, a setting of certain delusional beliefs and experiences in the context of others (since, as Jaspers has it, 'such understandable connections . . . play a part . . . in psychoses so far as content is concerned'[53]). Or perhaps an answer which refers to a pre-delusional context (Morag had, let's imagine, been performing yogic sun salutations each morning before she became ill) will be apt (psychosis often inverts agent and subject – so here an action originally done in response to the sun now becomes, in the patient's mind, an action having an effect on the sun).

What's not so clear – to return to the interventionist's suggestion – is what our questioner would have to be after such that an answer mentioning (that mere causal factor which is) Morag's amygdala activity would in any way satisfy his enquiry into why she's come to think the cosmos may be mended with arm movements. We may get some of the way there by imagining our questioner and the psychiatrist to be talking in an interdisciplinary neurology and psychiatry seminar; even here, however, the response is too coarse to adequately answer the question. The point of this mention of different questioners' interests has been to demonstrate that questions and answers about causes arise and enjoy their sense only within particular contexts of enquiry. Whilst the technical notion of a 'causal factor' may be designed to prescind from any particular such context, the same just isn't true of our use of ordinary causal concepts in the midst of sundry psychopathological and therapeutic contexts.

With respect to the treatment context, what interventions shall count as viable treatments also requires contextual situation. Perhaps, for example, a pharmaceutically-achieved reduction of amygdala activation leads to the cessation of Morag's delusion – but only at the general cost of her existential vitality. Such a 'chemical cosh' could be considered treatment only in a trivial and ethically debased sense – i.e. only in that sense in which whatever reduces a symptom is now to be considered treatment, regardless of whether this occurs in the context of enabling a patient to live her life.

The promise of interventionism resided in the simplicity of its criterion for distinguishing valid from invalid aetiologies and treatments. Is some putative difference really one that *makes* a difference? – this is its laudable, simplifying focus. Yet what it thereby risks losing sight of, because of its simplifying ambition, because of its mere focus on whether or not some phenomenon simply obtains, is the significance of those ontological, epistemic, and existential contexts which give meaning in the first place to the majority of our questions and answers about mental illness.

To what should we attend in order to understand why Morag developed her bizarre delusions? Once we've established that they obtain in the context of a mental illness, our enquiry does well to attend to her vulnerabilities, the context of her life, her preoccupations, and her suffering. Unless we're in the niche context of a neuropsychiatry seminar, we'll probably be uninterested in matters neurological. And entirely general answers (such as 'stress') are unlikely to satisfy anything but the most cursory and non-patient-centred curiosity. Hopefully we'll also want to know not just the external precipitants of Morag's delusion, but what it was about them that Morag found unbearable. Hopefully too we shall have an interest: in what exactly is compromised in her internal resources; in what latent amplifying fearful expectations (e.g. of how others will treat her) are aroused in her when she becomes overwhelmed; in what gets in the way of her being able to self-soothe; and in what in her inner terrain renders motivationally intelligible the shift to bizarre delusion. Similarly too for treatment: to focus on symptom reduction, uncontextualized by a concern with helping Morag better tolerate painful situations and then flourish in such ways as may then become possible, amounts to substituting a merely managerial for a genuinely therapeutic approach.

Conclusion: Incomprehension as a route to understanding

The argument of this chapter has been that to acknowledge Morag to truly be deluded is in part to grasp that such thought as her delusion embodies is not rationally or, in Jaspers' terms, 'empathically' intelligible. The question 'how *could* she think *that*?', if meant as an enquiry into reasons rather than causes, must accordingly remain rhetorical rather than receive an answer.

It's all too easy to consider this a merely negative finding – as if it provided a license to do nothing but see Morag's delusion as but the product of a broken biological mechanism, or to now take her for an It rather than a Thou. Return for a moment to the above-mooted concern that, if rationality is essential to the human form, and if to be psychotic is in part to be ununderstandable because irrational, then to be psychotic is to be less than fully human. The inference may appear sound, but what it misses is the sense in which rationality is essential to humanity. To bring this out, consider how it belongs to *the* cat to have four legs, or that it's in *the* beaver's nature to build a dam. *A* cat (or any number thereof) deprived of a leg, or *a* (bevy of) beaver(s) in want of building skills, is not thereby any less cat or beaver.[54] In fact, it's only because we know the cat to have four legs that we can say, of any particular cat, that it's lacking. So too with delusion: it's only such creatures as are essentially characterized by reason that may suffer its loss in delusion. For Morag to be delusional precisely is, then, for her to be a bona fide member of the species 'rational animal'. In this way, we might say that, far from impugning her human form, acknowledging the fact of her delusion instead reinforces our grasp of her humanity.

In a less abstract vein we may think too on the significance of the pain engendered by banging our head against understanding's limits. For anyone whose sensitivity has not been dulled, the experience is deeply disturbing, disorienting, jarring – is 'not only a puzzle: it makes us shudder'.[55] By attending to it carefully we learn not just something about our own frustrated impulse, but something significant about Morag.

Here our approach must be not positive or 'cataphatic' – as in (i) and (vii) above – but instead negative or 'apophatic'. As Jaspers suggests, we grasp the significance of Morag's delusions

ix)   … not through any positive understanding of them, but through the shock which the course of our comprehension receives in the face of the incomprehensible.[56]

Morag, we thereby appreciate, has suffered an inner catastrophe. And since this takes the form of mental illness, and indicates that something unthinkable has 'come to life in the very core of [her] existence',[57] we also grasp that here we are standing at the site not only of the terrible but also of the intolerable. Indeed, Morag has in her illness found life so unbearable that madness has been seized upon 'as the last means of saving' it.[58] Delusional reality and delusional meaning are now substituted for the unmanageable alternative of reality as Morag found it. The 'shock' and 'shudder' we experience – the unthinkable difficulty of reality which delusional experience presents to us – is accordingly one of our best clues as to the depth of Morag's disturbance. The apophatic moment alerts us to the character of her brokenness: through it we grasp that here we can't fall back on any assumption of, underneath it all, rational business as usual. We do well then to stay with it rather than rush off to other, positive, forms of understanding, since those cataphatic forms are as such unable to furnish the kind of recognition which may be offered to someone in the depths of her brokenness, and engaging in them makes for deflection from the difficulty of reality she suffers. Or, in Jaspers' words, 'Connected with all the attempts to understand schizophrenia we find the tendency to deny the facts of the process in their specificity.'[59] To inadequately recognize the ununderstandable is, therefore, to fail to show understanding to the psychotic subject.

So what is it that Morag cannot bear? In her autobiographical *Beyond All Reason* she tells of a young girl with an unlovable mother, of parents largely unable to contain her childhood terrors and pains or offer recognition to her in her emotional distress, of an early fear (reawakened later in her psychosis) of absolute destruction and annihilation, and of boarding school from eight years proving a relief from the home environment. Further on she notes for us her lack of sexual experience – her first kiss was at 27 – and her failure to integrate her sexual experience into her self-understanding. She comments too on her powerful and destabilizing unrequited romantic passions and their complex sublimation in vacillating religious passions and sometimes devastating collapses of faith. Later she's able to tolerate, and so to think through, a profound depression in which she registers her regret over fourteen wasted years of her life.

Further clues as to the underlying difficulty of reality she faced are revealed by her path to sanity. For along the way Morag encounters a Dr Upton, a psychiatrist and psychotherapist, and finds the courage to experience him as loving, as trusting, as dependable. She goes to see the film *David and Lisa* (1962), a moving drama about the relationship between a highly disturbed teenage boy and girl in a school for highly disturbed adolescents:

> The opening shots reminded me of my own horror of the mental hospitals I had been in, but I soon forgot that and became absorbed completely by the personal human drama – tense, beautifully acted, and at times deeply moving. The central characters were presented with a reality that struck me as perfectly authentic, and with a sympathy that implied absolute acceptance. So, by involving myself in their experience as I did, I was not only accepting my past sickness, but feeling it accepted too. . . .
>
> [Later] I walked slowly along the river bank, and let the chattering groups pass me by. . . . And a planet shone out in the clear sky above, as piercing in its light as a single sharp note of music, and the lights on the far bank were gay with a warming brightness, and I myself was feeling human and humane. . . .

I climbed up some steps onto the bridge, and as I did so it dawned on me what this new-found impulse meant. I had at last forgiven my sick self. . . .

I remembered the terrors of infancy which had been revived for me in my last time at hospital. I began to reach down towards the root of a forgotten fear of absolute destruction and annihilation. . . .

But this was something that I could not have done alone. I was thinking of Dr Upton at the time. . . . [I]n spirit I took him by the hand with the same confidence and comfort that a child holds someone's hand when retracing their steps to the place where they have had a terrifying accident. I pressed down into the darkly bright intensity of my hidden life and broke through to the perilous secret that my adult defences had guarded me from coming near. Dammed up and firmly sealed off down inside myself my primal, urgent need was still intact. And somewhere, in the uncharted time of early infancy, I had given myself and taken in return; I had needed and enjoyed and later felt that I had lost a mother's love. The sudden, living sense of need and loss came upon me so strongly that I wept. And then, refreshed as by a sudden storm of rain, I fell asleep.

During the next few days a tremendous emotional upheaval took place. I was able to recover into consciousness and to assimilate the terrifying feelings that stemmed from my first relationship in infancy. The barrier against them had been so strong that, except during periods of acute psychosis, it had never lifted until now. And it could not have lifted without disaster or destruction if there had not been a new relationship to take its place. It did not matter feeling I was an infant in dire need – I could need Dr Upton now. And need him I did, quite unrestrainedly. I just didn't mind. . . . Dr Upton was my safe anchorage. I could let my feelings free. . . . Mind, body and spirit were now at peace with one another. I had been made whole.[60]

In one sense, something ununderstandable gives way here to the understandable as Morag is able to trust in an other and – for the first time whilst sane – to experience, understand, and assimilate the terrors which have previously broken her mind. Aided both by the film director's and by Dr Upton's sensitivity and acceptance, she begins to tolerate knowing about the human connection she had been missing and to accept rather than judge herself in her vulnerability. Yet in another sense the ununderstandable delusion gives way to another ununderstandable phenomenon – that which Morag really is in herself. In what remains of this chapter, I shall explain what I mean by this.

So far we've seen how Jaspers invokes the notion of the ununderstandable in the context of true delusion. Yet he also notes how the 'ununderstandable is as much present in all normal life as it is in morbid states and processes', singling out three forms of it:[61]

i)   As discussed above, understanding 'halts before the *reality of organic illness and psychosis*, before the elementary nature of these facts'. When we grasp that someone is ill we can empathize with the person and show him understanding when he's unable to function as normal. Yet illness cannot itself be met with empathic understanding: a sigh or groan is intelligible as such, but not a fever.

ii) Understanding also halts 'before the reality of the *innateness of empirical characteristics* [which are] impenetrable and inalterable'. Attempts to say why someone reacts as he does come to an end at some point. This is so not only for non-psychological characteristics (hair colour, etc.) which as such do not yield to empathic understanding, but also for various matters of characterological constitution. Newborn babies, for example, have different temperaments: little Emil is placid while his twin brother Eugen is more agitated. We may only explain from the outside (*Erklären*) but not understand from the inside (*Verstehen*) such matters of temperament (*Anlage*).

iii) Finally, understanding 'halts before the reality of *Existence itself*, that which the individual really is in himself'. Here to *not* attempt to understand someone becomes an ethical imperative, otherwise one shall risk 'totalizing' her – which is to say, risk reducing her to another version of oneself.[62]

The risk of 'totalizing' attendant on attempts at understanding what Jaspers terms another's 'Existence' may be demonstrated even for the simplest of matters such as taste. Ilse prefers light chocolate; Morag, dark. If Ilse were to ask of Morag 'but *why* do you prefer dark to milk chocolate?', Morag may begin to feel aggravated, may begin to feel that she's not being met with as the individual she is. 'I just do' might now be her proper response. In not ceding her quest for understanding, Ilse has most likely taken her own preference as the self-evident model for anyone's preference. Deviations from this imposed norm would then naturally seem to require explanation. Yet should Ilse be able to accept that there's nothing about Morag's preference that needs understanding, no accounting for herself that is required from Morag, this itself would amount to an instance of offering recognition to her. Accounting for oneself stops on reaching the bedrock of one's Existence, on reaching that point where one might say simply: 'This just is who I am.'[63] Holding another accountable in her actions remains part of what it is to offer her recognition as a person, but honouring the unaccountability of another in her Existence will be the greater part of moral recognition's provision.

In psychosis we meet the ununderstandable at an unexpected juncture – which is why delusion brings us up short. We meet the ununderstandable not only in the sufferer's Existence which, as for any of us, undergirds all her intelligible discursive acts, but rather, and to our shock, at such junctures of expressive performance as would normally reward rational probing. Whereas we can all accept with Angelus Silesius that the 'rose is without why; she blooms because she blooms', we shudder on finding the same why-less-ness in the midst of seemingly well-organized talk. Attempting to retrieve speaker's meaning from Morag's delusional talk may well then be tempting for us. Yet it's precisely in persisting with this that we now fail to offer her acknowledgement in the depths of her predicament, fail to recognize that she's no longer in that world which is intelligible because shareable, fail to understand that she's now in an unthinkably lonely 'world of her own'.

What it means to be in such a world is the topic of the next chapter. To conclude the present one, consider what both Jaspers and Morag have to say about the dependence of all that is intelligible and valuable in life on its ununderstandable substrate. First Jaspers:

I'm to be counted genuinely rational only if my whole reason is truly both grounded upon unreason and acknowledged by me to be thus grounded.[64]

By 'unreason' here Jaspers refers not to the irrational, but to the non-rational, nature of Existence itself. The same consideration is offered by Morag – so long as we read her talk of the 'irrational', as we surely must, as also intending life's essential non-rationality. Here she is, in the final sentences of *Beyond All Reason*, writing about her recovery:

I have regained and strengthened my faith that life has a purpose and a meaning. I can honestly say I now have every reason to believe that living is worthwhile. Is that an irrational belief? Of course it is. Reason is a tool; a valued tool which it is our pride and privilege to use as best we may. But life and love and loveliness, whose existence reason confirms and must accept, are in themselves beyond all reason.[65]

3

Reality Contact

Introduction

What is it to lose contact with reality? It's to this question that our enquiry into mental illness (Chapter 1) and the limits of understandability (Chapter 2) has been headed, and it's from its answer that the subsequent chapters – on being in one's own delusional world (Chapter 4), self-alienation (Chapter 5), self-other confusion (Chapter 6), hallucination (Chapter 7), and formal thought disorder (Chapter 8) – take their bearings. Mental illness exists which involves, at most, a partial, less profound, loss of reality contact – illness such as 'neurosis', 'anxiety disorder', 'non-psychotic depression', etc. Yet it's only with the psychoses that we meet with such a loss of reality contact as compromises 'reality testing' (Chapter 4).

What follows develops an 'apophatic' approach to the nature of 'lost reality contact' by way of understanding the limitations of two 'cataphatic' – i.e. intelligibility-recovering – accounts. The first attempts to theorize lost reality contact as thought the failing of which can be properly articulated in terms such as 'falsity', 'atypicality', 'poor reasoning'; thought which can therefore be found intelligible in the same way we find mistakes intelligible. The second accepts that the applicability of such terms as 'falsity' presupposes what here is absent – namely, thought's normal sanity-constituting foundation. It nevertheless still aims at the recovery of intelligibility by suggesting that delusional thought rests on an *alternative* thought-sustaining foundation, and so allegedly becomes intelligible if read against this alternative backdrop.

The chapter's later sections ask what is it for the gate of the mind to become unhinged from the gatepost of the world when beset by such storms as sometimes beset the psyche. We intuitively grasp that the psychotic mind attempts to patch over its damage with those ersatz groundings which in all their (affective, cognitive, conative, and perceptual) forms we call 'delusion'. We also intuit that something of the mind's essential nature is torn away when it becomes untethered, and that it therefore can't truly return to itself without also returning to reality. But what is this reality contact which nourishes the mind and without which it cannot be itself?

Reality lost and found

To keep ourselves attuned to the real phenomenon, let's begin by considering the *Autobiography of a Schizophrenic Girl*.[1] The book's co-authors are Louisa Düss ('Renée') and her psychoanalyst Marguerite Séchehaye ('Mama'). In chapter one – 'Appearance of the First Feelings of Unreality' – Louisa recalls the initial signs of her psychosis. Here she is but 5 years old, on vacation with her family in the countryside, 'going for a walk alone, as I did now and then':

> Suddenly, as I was passing the school, I heard a German song; the children were having a singing lesson. I stopped to listen, and at that instant a strange feeling came over me, a feeling hard to analyze but akin to those I later knew all too well: unreality. It seemed to me that I no longer recognized the school, it had become as large as a barracks; and all the singing children appeared to me as prisoners compelled to sing. It was as though the school and the children's song were set apart from the rest of the world. At that same moment my eye encountered a field of wheat whose limits I could not see. And this yellow vastness, dazzling in the sun, bound up with the song of the children imprisoned in the smooth-stone school-barracks, filled me with such anxiety that I broke into sobs. Then I ran home to our garden and began to play 'to make things return to how they usually were,' that is, to return to reality.

In chapter two – 'The Struggle against Unreality Begins' – we encounter her having just started at secondary school, where she finds herself disproportionately terrified by the non-academic lessons:

> It seems that I had a very pleasant high soprano voice and the teacher counted on me for solo parts in the choir. But he noticed pretty soon that I sang off key, singing sharp or flat as much as a whole tone or two when I wasn't paying attention. Furthermore, I was unable to learn sol-fa, beat the measure, or keep in time. These lessons aroused an immeasurable anxiety quite disproportionate to the cause. It was the same for drawing. . . . I seemed to have lost a sense of perspective. So I copied the model from a school-mate's sketch, thus lending a false perspective from where I sat. In gymnastics I didn't understand the commands 'on the left' and 'on the right' which I confused. As for the sewing lesson, it was impossible to understand the technique of placing patches or the mysteries of knitting a sock heel. Varied as these subjects were, they presented similar problems, so that more and more, despite my efforts, I lost the feeling of practical things.
> . . . I once again experienced the sense of unreality. During class, in the quiet of the work period, I heard the sounds of the street: a trolley passing, people talking, a horse neighing, a horn sounding. And it seemed to me that each of these noises was detached, immovable, separated from its source, without meaning. Around me the other children, heads bent over their work, were robots or puppets, moved by an invisible mechanism. On the platform, the teacher who was talking, gesticulating, rising to write on the blackboard, also seemed but a grotesque marionette. And always this ghastly quiet, broken by noises coming from afar, the implacable sun heating the room, the lifeless immobility. An awful terror bound me.

By chapter six Louisa is now a teenager and

Unreality ... reached such a point that even Mama could no longer make contact between us. For some time I had been complaining bitterly that things were 'tricking me' and how I suffered because of it.

Yet these things weren't doing anything special; they didn't speak, nor attack me directly. What made me say they were 'tricking me' was their very presence. I saw things, smooth as metal, so cut off, so detached from each other, so illuminated, so tense that they filled me with terror. When, for example, I looked at a chair or a jug, I thought not of their use or function – a jug not as something to hold water, a chair not as something to sit on. No! They had lost their names, their functions and meanings. They had become 'things'. And these 'things' began to take on life, to exist.

By chapter eight Louisa has, except when with Dr Séchehaye, completely 'sunk into unreality':

Sometimes I felt a force in me urging me to sing, to shout at the top of my voice; or I made elaborate plans; to manufacture, for example, a super-comfortable baby carriage in which the infant could travel without inconvenience; or I imagined that everybody had died, except me, and that I was the earth's only inhabitant, with everything at my disposal.

Because I no longer struggled against it, I suffered less from unreality itself. I lived in an atmosphere of emptiness, of artificiality, of apathy. An invisible, insuperable wall divided me from people and things. I saw few people and wanted only to be alone. To that end I hid in the cellar where, sitting on the coal pile, I remained quiet, unmoving, my gaze fixed on a mark or a gleam of light.

She now spends months in restraints to stop her from self-harming or killing herself. By chapter eleven her descent deepens into frank delusion:

I was extremely unhappy. I felt myself getting younger; the [delusional] System wanted to reduce me to nothing. Even as I diminished in body and in age, I discovered that I was nine centuries old. For to be nine centuries old actually meant being not yet born. . . .

More and more a criminal guilt weighed me down. Now my punishment consisted in the transformation of my hands into cat's paws. I had a dreadful fear of my hands and the conviction that I would be changed into a famished cat, prowling in cemeteries, forced to devour the remains of decomposing cadavers. . . .

I wept and cried for hours, trembling when anyone knocked on the door and called, certain that the police were coming for me to put me to death. In the far corner of the room the voices, derisive and harsh, tormented me with taunts and threats.

We're finally grateful to read in chapter sixteen – 'I Become Firmly Established in Wonderful Reality' – of how Louisa has been able to use Séchehaye's needs-adapted psychoanalytic psychotherapy to work through her unbearable and overwhelming conflicts, leave behind her regressive defences against her fragile self's terrifying vulnerabilities, mature emotionally, and restore an ongoing and nourishing contact with reality. The harrowing, unbearable sorrows of her life no longer exceed her strength; her mind no longer has to seize upon madness to save itself, no longer needs to patch over the rents in its fabric with delusion.

Misrepresentation

The concept of 'reality contact' has rather fallen out of use in contemporary psychopathology. One sometimes gets the impression that, to the extent it's considered at all, 'disturbed reality contact' is seen as a metaphor for a failure of thought to be factually correct or well-reasoned. This, perhaps, is not surprising since our everyday ways of evaluating thought's cogency involve assessing its truth and well-reasonedness. So familiar are we with (what shall here be called) such *representational* measures of thought's fitness that we habitually apply them even when attempting to grasp such thought as is more radically *outré* than they can accommodate.[2] The deeper possibility that reality contact may be not a failure of representational thought but rather a failure of such thought's conditions of possibility is accordingly lost from view.

Correlative with this tendency is a conception of the mind as able to remain utterly itself even when not communing with that reality which in any case is now imagined to lie quite outside it. On this conception the mind isn't to be thought of as, say, a tree – which, since it's well rooted in the world's soil, may at least in its upper branches bear representational fruit. It's rather considered a butterfly floating quite free of the earth; a butterfly which, despite its ungroundedness, can, quite from within itself, somehow still find the steadiness to represent inwardly what lies outside it. Being 'in touch with', 'in contact with', 'communing with', 'moved by', 'rooted in' reality will now appear at best as crudely haptic metaphors for what, we're asked to believe, is in truth a more abstract, purely representational, matter. We inwardly represent – in perception, thought, or imagination – what currently obtains outside, or use inferential reason to reach beyond the present to what has been or will be. If it is imagined that reality contact can itself be understood in these representational terms, it's no surprise that losing touch with reality should also now also be theorized as a failure of representation. Of a piece with this are Anglophone psychiatry's tendency to corral all delusion into the category of 'delusional belief', Anglophone psychology's assumption that delusional disturbance is due to a disturbance in what it describes as 'normal processes of belief formation and maintenance', and the tendency of both to eschew non-empirical reflection on the form of psychotic experience.

Consider, by way of an example, the role such representational assumptions play in the extensive literature on the 'doxastic conception of delusion'. This literature debates whether the disturbances in a delusional belief's formation, coherence with other beliefs, and guidance of action is too profound for us to consider delusion genuine as opposed to ersatz belief.[3] Here's an extract from the work of a prominent theorist:

> The delusion that I am dead is very different from the belief that the supermarket will be closed on Sunday, but this does not show ... a categorical difference between

delusions and beliefs. Here is a challenge. For each delusion, I'll give you a belief that matches the type if not the degree of irrationality of the delusion.... [P]aranoid beliefs are badly supported by the evidence, and sometimes are also as resistant to counterevidence as delusions of persecution. The delusion that I'm dead is often justified in a viciously circular way, not dissimilar from the way in which prejudiced beliefs against a racial group are justified. The delusion that someone of a higher status loves me, or the delusion that my partner is unfaithful can be defended by mentioning facts that are apparently irrelevant. This is not so different from the strenuous defence of superstitious beliefs which seem to get confirmation no matter what happens. In many circumstances, the styles of reasoning that contribute to the irrationality of a delusion (externalization and personalization, self-serving biases, etc.) are common in groups of normal subjects, although normal subjects seem to have a better capacity to exercise reality checks on the beliefs they report.[4]

In the work from which the above is extracted the author does indeed show us that the irrationality of non-delusional beliefs can also be found in delusional beliefs. But what isn't demonstrated there is that the type of irrationality that marks delusion as such is also found in non-delusional beliefs. Take, for example, the delusion that one is dead: something has surely gone wrong if we consider its delusional irrationality to be but a function of its receiving circular justifications! Similarly with the paranoid, erotomanic and jealous delusions mentioned in the extract: such delusions may indeed be offered irrational justifications, not mesh well with their subjects' actions or experiences, or be rationalized in cognitively biased ways – just as non-delusional irrational beliefs may also be poorly justified or spuriously rationalized. Yet none of this shows that their distinctly delusional irrationality is itself helpfully construed in such terms. What instead it shows is that delusional thought may be irrational both according to everyday representational standards and in that deep and distinct way we articulate in terms of lack of reality contact and which we have yet to reflectively comprehend.

One clue to the fact that reality contact is not well theorized as the non-accidental matching of representation with fact is that, were that so, it would become hard to grasp why any failure in its accuracy or inferential rectitude should by itself also amount to the mind's loss of itself, and hard to grasp how a mind which finds itself also, in that very moment, once again finds reality. Our ordinary beliefs after all remain what they are regardless of whether they correctly or incorrectly represent states of affairs. Yet it's one of clinical reason's foremost intuitions about the psychotic mind that its disconnection from reality results in representations that are now not *ordinarily* but rather *pathologically* false (or in some sense ersatz).[5] Furthermore, both psychopathological and phenomenological reason have long considered ordinarily false thought to presuppose, rather than negate, reality contact.

A representational conception of reality contact will be shown to be inadequate to the task if it can be shown that representation presupposes, rather than constitutes, reality contact. Equally, reference to failures in representation will be exposed as inadequate for theorizing lost reality contact if what is intuitively recognized as delusion may obtain despite the absence of representational failures. So consider the suggestion that I'm in contact with reality just so long as I form *true* beliefs about it. As against this we may recall from Chapter 2 the rare fact of a delusional person accidentally, as it were, having delusions which do in fact correspond to reality – i.e. which are in some sense true – but which for all that are nonetheless delusional. To avoid that cul-de-sac we may – as clinical psychiatry has indeed sometimes been tempted – specify that I'm to be counted in touch with reality if I have not only true but *culturally congruent* beliefs. Yet such a rescue attempt appears arbitrary, politically illiberal, and over-inclusive: now any number of sane eccentrics and visionaries will count as out of touch with reality just so long as one or other of their intellectual inventions turns out to also be false.

To avoid this further cul-de-sac the representationalist may attempt to reference not, or not only, truth and prevalence but the *rational* relations enjoyed between representations in his understanding of reality contact. A belief that betrays a lack of contact with reality – a delusion – is, he says, not simply an atypical false belief, but a belief not standing in sound inferential relations to other of the subject's beliefs, thoughts, and experiences. A difficulty here, however, is that a capacity for aptly reasoning from one thought to another may equally be put in the service of, rather than check, the development of a coherent delusional system.[6] Furthermore, it just isn't at all clear that the inferential relations between the beliefs (experiences, etc.) of the delusional subject are any more wanting of cogency than those between the beliefs (etc.) of the non-delusional subject.[7]

The phenomenological psychopathologists have drawn our attention to the fact that delusion enjoys features which suggest it is not always well formulated as empirical belief – i.e. as not always playing a fact-registering or action-guiding game.[8] One such feature is the phenomenon Eugen Bleuler called 'double registration' or 'double bookkeeping':

> Kings and emperors, popes and redeemers engage, for the most part, in quite banal work, provided they still have any energy at all for activity. . . . None of our generals has ever attempted to act in accordance with his imaginary rank and station.[9]

We ascribe the delusional belief to the double bookkeeping patient on the basis of some of his utterances – yet his actions simultaneously count against such ascriptions.[10] Judge Schreber suffered the delusion of being changed by the action of divine rays into a woman so that he could, following sexual union with God, redeem the world by giving birth to a new human race. Of this belief he wrote:

> I have to confirm … that my so-called delusional system is [maintained with] unshakeable certainty, with the same decisive 'yes' as I have to counter … that my delusions are adequate motive for action, with the strongest possible 'no.' I could even say with Jesus Christ: 'My Kingdom is not of this world,' my so-called delusions are concerned solely with God and the beyond, they can therefore never in any way influence my behaviour in any worldly matter …[11]

More recently, Sass and Pienkos report the sometime delusional Sophie telling us that:

> I often feel that many of my aberrant pseudo-perceptions feel the way they do because I am actually perceiving them taking place in a parallel reality that only partly overlaps with this one.... For instance I can feel absolutely certain that space and time (and hence physical reality) no longer or never did exist, and yet understand that in order to get to a psychiatry appointment I have to walk down the street, get on the train, and so on (in other words, physically navigate or move through the 'objective' world). Or I can feel certain, even as I am talking to my psychiatrist, that I killed him five minutes earlier (fully aware that he is sitting a few feet from me talking). The strangeness is that both 'beliefs' exist simultaneously and seem in no way to impinge on one another ...[12]

None of this is to say that patients do not also sometimes, perhaps even often, act on their delusional beliefs. A young man believes his girlfriend has become possessed by Satan and so stabs her eighteen times; another, believing he can fly, jumps off a building. Such dismal outcomes have been offered as reasons to doubt the phenomenologists' claim that delusional thought is not connected to reality in the manner of ordinary representational thought. This, however, is far too quick. Somnambulists sometimes act out their dreams – yet this doesn't, and shouldn't, incline us to think that at the time of their sleepwalking they're more in touch with reality than is the non-somnambulistic dreamer.

Now, the phenomenological psychopathologists typically take one of the 'books' of the double bookkeeping patient to detail the accounts of her interventions in our 'consensual reality', and the other to contain a ledger of her transactions in an 'alternative reality'. As Jaspers puts it, for the psychotic patient 'a new world has come into being'.[13] And since, for the phenomenologists, to talk of a 'world' is ipso facto to talk of an indwelt and enacted structure of meaning, this alternative world must itself be intelligible, albeit not in an ordinary manner. From this point of view, what stops the psychiatrist from understanding his psychotic patient is his fallacious insistence on hearing the patient's utterances as if they were taking place in the consensual world. What he must learn to do is to bracket such assumptions so he can instead come to terms with those alternative assumptions which provide the meaningful structure of psychotic reality. Needless to say, such talk of 'alternative worlds' or fundamentally different 'structures of meaning' remains metaphorical and, therefore, non-elucidatory – until the metaphor has been cashed out. In what follows I consider a cataphatic attempt at cashing it out, one making use of Wittgenstein's notion of a 'hinge proposition'.

On being hinged otherwise

In *On Certainty*, Wittgenstein considers the status of such utterances the truth of which one would normally, as we say, 'have to be mad' to doubt. These utterances may, in relevant contexts, include 'here is one hand', 'my name is Richard', 'that's a book'. When we raise meaningful doubts, we do so against a background of the kinds of certainties articulated in such utterances.[14] You're watching me eat my dinner and ask if I'm left or right handed; that *these are my hands* is not in doubt. Outside the philosophy classroom such certainties typically go unformulated, instead showing themselves only in an unhesitating confidence of action and expectation. To even speak of certainty here may surely seem peculiar, since where doubt is unintelligible, certainty – in that ordinary sense which involves confidence in the warrantedness of one's judgement – is so too. (Wittgenstein accordingly speaks of 'objective certainty', the antithesis of which is not doubt but madness; I will speak instead of 'living certainties'.) My assuredness that I have hands and am writing a book, for example, shows itself primarily in my just getting on with that task by typing (with my fingers).

A central idea of Wittgenstein's text is that our confidence in the truth of what we say, when we voice our living certainties, doesn't stem from our taking ourselves to have good, or any, grounds for their assertion. For with such certainty we're already at that locus he calls 'bedrock', where the provision of grounds or justifications has, in relation to the inquiry in question, run its course.[15] Yet it's only because we have such a bedrock to our thought that our genuine doubts, queries, and inquiries make sense. For this reason the verbal articulations of our living certainties have been called *hinge* or *framework* propositions: 'the *questions* that we raise and our *doubts* depend on the fact that some propositions are exempt from doubt, are as it were like hinges on which those [questions and doubts] turn'.[16] And yet our acceptance of what such propositions articulate shows itself primarily in our living certainties themselves. We may voice them for philosophical purposes, or when teaching the meaning of our words ('This is a "hand"'), but such articulations have little other place in our days.

Our enjoyment of our living certainties, then, is not a function of our explicitly or tacitly cleaving to hinge propositions. Rather, our ready assent to hinge propositions is a function of a 'common sense' that has its roots not in our assent to propositions but in our assured action tendencies.[17] It's hard to see how I could even maintain my entitlement to claim I actually know what 'hand' means if, in this perfectly ordinary situation of sitting here typing, I start to wonder whether what I'm typing with is indeed my hand. My questioning here falls apart on itself in a way indicative of madness, and philosophical scepticism ('can I really be sure that I have hands?') thereby saws off the branch on which it sits. In extraordinary circumstances – perhaps following a bomb blast – we may imagine a use for a phrase like 'this is my hand' which conveys other than merely semantic information and which could be justified by appeal to grounds ('it's got my ring on it'). On the whole, however, my confidence that I have a hand is due not to my having grounds for believing, but rather in my having no cause to doubt, that I have hands – along with my having mastered some basics of the English language ('hand', 'this', etc.). Our sanely going about our business ultimately hinges, then, not on propositional belief but on living certainty.

We will return later to the significance of such certainties for our understanding of lost reality contact. First let's consider the suggestion that delusional beliefs function as alternative hinge propositions. Salient about the psychotic subject is the confidence and intransigence with which she cleaves to her delusion. This has led some to suggest that we might usefully model delusional certainty on the confidence we have in the truth of hinge propositions.[18] One author puts it like this:

[A]n obvious question to raise about delusions is whether the delusional beliefs do not have, for the subject, the epistemological status of Wittgenstein's framework propositions. The kind of status that we ordinarily assign to propositions like 'The world has existed for quite a long time' or 'This is one hand and this is another' is assigned by the deluded subject to propositions like 'I am dead' or 'My neighbor has been replaced by an impostor'.[19]

The approach is 'cataphatic': it aims to help us make sense of the delusional person's saying what she does by casting her expressions of delusional beliefs as instances of a class of expressions we understand perfectly well. The approach hopes to make intelligible how she's so enduringly sure about something we find preposterous: the delusion, despite its oddity, has become a fixed point around which all her enquiries turn, and isn't itself something which could be questioned. The delusion, that is, functions for its speaker like a hinge, albeit with a rather different content than is had by such hinges as reflect or enact what we call sane reality contact. This then provides a possible answer to our question as to what it could mean to live in an 'alternative reality' or a 'new world': it's to have delusions playing the role of hinges. What to a sane person appears simply preposterous – that the psychotic subject's boyfriend has become possessed by the devil – is, for the psychotic subject, now a mainstay of her world. *This* is not doubted; apparent evidence against it ('but he is so loving and kind!') is accommodated elsewhere in her system of belief ('because he's the devil he can make a devious ploy of being loving and kind').

A comparison between delusions and hinges reminds us of the fact that the delusional subject reasons – or at least rationalizes – in this way. To *really* doubt one's own delusion is impossible: to the extent that delusion becomes dubitable, it thereby becomes less itself. Perhaps to recollect and acknowledge this well-known fact was all we wanted from the comparison between delusions and hinges. Yet we might have hoped for rather more – for identity rather than analogy, for explanation rather than description. We can all acknowledge that the delusional person *treats* her delusions rather as we treat hinge propositions; she reasons from – and not to or about – them, treats them as axiomatic, etc. Yet we can also note that, whilst chalk is not cheese, somebody so minded may yet wrap it in clingfilm, store it in the fridge, put it in a sandwich – or may, for that matter, smear cheese on the blackboard. In short, mere analogy is too weak for our needs; what we must instead pursue is the question of whether articulations of delusions could actually *be* alternative hinge propositions.

So let's consider how framework propositions are identified. They are, as described above, the verbal form we give to certain practical sensibilities – our living certainties – and we discover them by coming to understand where our search for further grounds gives way. A key signal that we're at such a bedrock of justification is when whatever we're moved to offer as justification for a claim is less certain than the claim itself. All of this presupposes, of course, that we can not only imagine a meaning for the propositions in question when considering them in the abstract, but more importantly also grasp what is meant by them in their speakers' mouths. Furthermore, framework propositions are unlike expressions of ordinary true beliefs since their truth and their meaning are of a piece. 'The earth is very old indeed': this is more an explication of the meaning of 'very old' (if something's very old, it's as old as the earth is old) than it is the expression of a belief that could conceivably be wrong.

Let's now consider delusions. Unlike framework propositions, it's not at all clear which living certainties delusions articulate. In fact, what we find in the double bookkeeping of various delusional subjects is a striking disjunction between such practical certainties as guide their action and the delusional certainties that affect their thought. And unlike framework propositions, it really isn't clear that we can truly understand delusional expressions. (It was to help us understand delusions that the concept of framework propositions was invoked. If, however, we can only identify such propositions through our understanding, it's hard to see how the notion can really help us here.[20] We might even say that whereas framework propositions provide paradigms of sense, delusions provide paradigms of nonsense.) Finally, far from delusions sharing that feature of the framework proposition that their truth and meaning are of a piece, nearly all delusions are false.[21] In short, we're not really any clearer about what it means to say that a delusion codifies an alternative hinge proposition than we are about how to understand a delusion. True, a delusion may, in the manner described above, play a similar role to that played by a hinge proposition in what we might call a psychotic subject's 'cognitive economy', just as a replica of a Vermeer may play a similar role to a real Vermeer (be hung on the wall, admired, be made of similar material, etc.). Yet a delusional proposition is itself no more an actual hinge proposition than a fake Vermeer is an actual Vermeer. And so, despite any number of formal similarities between articulations of delusions and articulations of hinge propositions, it's hard to understand what's really being suggested when we're invited to view the former as instances of the latter.[22]

Against the above it might be argued that a delusion 'makes sense to the delusional subject, if not to others'. Perhaps, then, it's only our being differently hinged from one another that stops anyone other than the delusional subject understanding what he's saying? To evaluate this suggestion we need to ask what criteria for something making sense to someone are here in play. And the difficulty is that it's hard to think of any that aren't at the same time criteria for a delusional expression making genuine sense to someone other than the delusional subject. Naturally we must grant that it *seems* to the deluded person that he's making sense. Yet such 'seems' talk is used either to indicate the mere absence of demurral (the delusional subject, when thinking his delusional thoughts, notices nothing rationally *outré* about them) or to register a contrast with what's actually the case (i.e. with actually making sense). What it doesn't do is open up a way from appearance to reality; it doesn't of itself help us understand what it could be for a delusion to truly make sense to its sufferer. It's worth noting, too, that those who recover from psychosis are often as baffled by their recent delusional thoughts as are others. The question they ask themselves – 'What was I thinking?' – awaits no answer. Similarly the person who says 'You'd have to be mad to think that!' is not well understood as implying that if you only became psychotic, then the thought in question would become genuinely intelligible to you.

A comparison with dreams may help. Consider the fact that we often only notice the nonsensicality of various elements of our dreams (the things we sometimes say and do in them, for example) when recalling them on waking. If we insisted that 'in our dream these things really did make sense', what could we mean – other than that we didn't also dream of baulking at the cogency of our dream's content and structure? But the stronger claim we're stalking here – the suggestion that the dreaming or delusional subject *is* making sense, if only to himself, if only within an 'alternative reality' supposedly pivoting on alternative hinges – depends upon our locating and preserving a distinction between cases in which we merely seem to ourselves to be making sense and cases where we really are making sense to ourselves. Without such a distinction in play, our claim that 'the delusional subject makes sense to himself' really does collapse into the bland assertion, news to no one, that he doesn't, when in his delusion, baulk at its strangeness.[23]

We are, at this juncture, in the territory of what philosophically informed readers will recognize as the 'private language argument'.[24] We can easily find ourselves tempted by the idea of what Kant calls 'logical private sense': the idea that we could substitute, for the public accountability required of any genuinely meaningful use of language, a kind of inner self-ratification or 'subjective justification'. Thus Wittgenstein invites us to consider whether we might have an imaginary dictionary, reference to the definitions in which could genuinely serve to justify our uses of our terms.[25] His immediate objection to this possibility, however, is that 'justification consists in appealing to something independent' – whereas (i) justifying your judgement that a certain use of a term is correct, and (ii) imagining the term's definition, are not independent acts. At this his imaginary interlocutor demurs: 'But surely I can appeal from one memory to another. For example, I don't know if I have remembered the time of departure of a train right and to check it I call to mind how a page of the time-table looked. Isn't it the same here?' Wittgenstein's response is to remind the interlocutor that what makes it possible for us to describe either of these memories as 'correct' is the fact that there is, somewhere, a time written on an actual definitive timetable. Yet it's just this that's absent in such cases as enjoy no instantiation outside of the mind of the thinker.

The upshot of all of this is, once again, that it means nothing, other than affirming the absence of baulking, to say that 'the delusional or dream thought made sense to its thinker, if not to anyone else (including the subject when awake and sane)'. If a sentence makes sense, then there shall be such a thing as correctly or incorrectly understanding it. But although we know how to contrast seeming to understand something in a dream with actually understanding it in waking life, we don't know what is meant by raising that distinction purely within the context of dreaming. As Wittgenstein sums it up, 'One would like to say: whatever is going to seem correct to me is correct. And that only means that here we can't talk about "correct".'[26] The suggestion that expressions of delusions at least make sense to the deluded person fares no better than the suggestion that they're a deluded person's alternative hinge propositions: these philosophically motivated suggestions are themselves no more intelligible than the phenomena which they're being mobilized to explicate.

Perhaps it be urged that delusions can, after all, be seen as genuine hinges if we 'radically interpret' what the delusional person says – i.e. if we take his words in *whatever* ways are required for making what he says, when he's in his delusion, come out as true and meaningful.[27] Now the delusional person is considered akin to a speaker of another language, albeit a language largely coextensive with our own and by and large with the same words. Yet the difficulty with this suggestion is that we lose our sense of what's delusional about our speaker's utterances to the extent that we see her as merely suffering from an atypical aphasia – i.e. as involuntarily speaking in code. Are we imagining that she intends some of her words to carry different meanings than normal? At least when she's in her delusion she doesn't acknowledge this. Or are we imagining that she uses words in new ways – in ways which, if they're akin to hinge propositions, in fact constitute new paradigms of meaning – whilst failing to recognize that this is what she's doing? But how could this possibility be made out? If our subject truly is unable to say what she means by what she says other than by repeating the delusional utterance or by offering equally delusional paraphrases, it's unclear with what right we should maintain that she's using her words to mean much at all, let alone voicing hinge propositions with them. And a clear risk of our offering such a 'radical interpretation' of our delusional speaker's words, so that *we decide* to take them as instancing new paradigms of meaning – i.e. as new hinges – is that we fail to actually offer her any genuine recognition. Far from this semantic rescue effort constituting the provision of genuine understanding, it instead involves us not only in failing to offer acknowledgement to her in her psychotic brokenness, but also in usurping her role as authority regarding what she means.

Let's recap. We started by noting that delusions are not well understood as *misrepresentations* of facts; in truth, the notion of misrepresentation presupposes, rather than constitutes a failing in, contact with reality. An alternative, deeper, conception of reality contact was then offered, a conception in which reality contact consists in such living certainties as philosophers may articulate with 'hinge propositions'. Expressions of delusion were then suggested to be *alternative hinge propositions*. The difficulty for this proposal was that hinge propositions are of their nature both true and meaningful, whilst delusions are prima facie usually neither. The further suggestion was then made that delusions are meaningful 'to the delusional subject, if not to others'. However, the only coherent reading of this appears to be the negative one, itself news to nobody, that the delusional person doesn't herself baulk at her peculiar thought.

What follows presents an alternative, apophatic, understanding of delusion which attempts not to assign it to an intelligible epistemological genus, but instead to grasp it negatively – as manifesting a disturbance of such living certainty as constitutes a condition of possibility for meaningful thought. On this alternative understanding delusional thought is to be understood not as otherwise, but as un-, hinged.

Reality contact as readiness

An everyday experience of events in constant conjunction spontaneously gives rise in us to diverse expectations of or readinesses for what we shall now or later encounter. Only rarely does this involve something we should want to call 'reasoning'; only rarely do these expectations manifest in such thought as warrants the designation 'reflection' ('consideration', 'cogitation', 'reasoning'). Yet thought (judgement) it is that's here met with, at least in that sense of 'thought' which is properly self-ascribed by he who, stopped before a door and asked why he didn't push it open, replies: 'I *thought* it was an automatic door like the others.' Whilst not in any sense giving us something that, whether well or barely formulated, came before his mind, this man is still 'telling us what he thought'. Thought (judgement) permeates our unreflective immersed coping with our worlds; it's nothing other than that coping's intelligible form, and is not helpfully considered to be, say, a conscious or preconscious process lying behind it. Driving to my office, cogitating on nothing but the problem of delusion, I knock my wing mirror against yours. You rightly challenge my driving skill but don't do well to question my claim that I *misjudged* the available space.[28]

To be replete with such expectations or readinesses is to enjoy such thought as indexes our reality contact. And these expectations typically arise not from reasoning but from conditioning. Having this facility of becoming conditioned in our expectations directly by our experiences means that we're spared the vast and perhaps impossible task of reasoning our way from past to present or future.[29] Our reality contact here is far more securely shown by such expectation and activity as is a product of such conditioning than by any reasoning – reasoning which in any case has here been obviated by the conditioning.[30] Yet the irrelevance of reason *qua* act of thought (*reasoning*) to our aptitudes for apt readiness ought not incline us to take contextually apt expectations as themselves other than instances – indeed as foundational forms – of *rationality*. An apt expectation may not be a product of reasoning, but this doesn't prevent it from being one of reason's exemplifications – perhaps even one of its paramount paradigms. The notion of 'reality contact' nicely captures the nature of this basic form of rationality: we're looped into, are in contact with, reality when our expectations are directly conditioned and reconditioned by it in the course of our ongoing capable encounters and engagements.

The consideration that rational expectations arise from conditioning shouldn't be mistaken for the consideration that a self-standing 'inner' domain of ideas is kept in harmony by the causal impact of a world external to them. Hume's thesis that the 'transition of thought from the cause to the effect proceeds not from reason' but 'altogether from custom and experience' is germane to our own. But his consideration that such custom and experience establishes a 'harmony between the course of nature and the succession of our ideas' is too suggestive of the possibility that bona fide ideas could be entertained which were not thus conditioned.[31] Yet it's not 'ideas' *qua* cogitations, but our reactions and readinesses, which are conditioned by our experience. And, as a rule, only such reactions and readinesses as are thus conditioned will properly be taken to enjoy the form of thought or, to put it otherwise, properly be taken as genuinely expressive of 'ideas'.

So entrenched in theoretical thought is the assumption that one's reason must be made for by, and grounded in, acts of reasoning that it can be hard to clearly grasp the above-articulated possibility. Accordingly, it has sometimes proved tempting, for philosophers and cognitive scientists, to imagine that such behaviour as manifests reason (rationality, thought), whilst yet not preceded by conscious cogitation, simply *must* be a product of something called 'tacit reasoning' ('subconscious thinking', etc.). Against that may be cited the fact that it's hard to know what to offer by way of criterion for 'tacit reasoning' other than the overt utterance or act which the alleged reasoning is supposed to explain. Which in turn must surely cause us to doubt the explanatory power of such appeals to the tacit – and ultimately to doubt that concept's utility and substance here. Or perhaps an appeal will be made to brain processes as the real referents of such attributions of tacit reasoning. Yet that the brain is always humming in ways which subserve action is undisputed by all. The issue on the table, however, concerns the warrant for identifying some or other brain process as itself an instance of tacit reasoning. In particular, the pundit of 'tacit reasoning' must explain to us how she's offering any more than the vacuous: 'the behaviour may be counted as a manifestation of reason because it was produced by such brain processes as are themselves identified as instances of "tacit reasoning" by way of their resulting in such behaviour'. Here we encounter a vicious circle from which no number of brain scans can secure us exit.

So far we've considered how expectation may instantiate such reason as constitutes reality contact, but have as yet said little about what it is to enjoy such expectation, or about what it is for it to count as reason's instance rather than product. The expectations here under discussion make themselves known by a combination of our *absence of surprise* at certain events and our largely unreflective capacity to deal with or *get to grips with* them.[32] My anticipation that the ground will not collapse as I walk across the room rarely manifests in my thinking; it rather shows itself directly in my confident stride and in my absence of surprise at the ground's stable resistance. My expectation that the sun shall soon set manifests directly in my surprise if this doesn't happen, in my lack of surprise when it does, and in the relevant adjustments I now make to my activities and intentions (taking a torch on my walk, getting on right away with the remaining gardening tasks).

Perhaps it will be suggested that a justification or rule is here required – one which explains why it's legitimate to form those expectations we count as rational, and illegitimate to form those we count as irrational. And perhaps, by way of such a justification, we're given 'it's rational to expect B to now follow A if, in one's prior experience, B has indeed followed A'. Yet whilst this may, on some particular occasion, work as a reminder that reasons ought to be provided if we're to be counted rational in *not* expecting B to follow A, it doesn't tell us *why* we ought to expect B to follow A. Once we (erroneously) accept the notion that bona fide reason must always be either produced or justified by reasoning, then we've already made it hard to bring into focus that form of rationality meant by 'reality contact'. This is because a question such as 'wherein the rationality of the expectation?' itself rather encourages us to believe that rationality is *not* met with in the expectations themselves – i.e. it presupposes that to expect thus-and-so is *not* well taken as itself constitutive of what being rational here amounts to.

By contrast with the thought that all bona fide rationality must be instanced by reasoning, the thought here on offer is that we simply take the panoply of expectations which constitute our grip on the world as constitutive and *sui generis* instantiations of rationality. A rational expectation of the sun, in this context, is that it shall soon set; in another context, that it will shortly disappear behind the cloud. And the same goes, too, for the millions of expectations which structure our every world-engagement. To be sane, to enjoy reality contact, is in part to anticipate here in *this*, there in *that*, later on in *this other*, way and to act in accordance with such anticipations.[33] And such anticipations are directly met with, first and foremost, in our utterances and actions.

Perhaps it will be suggested that, without a principle to be appealed to in order to distinguish them, it betrays nothing but prejudice to count one person as sane and another as having lost reality contact. Here we're straying onto the final chapter's topic, so must leave the bulk of discussion for then. For now I simply stress again that to make a determination without justification does not, when determining in some particular way *is itself constitutive of what here counts as* justifiable, amount to making an unjustified determination.[34] To suppose otherwise not only betrays a generalist prejudice which itself lacks a compelling principle; it also risks ignoring the fact that, in *any* chain of justification, we shall come to a point at which we say 'behaving (judging, thinking) thus *just is* what being rational here amounts to'. It may disappoint the rationalist to find that decisions on the reasonableness of our expectations are not always properly referred to the court of principles – i.e. it may be disappointing for him to learn that, in the justificatory procedure, his 'spade is turned' quite so soon.[35] But we may remind him that rules themselves require application, that what shall count as the correct application of a rule can hardly always depend upon some other rule without our being lost to an endless regress, and that without demur we allow deductive inferences their validity without referring to yet further principles. It may also help here to think on other cases of exemplarization as when we: use colour samples as paradigms; refer back to certain works of art, or items of apparel, or buildings, to keep a clear fix on the meaning of aesthetic and stylistic terms; refer to a particular saint's reactions as sense-providing paradigms for a particular moral quality; and fix the meaning of substance terms by ostensive – rather than by formal, lexical – definition. In none of these cases does it make sense to ask for justification as to why the example should be taken to *fit* the definition, and this is because the example itself partly *constitutes* the definition.[36] One might as well ask how it is that, in the symbol ending this sentence, the white disc fits so perfectly inside the black circle: **O**.[37] The question is misplaced precisely because the one defines the other. So too, the thought goes, when we're considering those situated expectations which constitute paradigms of that rationality instanced by reality contact.

Reality contact as engaged activity

So far we've mainly considered our expectations of how the world shall turn about us, but leaving matters focused there risks an all too passive conception of reality contact. For it's not primarily in our expectations of how matters independent of our agency shall unfold, but in our actions and interactions, that we keep in touch with reality. The expectations I have of how things shall behave come not simply from my past witness of, but also from my past interactions with, them. I expect water to come from an opened tap, but I also expect the tap to turn when I manipulate it thus. These expectations too are not first and foremost registered in reasoning – but, rather, have their life within my bodily comportment. When I see an escalator I expect it to behave differently than a flight of stairs, but I also expect it to affect my bodily balance in particular ways when I take it. This expectation has its life not in my deliberations but in the automatic postural compensations I make as I embark on my escalator journey; it resides in my differential muscular tensions and readinesses, and of these I should struggle to give a precise verbal articulation. Yet despite their non-cogitative nature they're still properly the subject of avowals, as when, stumbling on mounting a surprisingly fast-moving escalator, I truthfully say: 'I expected it to be slower moving.'

A vast range of such sensorimotor expectations are of a piece with my visual, tactile and auditory reality contact – expectations that have been explored in detail by the phenomenologists.[38] So profoundly constitutive are they of the background of my coping with the world that they usually become a matter of thematic appraisal only when thwarted. I expect a vast array of occlusions and revelations to obtain as I walk across a scene with eyes open; I anticipate a change in what of the scene is visible when I simply turn my head. Our mastery of any corporeal skill – writing, pouring a glass of water, flushing the loo – involves the bedding in of a gamut of corporeal expectations that sensory stimulation will co-vary with bodily movement in particular ways. Such expectations are manifested in, and constituted by, my capacities for coping in environmental interactions.[39] And, once again, the index of such sensorimotor expectation is not primarily what I can avow, but rather what does and doesn't surprise me, and more generally how I ongoingly cope with what I encounter in the course of pursuing the goals that both pre-date, and arise during the course of, my activity.

The rationality evinced by such sensorimotor world-negotiations is dual. On the one hand, we encounter (i) that rationality which can be ascertained by comparing some stretch of behaviour with some avowed or otherwise ascertained goal. You said, sincerely, that you wanted to drive to London, but I've just seen you head the wrong way down the London road. It turns out you 'weren't thinking', were distracted, were 'on autopilot' – and so failed to act in accord with your own plan. It's important here that we have such explanations available since they preserve our sense of your yet having – to give now the other hand – (ii) that deeper rationality which appertains to the having of intelligible goals as such. This deeper intact intelligibility provides the context for our judging the particular behaviour to be irrational: it's against the context of an intelligible goal, safely ascribed to you, that your action is judged as failing to cut the rational mustard. You did want to go to London – my taking your utterance about going there for an intelligible avowal of such a goal is often not defeated even by such behaviour as manifestly goes against it. But push this charitable latitude too far and we start to encounter that second, deeper, kind of irrationality that here is our particular concern: the kind manifest in the 'double bookkeeping' mentioned above. Now we meet with the 'patient who claims that the doctors and nurses are trying to torture and poison her' but who will 'nevertheless happily consume the food they give her', or with the 'patient who asserts that the people around him are phantoms or automatons [but] still interacts with them as if they were real'.[40] Now, and despite your engaging in behaviours or utterances which to all appearances seem like intentional acts, avowals, etc., the surroundings to them are in fact not such as to secure our judgement of them as such. You deny having been distracted or on autopilot, give no other reason for having driven in the opposite direction, yet when asked still say your intent was to drive to London. At precisely this point, when I'm unsure whether I can still treat your apparent avowal of an intention as such, I start to wonder whether you're 'ill', 'not in your right mind', 'out of touch with reality'. For now I seem to no longer encounter intelligible action or utterance; now talk of your making a mistake is not so clearly apt.

Perhaps at times I pick up pieces of your behaviour or utterance and, tacitly assuming an implicit backdrop of humanly intelligible action or discourse, take them, and you in them, to manifest a sane intelligibility. But then, let's imagine, I'm jolted out of my presumption of your sanity by recalling your having also recently said or done things which go against my current understanding of you. Or perhaps I'm instead shocked out of my presumption by what you next go on to say and do. After all it's only against its surroundings – the environmental context, the personal history, the individual's behaviour and talk before and after – that a locution or action can be said to enjoy a sense. My grasp of your meaning is made for by my implicitly reading you against such contexts.[41] My default presumption is, or at least should be, a presumption of your sane intelligibility, and failures of understanding on my part ought to inspire a further reaching out on my behalf. But I should be showing a lack of courage in facing the terrors of madness, failing to offer you recognition in your suffering by failing to recognize your mental devastation, if I'm unwilling to cede this presumption when appropriate.

Reality contact as synchronized interaction

When judging that someone's out of contact with reality we consider the coherence of her interactions not only with her utterances and her surroundings but also with ourselves. Your reality contact, for example, is manifest directly in the form of your empathic reaction to my visible suffering. Here again the sane rationality of your engagement with me is often shown not by your reasoning but by your acting without need of reasoning: to expect any thinking at all from you, before you're moved to react empathically to me in my distress, would usually be to expect 'one thought too many'.[42] For unless we're considering, say, the actions of a surgeon forced to operate without anaesthesia, it's when someone fails to respond empathically to another's distress, or when she tends to another's pain but in a calculative manner, that we find her disconnected from reality. A spontaneous apt responsivity, by contrast, partly constitutes, and so does not itself track or index an otherwise assessable, reality contact.

The psychopathological investigation of schizophrenic psychosis is particularly helpful for discerning what in our non-psychotic interactions speaks of true human connection. In particular, it helpfully steers us away from matters of intellectual performance for, as Bleuler writes, 'One can often feel much more connected with a severely retarded individual, one who does not speak a word, than with a schizophrenic person, who might still have his intelligence, but is affectively inaccessible.'[43] The schizophrenic subject may suffer an unnatural rigidity of mien and prosody; his expressions may fail to hang together. His interactions may be marked by: a disturbance of rhythmic and empathic resonance and conversation-sustaining synchrony, a reduced spontaneous imitation of conversational head movements, an impairment in handling conversational turn-taking markers (filled and un-filled pauses in speech), a diminished ability to coordinate attention with others to shared objects, a reduced susceptibility to contagious yawning and laughter, a difficulty in reading others' body language and facial expressions, a tendency to conflate ironic and non-ironic discourse, and a difficulty in intuiting others' intentions and understandings.[44] For all these reasons we struggle to find our feet with the schizophrenic subject, especially when he's in his psychosis, since his own feet are not on common ground. We find him irrational – which is not to say that we doubt his reasoning, but rather to note that his interactions themselves embody sense in a more precarious, and sometimes disrupted, manner.

On being unhinged

For expository purposes, the above divides reality contact into expectation, personal activity, and interpersonal interaction. In truth, these are not three separate phenomena but different aspects of a person's unity or disunity, many of our interactions, from infancy onwards, being both triangular and triangulating. (Triangular: interacting with other subjects whilst attending to objects also understood as objects of others' attention. Triangulating: our ongoing participation in situated self-other-object encounters enables our utterances and other actions to remain trued up to those praxical canons that define thought, meaning, coherence, reason.) In such ways is our reality contact constantly enacted and entrained. Instinctual sensibilities and expectancies are corralled by custom, we participate in the order of sense, and in our living dispositions we become both guardians and living icons of mind's humanly meaningful hinges to world.[45]

At its hinge our mind shares in – is in communion with – what we may call the world's 'flesh'; at the hinge the world itself informs or is 'fused into' our words' and actions' meanings.[46] We do not first learn our words – 'tree', 'love', 'promise' – in abstraction from the world, a world to which we then apply them like templates applied to objects in a scene. Our understandings are not first of all 'abstract ideas' to be grasped in abstraction from our world-involvements and which we hope will nevertheless go on to find concrete application in our lives. Instead, language is born and lives in our situated interactions with others and objects, the meanings of our terms not being anchored to extra-worldly ideas but rather being a function of their use – their use, for example, in identifying trees, or in acts of love, or in the performance of promises. Such interactions are made possible by the entrainment of our sensibilities to our situations and to the sensibilities of our neighbours. At its participatory hinge, thought's form is of a piece with its objects. Our lived certainties are formed and maintained by interaction with the objects to which they pertain. There is, therefore, no such thing as being wrong about that of which a hinge proposition speaks. The proposition is simply a way to voice the living certainty that obtains in our interactions with our world. The certainty of thought's hinges is nothing other than our utterances' tight entrainment to paradigmatic situations of their apt deployment. I 'should have to be unhinged' to doubt or entertain the negation of the hinge proposition – which is to say that it's only when words and world come apart, so that the meaning of the former is no longer entrained by participation with the latter, that I could be imagined to 'doubt' – i.e. for acts of thinking to become unmoored from – such self-evident truths. The situation here is easily disguised from us by our habit of taking truths to either be analytic (meaning-stating) *or* world-involving, a habit which ignores the way in which hinge propositions are analytic articulations which secure their sense through our participation with their worldly objects.[47]

Now, it shouldn't matter a jot for your sanity if you never encounter a hinge proposition in your life. As described above, it's not the mastery of such propositions that hinges mind to world, but rather our indwelling of, and our thought's entrainment to, the situations of a shared world. Being unhinged accordingly consists not in our 'doubting' of hinge propositions, but in our words and thoughts no longer being entrained through a steadying communion with other language users and with the situations of our lives. At the pivot point of its hinge, mind is not other than world, is not stood back from it, appraising it, representing or misrepresenting it. At the hinge we lend our expressive voice to – or rather, do not refuse to share it with – the world itself. Thought is not here, any more than when we express our feelings, in the business of getting anything right or wrong.[48] But sometimes our experiential grip on our situations, and our words, become unsteady. Sometimes, escaping its gravitational pull, thought escapes the world's sense-readying orbit. Thus unanchored, language-in-use becomes unconstrained: the psychotic mind no longer automatically rules out as unintelligible such locutions as fail to express genuine possibilities. In this fashion sense and nonsense are levelled. The stability of our bodies' form itself conditions the meaning of our talk of sex, but now my words detach from their bodily anchor and I confidently proclaim that my body is spontaneously changing from male to female. Or you tell me that, despite already being dead, you should yet appreciate a continental breakfast in the morning – showing no awareness of the communicative obligation you're here under to provide and demonstrate a sense for such an extraordinary combination of words. With your feet no longer on common ground, your head now resides entirely in the clouds.

The person with a schizophrenic diathesis has an intrinsically vulnerable grip on reality. Their assuredness is vitiated; their 'natural attitude' is lost and questions usurp the reign of unthinking certainty; what 'goes without saying' is no longer self-evident.[49] As a young woman put it on admission to Freiburg University Psychiatric Clinic: 'What is it that I am missing? . . . I find I no longer have a footing in the world. . . . It seems I lack a natural understanding for what is matter of course and obvious to others. . . . I am missing the basics. . . . It is not knowledge . . . It is the kind of thing you just get naturally. . . . My soul is sick.'[50] And yet pathognomonic of mental illness is not merely reality contact's fragility, but its ongoing loss when the mind is flung out of reality's orbit by affect too painful to bear,[51] now circling an alternative, delusional, safer but un-nourishing sun. As R. D. Laing puts it, 'In its dread of facing the commitment to the objective element, [the self withdraws] to preserve its identity; but, no longer anchored to fact, to the conditioned and definitive, it comes to be in danger of losing what it was seeking above all to safeguard. Losing the conditioned, it loses its identity; losing reality, it loses its possibility of exercising effective freedom of choice in the world. In the escape from the risk of being killed, it becomes dead.'[52]

Consider again Louisa, whose 'feelings of unreality' first occurred to her when *disengaged* from the world – when she 'stopped to listen' to the sounds of singing children, when sitting at her desk 'in the quiet of the work period'. She pauses thus when anxious: when (as a mere 5-year-old) walking alone in unfamiliar surroundings; when struggling with her practical school lessons; when overwhelmed by her responsibilities at home. Now that the passive recurrent syntheses of her meaningful experience are thwarted by anxiety, now that mind and meaning are no longer enacted by truck with reality, Louisa is thrown out of living contact with it: 'It seemed ... I no longer recognized the school ... as though the school and the children's song were set apart from the rest of the world.'

At first Louisa can return to familiar surroundings and there can 'play "to make things return to how they usually were," that is, to return to reality'. 'What saved me ... was activity. . . . To move, to change the scene, to do something definite and customary, helped a great deal.' Movement in familiar scenes enables the enaction of a stable and stabilizing mind-world relation. But if these interactions are themselves too challenging, or if Louisa is too disturbed, entering into them itself becomes disturbing. Striking about Louisa's narrative is the absence of other people as trustworthy stabilizing sources of certainty. Rather than find her feet in the world through participating in it alongside the containing balm of an accommodating other, Louisa – this little girl who we first met aged only five 'going for a walk alone, as I did now and then' – is left to face the world solo. But now her situations overwhelm her; she can no longer gain or keep her bearings: cannot learn sol-fa, beat a measure and keep in time, draw with a unitary sense of perspective, coordinate her body in gym, coordinate her sewing. Without the steadying horizon of the world being available for calibrating her experience, she and it fall apart: 'my eye encountered a field of wheat whose limits I could not see. And this yellow vastness ... bound up with the song of the children ... filled me with such anxiety that I broke into sobs'. She loses 'the feeling of practical things'. Each sound from the street becomes 'detached, immovable, separated from its source, without meaning'. Objects were 'tricking' her. Once-familiar items – jugs, chairs – become mere things which have 'lost ... their functions and meanings'. Once-familiar people – other children, the teacher – become uncanny, unpredictable, like robots or grotesque puppets. In short, such expectancies as constitute stable reality contact, that give structure to experience, have for Louisa become radically compromised. She no longer knows what to expect of the world; her body no longer thrums with such consistently and automatically updated expectancies as constitute stable reality contact. She no longer remains selfsame by automatically adapting her experiential expectations of the world as she and it move in relation to one another; her sensorimotor relations no longer continuously embody the requisite invariances across transformations to make for stable reality contact.[53] As a result, when she gives up the struggle of attempting to stay connected to reality amidst the flow of life, she opts for the simplicity of solitude and stasis: 'I saw few people ... wanted only to be alone ... hid in the cellar where, sitting on the coal pile, I remained quiet, unmoving, my gaze fixed on a mark or a gleam of light.'

The cost, for Louisa, of trying to stay in touch with reality is confusion, chaos, and the terror of falling apart. Yet the cost of giving up on reality contact is also high: by 'sinking into unreality' she becomes vulnerable to frank delusion. Without reality contact her thought becomes unmoored, and delusion must now provide for it an alternative, ersatz mooring. But for delusion to successfully bind her mind's wounds, it must be up to the thematic task, and this task may require thought which itself is terrifying. Threatening content may be less unbearable than the shattered form it replaces – persecution may be less intolerable than dissolution – but for anyone with the ears to hear it, the echo of the latter is ever audible behind the noise of the former. Everyone 'had died, except me', Louisa tells us, and her 'punishment consisted in the transformation of my hands into cat's paws.... I would be changed into a famished cat, prowling in cemeteries, forced to devour the remains of decomposing cadavers.' The 'police were coming for me to put me to death'. In fact, something similar may be said of compensatory delusion: the erotomanic or grandiose wish-fulfilments that disguise from the patient her devastating shame are, for any psychiatrist in the game of finding a common humanity in his patient, ever redolent with that shame's pathos.

How, when embodied living certainties are no longer available, disembodied delusional certainties take their place, so that the psychotic subject now dwells in a 'world of her own', is the topic of the next chapter.

4

A World of One's Own

Introduction

On meeting someone actively psychotic we find her 'living in her own world'. By that is here meant, in part, her preoccupation with hallucinations, but also her absorption in delusional thought. In *Operators and Things: The Inner Life of a Schizophrenic*, Barbara O'Brien describes for us an unusually vivid stretch of near-continuous hallucination and delusion. She starts by recounting the moment of her apophany,[1] which is to say, the moment a delusional world was born for her, the basic character of which was for her as obvious and unquestionable as the fundamental facts about non-delusional reality are for the sane:

> I awoke one morning, during a time of great personal tension and self-conflict, to find three grey and somewhat wispy figures standing at my bedside. I was, as might be imagined, completely taken up by them. Within a few minutes they had banished my own sordid problem from my mind and replaced it with another and more intriguing one. They were not Men From Mars, but the Operators, a group in some ways stranger than Martians could be. I listened to what the Operators had to say, weighed the facts which they presented to me, and decided that there was wisdom in following their directions. I packed some clothes and mounted a Greyhound bus, as they directed, and followed them. Riding off in the bus, I left safely behind me a mess of reality with which I was totally incapable of coping.[2]

An Operator, Barbara explains, is a 'human being with a type of head formation which permits him to explore and influence the mentality of others', whilst a Thing is a 'human being without the mental equipment of Operators'.[3] Barbara's otherworldly Operators include Nicky, Sharp, Hinton, and Burt:

> The boy [Nicky] was about twelve years old, handsome, and with a pleasant, relaxed smile. The elderly man [Burt] was impressive: solid, conservative, a reliable man with built-in rules. The third [Hinton] was a real weirdo with hair three inches too long, black, straight, and limp, and with a body that was also long and limp. The face didn't belong with the body or the hair; the features were fine and sensitive, the expression, arrogant and unbending. . . .

Burt explained.... I had been selected for participation in an experiment. He hoped I would be cooperative; lack of cooperation on my part would make matters difficult for them and for myself....

I thought: I have come upon knowledge which other people do not have and the knowledge is obviously dangerous to have; others would be in equal danger if I revealed it to them....

Burt cleared his throat. 'The one great difference between an Operator and a Thing is the construction and ability of the mind. Operators are born with special brain cells known as the battlement. With these cells, an Operator can extend and probe into the mind of a Thing. He can tap the Thing's mind and discover what is going on there, and even feed thoughts to the Thing's mind in order to motivate it. The mental difference is one of ability, not one of quality. Operators, like Things, may be stupid or intelligent. But that one difference permits the Operators to rule the Things.'...

I was on my second cup of coffee when the council Operators returned. Their voices shaking with indignation, they handed down an ultimatum. Sharp and company had two hours to clear out. As soon as they had gone, a council Operator would take me over.

In the silence that followed the council's departure, the grey faces of Hinton and Sharp turned and looked at me steadily. Whether I knew it or not, Sharp said, I was in more danger from the council than I was from them. The moment they walked out, the council would return and destroy me.

'That's cloak-and-dagger stuff,' I told him.

Hinton sighed. 'At least, buy some nails and a hammer and nail down the windows. Because that's the way you're going to go. Wait until you have twenty Operators from the council in here, working on your mind, telling you to jump. Believe me, you'll jump. So far as the council is concerned, you're a monstrosity and a source of danger, something that has to be put out of the way.'

I evaluated the shock, horror, and anger in the voices of the council Operators, packed an overnight bag, went down to the bus depot, and bought a ticket for the nearest large city.

'We'll be in touch with you,' Sharp told me. 'We'll be in a car, following.'[4]

After six months Barbara is able to return from her own to the real world. Her narrative deftly describes these worlds, the psychodynamics and precipitants of her psychosis, and the symbolic representation of troublesome features of the 'mess of reality' within her psychotic unreality. We shall return to such themes later in the book. The question I'm raising now has, however, to do not with content or mechanism but with form. It is: What is this 'other reality'? What is it to 'live in a world of one's own' in such a way as counts as psychotic?

Schizophrenic autism

Eugen Bleuler (1857–1939) is remembered today for introducing to us his concept of 'schizophrenia' (1908) and for exemplary stewardship (1898–1927) of the Burghölzli asylum. Less well remembered is his authorship of 'autism', a term he derived from the Greek for 'self' (αὐτός). Today's Anglophone psychiatry follows the child psychiatrists Leo Kanner (1943) and Hans Asperger (1944) in using it to denote a developmental disability ('early infantile autism', 'autistic spectrum disorder'). Yet 'autism' began its lexical life as Bleuler's descriptor for that manner of being in a world of one's own we find in schizophrenic psychosis.[5] Schizophrenia, he tells us,

> is characterised by a very peculiar alteration of the relation between the patient's inner life and the external world. The inner life assumes pathological predominance (autism).... The most severe schizophrenics, who have no more contact with the outside world, live in a world of their own. They have encased themselves with their desires and wishes (which they consider fulfilled) or occupy themselves with the trials and tribulations of their persecutory ideas; they have cut themselves off as much as possible from any contact with the external world.... This detachment from reality, together with the relative and absolute predominance of the inner life, we term autism.... In less severe cases ... patients are still able to move about in the external world but ... everything which is in contradiction to their complexes simply does not exist for their thinking or feeling.... The autistic world has as much reality for the patient as the true one, but his is a different kind of reality.... In milder cases the real and autistic worlds exist not only side by side, but often become entangled with one another in the most illogical manner. The doctor is at one moment not only the hospital-physician and at another the shoemaker, ... but he is both in the same thought-content of the patient.... Wishes and fears constitute the contents of autistic thinking.... The autistic thinking is the source of delusions, of the crude offences against logic and propriety, and all the other pathological symptoms.[6]

Despite its central significance for the development of the cardinal schizophrenic symptoms, Bleuler construes autism as but one of several organizers of primary pathological processes. Yet by the time of Eugène Minkowski's seminal *La Schizophrénie*, psychopathologists had started to offer it as a central unifier of schizophrenic psychosis.[7] Manfred Bleuler, Eugen's son, describes how on this conception the very essence of schizophrenic existence becomes 'the turning away from the community and from reality, the submerging oneself into an autistic life'.[8]

We can discern three aspects of such existence as the Bleulers conceive it: (i) a *disconnection from reality* conditions the flourishing of delusional experience and thought, (ii) a distinctive *fantasy-involving form of thinking* elaborates this 'other reality' which the schizophrenic person now lives in, and (iii) there obtains a *motivated avoidance* of the unbearable anxiety arising when reality contact is overwhelming, and a *motivated retreat* to this other reality. What it means to (i) disconnect from reality was discussed in the third chapter, and (iii) motivation's general role in mental illness was discussed in the first chapter. The present chapter concerns the significance of (ii) fantasy and (iii) motivation in the creation of delusional worlds.

Autism and fantasy

The first thing we tend to suggest, when asked what 'living in a world of your own' means, is that publicly available reality has here been replaced by private fantasy. Thus Françoise Minkowska describes schizophrenic autists as 'patients who flee reality and who, instead of directing their activity toward real goals, create for themselves an imaginary world'.[9] Manfred Bleuler offers us this dictation from Elena, a young pianist and patient of Enrico Morselli:

> Now I am in the other life – in the other world – where I sometimes see angels and hear music. But I feel that it is not right, that it is something like the world of madness. I would not want to retreat from real life, but I am drawn by something that is stronger than I am. I seem to split and become two people, and I understand that I cannot live life that way, so I bury myself in the other one. In truth, I am closer to the soul, to Dante's Paradise in that world, but I feel removed from life, devoid of emotion, and detached from everything.[10]

And Eugen Bleuler himself typically characterizes the 'different kind of reality' in which the schizophrenic person lives in terms of substitutive and unassailable fantasy.[11] This disconnected and dreamlike inner world is part-constituted by wishes, and can both displace, or more curiously obtain alongside, reality relations (i.e. double bookkeeping). The draw of madness away from the pains of reality contact is well articulated by the poets under the guise of the faery folk's allure. Keats' *La Belle Dame Sans Merci* offers us a wish-fulfilling fantasy in which a 'knight-at-arms' is lured away from this world by 'a lady in the meads, full beautiful – a faery's child' with wild eyes, who 'all day long . . . would bend, and sing a faery's song', and 'sure in language strange she said – "I love thee true"'.[12] A similarly wish-fulfilling and misery-evading fantasy is offered in Yeats' *The Stolen Child*, which tells of the faery folk who lure a child away from a world 'full of troubles, and anxious in its sleep', a world 'more full of weeping than you can understand', to dance all night on moonlit shores.[13] (Think, too, of the common idiom of being 'away with the fairies'.)

And yet, despite its intuitive appeal, there is much amiss about a conception of autism as the substitution of the preferable contents of fantasy for the troublesome denizens of reality. Jean-Paul Sartre was one of the first to articulate these difficulties.[14] First, the conception of autism as withdrawal to private fantasy assimilates mentally healthy daydreamers to those Sartre called 'morbid dreamers' (primarily: schizophrenics).[15] Next, a good number of schizophrenia sufferers are, unlike Barbara with her 'Operators' and 'Things', fairly poor in their capacity to elaborate entrancing fantasy.[16] (If autism is really to be the central organizer of schizophrenic psychopathology, and if autism is to be characterized in terms of a preoccupation with fantasy, it's hard to see how there could be such a thing as a fantasy-poor schizophrenic.) Third, and as Sartre describes, this conception misses the psychological significance of autism's substitution, for reality-oriented thought, of formally altered thought. Morbid dreaming differs qualitatively from daydreaming:

a preference for the imaginary ... is not at all just a case of preferring one sort of object to the other. It must not be believed, for example, that ... morbid dreamers in general try to substitute a brighter and more seductive irreal content for the real content of their life, and that they seek to forget the irreal character of their images by reacting to them as if they were objects currently and really present.... One ... not only flees the content of the real (poverty, disappointed love, business failure, etc.), one flees the very form of the real, its character of presence, the type of reaction that it demands of us, the subordination of our conduct to the object, the inexhaustibility of perceptions, their independence, the very way that our feelings have of developing.... The morbid dreamer who imagines being king will not put up with an actual monarchy, not even a tyranny where all his desires would be granted. A desire is never in fact granted to the letter precisely due to the fact that an abyss separates the real from the imaginary.... Only ... irreal objects can be annihilated when the caprice of the dreamer stops, since they are but his reflection; only they have no consequences other than those one wants to draw from them. It is therefore wrong to take the world of the schizophrenic for a torrent of images with a richness and a sparkle that compensates for the monotony of the real: it is a poor and meticulous world, where the same scenes keep on being repeated, to the last detail, accompanied by the same ceremonial where everything is ruled in advance, foreseen; where, above all, nothing can escape, resist, or surprise.[17]

Within the autistic world there's no distinction between appearance and reality, no possibility of the contents of the imaginary world resisting one's will, disconfirming one's belief, or challenging one's sense of self: the confronting mind-independence of the world is subverted.[18] Within one's own world one is sovereign. As one of Manfred Bleuler's patients, who knew something of how to move between the worlds, said: 'In my world I am omnipotent; in yours I practice diplomacy.'[19]

A fourth difficulty with that conception of autism which focuses on the wish-fulfilling contents of 'another world' is that it ignores the costs as well as the benefits of living there. A detachment from reality makes it unavailable as a resource to check one's fears or to nurture and comfort the dejected soul.[20] The autistic world accordingly becomes lifeless, since desires can only be satisfied if they're first kept in play – which itself involves tolerating the knowledge that they're yet unmet. Autism, however, involves the dismantling of desire – not its enlivening satisfaction but rather its lifeless pacification and short-circuiting.[21] As with major tranquilizers, which diminish both terror and exuberance, so too the autistic state purchases invulnerability to loss and pain at the expense of nourishment and vitality.

Such costs are well documented by the poets. Keats' above-mentioned knight-at-arms sees previous 'death-pale warriors' as 'held in thrall' by the faery, sees their 'starved lips in the gloam'. He awakens and finds himself 'on the cold hill's side', 'alone and palely loitering, though the sedge is withered from the lake, and no birds sing'. And Yeats' 'stolen child' similarly finds himself starved of life: 'He'll hear no more the lowing, of the calves on the warm hillside. Or the kettle on the hob, sing peace into his breast. Or see the brown mice bob, round and round the oatmeal chest.' Even so, with a 'faery, hand in hand' he walks away from a world that's 'more full of weeping than he can understand.'

Minkowski – our most notable theorist of schizophrenic autism – describes the loss intrinsic to autism as a diminishment of 'contact vital avec la réalité'.[22] Its costs are well articulated by R. D. Laing in his account of his tragic young patient Julie:

> Reality did not cast its shadow or its light over any wish or fear.... Every wish met with instantaneous phantom fulfilment and every dread likewise instantaneously came to pass in a phantom way. Thus she could be anyone, anywhere, anytime. 'I'm Rita Hayworth, I'm Joan Blondell. I'm a Royal Queen. My royal name is Julianne.' 'She's self-sufficient,' she told me. 'She's the self-possessed.' But this self-possession was double-edged. It had also its dark side. She was a girl 'possessed' by the phantom of her own being. Her self had no freedom, autonomy, or power in the real world. Since she was anyone she cared to mention, she was no one.[23]

This takes us to the final limitation of an understanding of autism as retreat to wishful imagining. This is that it underplays the significance of intact reality contact for bona fide imagination: holidays of imagination must always be paid for by the labour of reality contact. The schizophrenic, because he's not a daydreamer but rather a morbid dreamer, does not so much retreat into fantasy as retreat into a state of mind in which the distinction between reality and fantasy no longer finds purchase. Fantasy, by contrast, ultimately presupposes, rather than negates, reality contact: it's only those who can properly be said to effect reality-oriented judgements who may also be said to imagine or daydream.[24] The schizophrenic subject, however, has, in her autism, suffered a collapse of the two domains. Whilst we do sometimes talk of her delusion as fantasy, this may be modelled on our talk of her delusion as belief: both descriptions merely emphasize the absence of thought with objective content; neither positively determines the nature of the psychopathology.

Loss of reality testing

We've now arrived at the second of what's here been styled the central 'apophatic' results of this treatise. The first, an apophatic understanding of reality contact and its loss in psychosis, was offered in Chapter 3. The second, which depends on the first, is an apophatic understanding of the pathological state we call 'schizophrenic autism' or 'living in one's own delusional world', or – if the focus instead be on the disability maintaining that state – of what's called 'impaired reality testing'.

In offering this new reflective understanding of autism – as a *state which, when it supervenes, renders inapplicable a conceptual distinction between (i) reality-oriented judgement and (ii) fantasy* – the intention is neither to develop an empirical theory or hypothesis nor to provide the term with a new meaning, but instead to sharpen, and accurately reflect on, its extant meaning. The assumption is instead that, whilst our use of the term 'autism' – and the soon-to-be explored concept of 'reality testing' – in psychopathological practice are in order, so that they pick out a significant and central psychopathological phenomenon, psychopathologists may hitherto have had an inadequate reflective understanding of how they intuitively use their own terms. (It is, as Plotinus and St. Augustine noted, one thing to correctly use a word such as 'time' – perhaps in sentences like 'What's the time?' or 'It's time to go!' – but quite another to say something sensible when asked to define it.[25]) The intention, then, is to develop our reflective understanding of what our psychopathological terms mean out of a reconsideration of what we intuitively grasp to be their proper use, and in the light of that clear reflective understanding, to further sharpen that use. Other theorists may take a different tack, tying the terms' meanings to their extant definitions and then, on that basis, employing or rejecting them as apt designators of psychopathological reality.[26] That, too, is of course perfectly legitimate – and so long as we track the tack in play we shan't talk past one another.

A clue to the character of this collapse of imagination and reality-oriented thought is found in Eugen Bleuler's original formulation. Bleuler writes that whilst the psychiatrist Pelletier has it 'that above all, the patient does not differentiate any more between reality and fantasy', this is only 'true in a certain sense' and does 'not get at the essence of' schizophrenic autism. The deeper suggestion he grasps for here is that in autism there is neither a substitution of fantasy for reality, nor a failure to distinguish which of one's experiences are genuine perceptions and which genuine fantasies, but rather an 'inadequate or absent distinction between fantasy and reality' themselves.[27] Freud similarly talks of the 'uncanny effect … produced' not by a person choosing to indulge in imagination rather than reality-oriented perception and thought, but 'by *effacing the distinction between* imagination and reality'.[28] Neither of these psychopathologists had available to them the philosophical resources for sharpening their point, but what I'm here proposing on their behalf is that we best understand the autistic retreat as a withdrawal not so much from reality to fantasy, or into a state in which a person is confused about whether in fact he's perceiving or imagining, but into a state in which there is no such fact to be determined, judging and imagining themselves now being confused. Or: into a state in which genuine imagination is itself as equally vitiated as is perceptual or cognitive contact with reality, since the constitutive contradistinction between judgement and imagination has here collapsed.

Freud's concept of 'reality testing' is often defined in terms such as 'the ability to see a situation as it really is, rather than as one fantasizes it to be'.[29] (The definition appears sound, albeit that the notion of seeing a situation through the prism of one's wish or fear requires elucidation.) However, it's also often explicated – as indeed Freud himself explicated it – in terms of a hypothetical activity underlying the said ability, an activity whereby an experience or belief is tested for whether it originated 'internally' (and so is to be counted hallucination or delusion) or 'externally' (and so is trusted to be genuine perception or veridical belief). Yet such an activity is mythical: reality contact is a precondition for, and not a product of, our testing of thoughts against reality. If I were not in contact with reality, then I couldn't enjoy thought which accurately or inaccurately represented it; only if my feet are already on the ground may I take my head out of the clouds.

A similar hypothetical task is often given to the patient who recovers 'insight': this patient has supposedly had to learn to see his currently disturbed thoughts as delusions and to know his hallucinations for what they are. The confusion attending this idea is easy to see: delusion into which one has insight has already ceased to be itself. Insight can therefore only be into the fact that one *has been* deluded. To recover insight, then, may more clearly be understood simply as (in and for some moment, and to some degree) both ceasing to be psychotic and recognizing that certain of one's recent thoughts and experiences were but 'symptoms of an illness'.

It's tempting to suppose that someone with compromised reality testing delusionally mistakes his hallucinations for true perceptions.[30] This, however, isn't quite right. What is true is that someone who can't reality test is unable to acknowledge that his hallucinations are hallucinations. But if someone has lost touch with reality, so cannot reality test, and so becomes delusional, then we don't meaningfully describe him either as merely imagining perceiving or as believing himself to be perceiving. To be sure his delusionality does (in part) consist in his failure to recognize that his experiences aren't (as we say) real; however, it doesn't consist in his taking them for real.

What of the suggestion that we can only know that we're hallucinating when we are hallucinating, and perceiving when we are perceiving, because we have the ability to test these experiences against reality? With respect to hallucination: the suggestion overlooks the possibility that some experiences may be so bizarre that anyone with intact reality contact will automatically take them for hallucination and quite legitimately not bother to check them against reality. And with respect to perception: our knowledge that we're perceiving when we are perceiving – just like our abilities to know we're awake when we are so, to know that we're exercising our imagination when we do, and know what we're experiencing – is what's called 'primitive' – which is to say, is properly taken as bona fide even when unevidenced. That it's not unreasonable to posit such knowledge as stands in need of no justification can be seen by thinking on the fact that we could, after all, in turn always ask, of any X offered by way of ground for our claim to know that we're perceiving or imagining, what the warrant is for our claim to know this X. And so, if we're not to court an endless regress, we do well to accept the 'I just do!' answer to 'how do you know right now that you're perceiving?' – i.e. do well to acknowledge that our claims to know either that we're perceiving or that we're imagining are in the normal case groundless, and perfectly proper despite this. In short: here we're innocent – i.e. allowed our knowledge claims – until proven guilty.[31]

Barbara woke one morning 'to find three grey and somewhat wispy figures standing at' her bedside. To sum up the moral of this section: the one question we don't do well to ask is whether Barbara *really believes* that the Operators are standing there. What makes for living in one's own world – i.e. for schizophrenic autism, for a failure of reality testing – is there no longer being a fact of the matter as to whether Barbara is here judging or imagining.

Any of us can easily (i) visually imagine (i.e. bring to mind) three wispy figures standing by our bed, (ii) recall how we would affirm the fact that we are indeed imagining them, and (iii) recognize that Barbara is disinclined to offer any such confirmation. For this reason, it's tempting to infer that she must instead truly believe that there are Operators standing by the bed. In a sense we may indeed say this, as of course may Barbara.[32] But that sense, as I mentioned above, has to do only with registering that here we don't have to do with objective thought. In another sense of 'believe', this inference – that Barbara truly believes there are Operators in her bedroom – is precisely the one we should resist if we want to understand what it really means to be living in a world of one's own in such a way as involves delusion.

To grasp the point with analogy's aid, consider the fundamental importance for a viable economy of the distinction between real and counterfeit money. Part of what enables a cash-based currency to maintain its value and fulfil its function is the fact that our concept of it is conditioned by a conceptual distinction between the genuine and the forged. Real money is minted by (say) the Bank of England; the counterfeit is made elsewhere. Should a future society abandon the distinction, such that there's no longer a point in talk of 'real' versus 'forged' money, anything being in some sense usable regardless of its provenance, then the concept of 'currency' is itself debased. Similarly, the thought goes, with that debasing of the distinction between judgement and imagination effected by schizophrenic autism. Here we confront no merely conceptual matter – as if what were at play were just, say, how the patient conceives of the status of his mental acts. Nor do we meet with someone using forged (imaginary) instead of real (reality-oriented) money (thought). What's rather at stake is the very determinacy of his mental acts and states of mind and the possibility of our continuing to classify them as either fantasies or reality-oriented thoughts. If we ask of our future society whether some piece of what still looks like money is, in fact, genuine or counterfeit, we should be guilty of projecting onto it a distinction that itself is now voided. So, similarly, when we encounter someone in his autism, we find a mind the very form of which no longer instantiates the distinction between judgement and fantasy.

This, in part, is what the age-old paradoxical characterization of psychosis as 'waking dream' picks up on.[33] Someone who fantasizes (i.e. daydreams) temporarily suspends her reality-engagement, but may return from imaginary to real activity at any point. Fantasy, we might say, is a holiday which can only be earned by the work-life of world-involvement, and it depends for its character, and its content depends for its determinacy, on the subject's continued capacity for reality testing. Someone who exercises her imagination is in essence fundamentally in contact with reality, even whilst dwelling on matters fantastic. Essential to our understanding of fantasy as the mind's idling is the condition that reality-oriented thought may supervene when required. But when we dream, that capacity for reality-oriented thought is no longer in play; when dreaming, there simply is no distinction between imagining something, and genuinely taking it, to be the case.[34] This is why Heraclitus tells us that 'the waking have one common world, but the sleeping turn aside, each into a world of his own'.[35] So too in schizophrenic autism: fantasy and reality-oriented thought here lose their constituting contradistinction, and so in the psychotic state itself there's no real place for talk of either. And so too is the psychotic subject in a world of her own.

Autism and motivation

Of the various characteristics of mental illness discussed in Chapter 1 – irrationality, suffering, a self-maintaining character, motivated avoidance of anguish – the last characteristic, motivation, was offered as essential but non-necessary. We can acknowledge cases of mental illness wherein madness is properly ascribed on the basis only of sheer overwhelm and self-maintaining rational breakdown. 'Mental illness', however, is a family resemblance concept, so we shouldn't take the mere possibility of non-motivated delusionality to mean that, when a mind becomes mad to avoid anguish, it isn't thereby manifesting an essential aspect of mental illness. In such cases, talk of 'mental illness' signals not only suffering and disorganization in the face of overwhelm, but also the supervening of an alternative organization wherein the mind sacrifices its primary tasks of maintaining intelligibility-finding (and hence intelligible) world-involvement and of sublating inner conflict (through emotional work and personal growth) to the end of self-preservation. Whilst the self-preservation met with in ordinary illness is properly described in *functional* terms ('killer-T lymphocytes *function* to destroy virally infected cells'), the self-preservation met with in mental illness is, as befits the psychological context, often properly described in *motivational* terms ('the mind ... *seeks refuge in* madness from the mental suffering that exceeds its strength' (Schopenhauer)). This mind isn't merely compromised; it's also compromising as it beats its retreat from unbearable overwhelm to a world of its own in which reality and fantasy have collapsed together.

On this conception, then, it's prima facie reasonable to think of someone's schizophrenic autism as at least sometimes a function of his psychodynamics – i.e. as a result of his motivatedly, if unconsciously, distorting his mind's own defining, reality-facing, form in order to manage his emotional equilibrium. Yet a somewhat different conception is offered us by Eugène Minkowski, the most profound of our post-Bleulerian schizophrenia interpreters, and nearly all of today's biological psychiatry follows in his lead. For Minkowski provides an extended discussion of the personally meaningful 'content of psychosis' only to proceed to deprecate the significance of painful predicament and its motivated avoidance in an understanding of the essential nature of the illness.[36]

Contending with predicament is of course often important, he opines, and naturally we owe a great debt to Jung's depth psychological investigations of psychosis, investigations which help us grasp the obscure meanings of various individuals' psychotic experiences in relation to their pre-psychotic predicaments.[37] Yet the essential autistic core of schizophrenia is, he suggests, far more clearly appreciated in terms of mere deficit or defect rather than in terms of psychodynamic processes.[38] We all, schizophrenics and non-schizophrenics alike, have our existential predicaments, and it's therefore only to be expected that these show up in the delusional life of the schizophrenic as also in the inner life of the non-psychotic subject. But understanding what makes definitively for a schizophrenic inner life, rather than just grasping what contingently is that life's psychology, is, he suggests, better pursued merely by reference to what now is damaged or deficient. Such damage or deficiency, he reasons, is after all what makes for illness.[39]

From the perspective of the present work, it's surprising to see Minkowski in effect reduce schizophrenia from a prototypical (suffering- and motivation-involving) illness to a mere disorder or disability. For sure, in doing so he follows a venerable psychiatric tradition associated especially with Emil Kraepelin. And there is of course nothing to stop anyone reserving the terms 'schizophrenia' and its cardinal trait of 'autism' for whatever disturbances of association, boundaries, and reality contact are intelligible only in non-motivational terms. What would be of concern, however, is if that decision led to core aspects of the psychotic experience being overlooked. When Barbara tells us that by 'Riding off in the bus, I left safely behind me a mess of reality with which I was totally incapable of coping' – or when she hallucinates the frightening Operators whose threats, unlike her real-world predicaments, at least have a thinkable and hence more manageable form – does this really just accidentally diminish her angst, or is it rather motivated by an urgent need for the angst's abating? And when we turn to some of Minkowski's own examples of lost reality contact, what we find is that rather than suggesting the irrelevance, they rather seem to suggest the significance, of motivation in our understanding of the loss of reality testing.

Consider first the man who, when out walking, 'was sometimes struck with the appearance of a woman. He would then return to his house, sit down on a chair, cross his arms and take up a position as symmetrical as possible to reflect on the event. He would try to solve the problem of why a woman's body made a particular impression on a man'.[40] What's striking is that, in his treatment of the case, Minkowski gives no thought at all to the natural understanding that here we find the intolerable emotional experience of frustrated sexual desire, and the practical problem of how to achieve sexual intimacy with women, being delusionally sublimated into the bizarre intellectual problem of why heterosexual men are attracted to sexually attractive women.

Or consider the case of Paul, a socially withdrawn seventeen-year-old schoolboy, whose morbid rationality and diminished vital contact with reality Minkowski again describes beautifully. Just before his autism set in, Paul 'seems to have been preoccupied with questions of a sexual nature; he would question his father and ask him for explanations, revealing a complete ignorance of the subject'.[41] At bedtime Paul would take over an hour ensuring the linen was perfectly symmetrical on the bed. He also spent hours in the bathroom, explaining this in terms of his preoccupation with: the size of a feather duster in there, the exact time he entered, and the size of the crack at the door's base and whether he may be seen through it – which latter thought, Paul alleges, troubles him not at all. Again, it's hardly a great leap to detect here a defensive intellectualizing retreat from various psychosexual troubles. Yet Minkowski opines that the 'sexual curiosity that appears at the outset of the illness, which could be considered for that reason a point of departure, can only be a precursory sign of the interrogative attitude that takes a firm hold afterwards. In any case, it is this attitude that must be rectified before attending to anything else.' Yet why might it not instead be that the deployment of this intellectualizing, interrogative attitude is a defensive reaction to a normal, but for this teenager utterly unmanageable, preoccupation with matters bodily and sexual?[42]

Consider, next, Minkowski's case of the schizophrenic woman who 'in an advanced stage of her illness, passed the time making hats for herself. She had made 16 of them. One day, she lost two of them. As a form of retaliation against this she decided to break two of her mother's 16 cups'.[43] Once again we're hardly going out on a limb if we here risk a hypothesis about the symbolic resonance of the hats, cups, and breakages – for example, that the patient made hats to provide herself with her own version of that which she enviously felt her mother to both cherish and unfairly withhold, so that, following her loss, she was driven to even the score by breaking two of mother's cups.[44] Of course, we don't know the details, so must indeed here be content with mere hypothesis. But what's evident, and what's already registered in Minkowski's mention of retaliation, is that matters motivational are not incidental to the case.

Throughout his text Minkowski keeps a careful eye on the distinction between delusion's motivated, symbolic, content and delusional form so as to not lose sight of the latter. Yet whilst the distinction between content and form is important, what gets lost is the above-articulated Sartrean notion that it's in fact not just the content, but the form, of the delusional world that is sought by she who finds the discord between the real and the desired world too painful to handle. To live in one's own world becomes for Minkowski merely a matter of being detached from reality, and psychological functions such as wish or imagination, shame and guilt, repose and confidence become mere content-providers for a mind the alternative form of which is to be understood otherwise. Yet from the alternative perspective offered here, matters biographical and formal do not keep to their own enclaves any more for psychotic delusion than for everyday mood. To insist that they do is, far from exercising a clear-sighted restraint, to risk colluding with the delusional subject's efforts to dismantle his reality contact in the domain of his disquiet. For, as we already know, we often become moody when we fail to tolerate, process, understand, or get to grips with our specific emotional predicaments.[45] Our worlds are now encountered under a formally altered aspect, an aspect that resolves when (amongst other possible resolutions) we find a way to own, acknowledge, or fathom the specific significance of our situated encounters. When mood resolves, and we find a way to once again meaningfully suffer what we experience, predicament once more becomes thinkable in its particularity. Delusion can here be understood as a further step on from unbearable mood, the mood's form resolving not into thinkable content but into the merely ersatz thoughts of a quasi-dreaming mind.[46] Something like, but by definition not, thinkability in its specificity is now restored, albeit at the cost of reality contact.

Perhaps the principal reason Minkowski struggles to find a place for motivation in his understanding of autism is his tendency, widespread also in today's biological psychiatry, to judge the attribution of motivation to the schizophrenic autist to be too much of a stretch only because of a prior conflation of motivation with intention. He's surely right to think it wrong-headed to suppose that the overwhelmed subject typically intends to enter a delusional world. Even taken to it's extreme, the 'policy of the ostrich' – i. e. putting one's head in the sand – is not, as Minkowski notes, a good model for entering a delusional world.[47] But unconscious motivation is properly ascribed to subjects on the basis of the shape of their behaviour, thought, and feeling over time, rather than on the self-ascriptions they're disposed to make at the time. And the avoidance of anguish by flight to a delusional world is best understood as having a reflex character, and as motivated in a similar way to much animal behaviour. Retrospectively, however, the patient may be able to own the motivated character of her flight from reality; thus Minkowski himself cites a patient who reports of himself that, 'I suppressed feeling as I suppressed all reality. I dug a moat around myself.'[48]

Notwithstanding, it's plausible to suggest that the schizophrenic person's motivated autistic retreat exploits his schizotaxic disposition – i.e. his non-motivationally-intelligible weakened reality contact, loose cognitive associations, and unstable ego boundaries.[49] So too the bipolar patient's psychosis may exploit the abnormal ease with which his self-conception separates from his emotional life. And this in turn may explain why many can suffer hideous tormenting conflicts without yet going psychotic: their (non-schizotaxic) constitution ruling it out as a live option for them. Yet whilst such dispositions may be necessary for schizophrenic illness, they're insufficient (for we at least need suffering before we shall talk properly of mental illness), and they obtain also in those who haven't become ill. Furthermore. we have the observation (of Bleuler and Jung amongst others) that, when we're considering mental illness, autism and accessory symptoms such as delusion prevail in the ambit of emotionally charged complexes. In short, Minkowski does not provide good reason to doubt that the patient is not only thrown, but also takes flight, into his own world. And especially when we consider the retrospective testimony of the patient, and take note of his psychodynamics and the relief that delusionality affords his complex-ridden person, we can surely find a place for the motivational element within our understanding of his autism.

Against the above it might be suggested that to read motivational dynamics into the very core of our understanding of schizophrenic illness gives the psychological discipline of psychoanalysis an ontological promotion it hasn't earned; and that the autistic core of schizophrenia is in any case better explicated in 'basic' neurobiological terms rather than in terms of 'higher level' motivational factors.[50] Let's consider these in turn.

As for the first suggestion, we may counter that the concept of motivational dynamics belongs not first and foremost to the science of psychoanalysis, but rather to both our pre-psychoanalytic articulation of the more difficult moments of our daily lives and our psychopathological system quite generally. If psychoanalysis here builds on our insight into what we already latently grasp, then all well and good. But when it comes to our understanding of mental illness it takes a curiously blunted psychopathological sensibility to read the psychodynamics out of, and not any particular schooling in psychoanalysis to read them into, our intuitive grasp of what we clinically encounter.

As against the second consideration – that the fundamental nature of schizophrenic autism is such as to invite neurobiological rather than psychodynamic explanation – we may ask why these accounts should be thought to compete. After all, it's part of the design of such motivational concepts as the *drive* or the *need state* that they sit rather closer to matters physiological than do other psychological concepts. (They are, we may say, 'psychobiological' in character.) And the basic conflicts which psychoanalytic investigation tracks – to do with sexual desire, social affiliation, competition, aggression, attachment, etc. – and the basic affects here in play – of interest, lust, love, rage, fear, anxiety, terror, etc. – do not float free of the brain but are all – as affective neuroscience well describes – directly anchored in distinct neural circuitry.[51] Without taking a stand on matters empirical, it's surely at least imaginable that unless there is, say, sufficiently complex cortical activity to allow competing drive activations to be negotiated, then the clashing of such activations may constitute an overwhelming degree of that inner push–pull tension we call 'anxiety'. And if someone is sufficiently schizotaxic to not be inexorably tethered to the world, it's conceivable that such anxiety will propel him into orbiting a different, this time psychotic, sun. In short, shouldn't we need positive reason to suppose that matters neurological and affective are here *not* of a piece, rather than have that assumption of brain/affect dualism be our starting point and then have to justify a psychodynamic understanding of schizophrenic autism?[52]

Cataphatic approaches to autism

A thought offered us by Jaspers is that delusion proper 'shows itself as a whole primarily in the fact that it *creates a new world* for the deluded person'.[53] And Barbara O'Brien's describes her entry into a 'new world' replete with 'grey and wispy' figures called Operators who talked to her and responded to her unarticulated thoughts. It's time now to attempt a closer look at when it is that living in a new world of one's own amounts to suffering a psychotic illness. What follows first considers three 'cataphatic' approaches – i.e. attempts to define or explain what it is to live in such a world in positive, intelligibility-retrieving terms. When these are seen to crumble, attention will be turned to the 'apophatic' approach begun above (where autism was analysed not as the presence of anything positively intelligible but rather as the absence of the constituting contradistinction of fantasy and belief), prosecuting this through a consideration of the idea of the delusional mind's 'short-circuit'.

The first cataphatic approach has it that someone lives in his own world if he mistakes his imaginings for beliefs.[54] Barbara's delusional thought that she's at the mercy of the Operators is, this suggestion has it, after all a thought of an ordinary-enough, intelligible, sort; it's just that she's mistaken her fantasy for her registration of a fact. But the difficulty with this proposal is that it purchases the intelligibility of its conclusion (she was after all daydreaming) at the expense of the intelligibility of its conception of self-understanding. For our ordinary capacity to truthfully state, as the case may be, either that we know or are just daydreaming that three wispy grey Operators are talking to us isn't dependent upon our identifying what species of attitude we hold. Our knowledge of the form of our attitudes is instead brute. And when I tell you that I was daydreaming of Operators pursuing me, my say-so is criterial for it being daydreaming that I was engaged in. That's to say, one of the main criteria for properly ascribing daydreaming to someone is her say-so that this is what she's doing. Only if we reify daydreams or beliefs into entities which somehow float free from the actual grounds for their ascription could we think that someone mistakes their imaginings for knowledge. To say of Barbara, then, that she 'no longer knows that she's daydreaming' is, therefore, to say of her that there's no longer a fact of the matter about whether it's really daydreaming that she's doing – a loss we also register with the telling phrase: 'she's lost her mind'.

The second cataphatic approach has it that delusion is in part marked by the delusional subject relating to the world about him as if he were relating to his internal world. As one psychopathological theorist puts it, delusional statements are 'statements about external reality which are uttered like statements about a mental state, i.e., with subjective certainty and incorrigible by others'.[55]

Consider: the content of her thinking may be unusual, but we can imagine Barbara wondering if her neighbours were spying on her without thereby considering her deluded. It's instead when she's certain regarding matters about which we're sure that hesitancy is warranted, when she brooks no debate, when she provides no justification precisely where the strongest of arguments is needed, that we find her delusional. Were Barbara instead to be avowing that she had the nursery rhyme 'Ring a Ring of Roses' on the brain, we should be far more likely to count delusional he who insisted on Barbara providing evidence than we would Barbara herself. For in this latter case she'd be arrogating to herself an authority which is entirely appropriate in the circumstances. What isn't appropriate, however, is for Barbara to make claims about 'external reality' as if they had the unchallengeable character of articulations of the inner life. To claim thus, the suggestion goes, is in fact what makes for delusionality.

At first glance the idea appears promising. On further inspection, however, three objections present themselves.

First, we ordinarily consider delusional not only beliefs about 'external reality' (three Operators stand at the foot of my bed) but also a variety of inner experiences.[56] These include passivity ('made') experiences of action, impulse, emotion, and thought (thought insertion, withdrawal, and broadcast), and certain cenesthopathies ('electric currents and spirit beings are inside my neck'). To rule these out by insisting that delusional utterances be 'statements about external reality . . .' not only traduces the psychiatric lexicon but also misses the point of our talk of delusions as 'beliefs' – which is (not to distinguish them from experiences but rather) to register their essential non-objectivity.

Second, what criterion shall we use to determine whether a delusional utterance really is about either inner or external reality? There is of course its content – 'Operators are born with special brain cells known as the battlement. With these cells, an Operator can extend and probe into the mind of a Thing. He can tap the Thing's mind and discover what is going on there, and even feed thoughts to the Thing's mind in order to motivate it.' – but what does it mean to say that such content concerns the external rather than the internal world? We might ask Barbara, 'do you take these things of which you speak to obtain independently of you and your thought, or do they relate only to what you imagine?' Perhaps she'll give us an equivocal answer, or answer that she's not simply imagining things, or say that her thoughts truly concern 'external reality', or becomes too thought-disordered to count as expressing a clear stance. Yet regardless of her reply, what remains unclear is how we should here understand her words. For her radical unworlding is such that it in any case becomes unclear whether the usual distinctions – employed either by us or by her – such as 'subjective' and 'objective', 'unreal' and 'real', or 'internal' and 'external' – remain adequate to her experience.[57]

Third, consider what it is for a 'statement' to be 'about a mental state'. Such statements have the form of avowals: in making them we don't express judgements about how matters are with us but rather directly express those matters. (We don't say 'I take *myself* to have toothache, an ill temper, and a good mind to call it a day'; instead, we simply say 'I have toothache, an ill temper, etc.') And a statement being an avowal is criterial for it being 'about' a 'mental state' (so long as we include bodily aches as mental states). Such statements may be said to be logically 'incorrigible by others' since, not being correct or incorrect judgements in the first place, they're not open to correction. Talk of their being uttered with 'subjective certainty' presumably also indexes the same fact that we've little or no use for talk of doubt in relation to our knowledge of our mental states. (There is no such thing as your not being sure whether one of your mental states is either (i) knowing it's time for dinner or (ii) wishing that global warming weren't happening.)

The question now is what sense we can make of the idea of someone making 'statements about external reality which are uttered like statements about a mental state, i.e., with subjective certainty and incorrigible by others'. The way this is written – with its deployment of the seemingly univocal term 'statements' – might make it seem as if matters of doubt and certainty are merely epistemological, whereas the individuation of 'external' and 'mental' domains is a purely ontological matter. If that division of labour could somehow be made good, then the proposal might stand. But as soon as we acknowledge that the form of the statement (avowal, or expression of judgement) itself partly discriminates the domain (mental, or external), it becomes hard to know how to take the proposal. For now we feel rather as we would on being asked to accept that the reason why an intonation strikes us so peculiarly is that, despite being sung by a high-pitched soprano voice, it's actually a bass note. Or if it be said that what it is for Barbara to make a statement about the external world (such as 'the Operators are following the bus she's on in their own car') as if she were avowing a mental state is for her to be talking about erstwhile denizens of the external world whilst yet brooking no correction, then we seem to be no further forward. For people can be recalcitrant and overconfident – or for that matter be aptly firm and confident – in their judgements regarding the world about them without in this way acting as if they were avowing mental states. Perhaps in the end the only clear sense-making interpretation we can give of this second cataphatic approach has it that delusional people react to attempts to correct them just as non-delusional people do when others doubt their avowals of their mental states. This, however, leads us merely to an empirically false hypothesis, since we already know that delusional people typically don't, for example, say 'Who are you to doubt my *sincerity*?!' when their delusions are challenged.

The third cataphatic approach to understanding what it is to be in one's own world has it that the schizophrenic subject's very experience of, and not just his talk about, the outer world has, when he is in his autism, become subjectivized, whilst his experience of his inner life has correlatively become objectified.[58] The approach is cataphatic in the sense that its aim is to *shed light on* why the subject who has lost reality testing talks and acts as she does through aptly characterizing the experience which such acts and talk reflect – rather than its aim being simply to index the character of such talk and acts themselves.

Let's unpack this approach's subjectivizing and objectivizing moments in turn. By exemplification of its first (subjectivizing) moment, the schizophrenic judge Daniel Paul Schreber, author of *Memoirs of My Nervous Illness*, has been described not as experiencing 'his delusions as being literally true but, rather, as having a certain "subjectivized" quality – that is, as being in some sense the product of his own consciousness . . .'. The schizophrenic 'may perceive . . . the external world . . . [but] what

Pierre Janet called "le sentiment du réel" is lacking'. Insects which Schreber saw flying past, which 'would to the normal person have the quality of reality – existence independent of that of the self-as-subject – seem to have had for Schreber the ephemeral quality of something merely phenomenal'.[59]

With respect to the second (objectivizing) moment, the objectification of inner reality is said to obtain because of a preponderance of 'hyperreflexive' self-relations – i.e. 'forms of exaggerated self-consciousness in which aspects of oneself are experienced as akin to external objects'.[60] The body moves from being the tacit medium of world-directed perception and action, something in which attention is embodied and from which it's directed to the world, to being the object of the schizophrenic subject's attention. This backwards migration of attention's viewpoint objectivizes and alienates what it encounters, so that 'what might have been thought to be inalienable aspects of the self come to seem separate or detached. This may affect ... one's arms or legs, one's face, the feelings in the mouth or throat, the orbital housing of the eyes – even one's speaking, thinking, or feeling.'[61]

To turn now to critique of the idea of the first (subjectivizing) moment, we may ask what it means to say that the world is experienced as, or as if it were, part of the mind. Illuminating about the suggestion is its drawing our attention to matters not just of the content but moreover of the form of schizophrenic consciousness. It also brings to mind certain philosophical doctrines – of solipsism, of phenomenalism – and reminds us of the circumstances in which such doctrines may tempt us. Thus Louis Sass – author of the above-quoted remarks – follows Wittgenstein in describing how if we disengage from the world, stand stock still, and stare at what is before us, we may start to have an experience which we want to describe in such solipsistic terms as: 'what I see is nothing other than my experience itself', 'objects are now but images', 'only I and my experience exist'.[62]

Our difficulty, however, is that our wanting to say just these things doesn't mean that we're thereby articulating meaningful possibilities. Wittgenstein, after all, developed his critique of solipsism and phenomenalism precisely by showing such metaphysical doctrines to be nonsensical. And it's simply not straightforward to say what insight may be shed on one obscure phenomenon (schizophrenic experience) by analogizing with another (solipsism/phenomenalism) which itself has but the appearance of intelligibility.[63]

There are hereabouts difficult philosophical issues at play, issues concerning whether or in what sense we may be said to understand a philosophical doctrine that turns out to be nonsense, and what the value of developing the capacity to maintain clarity whilst engaging with compelling philosophical nonsense could be for the project of making sense of psychopathology.[64] Rather than follow such threads, let's consider instead what surely all will acknowledge: that the only criterion for Barbara having an experience which in some (or other, or no) sense is of the world being of a piece with her subjectivity is that we're inclined to describe it in such terms. We have here no independent criterion of correctness for describing the experienced world as subjectivized other than Barbara herself either talking of it as 'but an appearance', etc. or her now making such steps in her thought about the world as when sane she'd only make in her articulation of her experience. In short, the phenomenological psychopathologist's descriptions of schizophrenic experience don't here offer an explanation of, or articulate a further fact about, the structure of her experience. They provide a non-occlusive language for talking about it, they offer apt recognition to it – and these are powerful offerings. But they don't further a cataphatic ambition of retrieving sense from what appears incomprehensible. For sure, we may find ways to make that experience more relatable: we discover that we too want to articulate our experience of the world in subjectivized terms during our more dissociated moments (as when we stand stock still and stare). Even so, we only get so far, here, as an 'as if': 'it is for me as if I were the only subject who's ever existed'; 'it's as if the world's objects have become two-dimensional images'. And we may conceptually grasp how the step from here to delusion is a function of lost reality testing. And yet none of this allows us to retrieve sense from Barbara's delusional pronouncements. We no more understand what it is to really – i.e. not only 'as if' – take a tree to be but a perceptual image than we understand why Barbara might now talk about a tree as if she were talking about such an image, as when she says it will disappear if she blinks.

Let's now recall the other (objectivizing) moment of this third cataphatic approach: the claim that the inner life of the schizophrenic subject has become objectivized. You may surely make something of the idea of experiencing parts of your own *body*, and various of its movements and sounds, as mere objects. Yet what appears more relevant for understanding what it is to be in one's own delusional world is the suggestion that one's own *experiences* – perceptions, bodily sensations, emotions, and thoughts – may also be experienced as objects. On such an understanding, our thoughts, ruminations, fantasies, etc., constitute this alternative reality's furniture, and we have not only retreated away from parts of our now partially unlived body, but also somehow now retreated behind our own mind itself, now being but spectators of our own mental goings on.

As with the idea of objective reality's subjectivization, the objectivization of subjective reality is a notion easy enough to articulate but hard (or perhaps rather: impossible) to understand. A meditation manual may tell you to 'observe your own thoughts', but its doing so invites you to pay attention to the fact of your thinking (ruminating, fretting, daydreaming, etc.), rather than invites you into a potentially infinite regress of having thoughts about thoughts, or to attend to your attendings, or deploy a mythical inner faculty – one borrowing the title 'introspection' – with which, supposedly, thoughts may be made 'present to consciousness'. Perhaps it be insisted that we do after all feel our feelings, think our thoughts, and experience our sensations and emotions – and that reference to the inner faculty in question is nothing but an acknowledgement of this fact. Even so, the verbs just deployed (feel, think, experience) do not refer to modes of encountering that of which the nouns speak (feelings, thoughts, sensations, and emotions), since to feel, experience, or think a feeling or sensation or thought just is to have it. We could here decide to follow those in the philosophy of mind who, in constructing for us a curious range of gerunds ('believings', 'imaginings', 'cogitations', etc.), seem to hope to reference a domain of inner 'goings on' populated by these putative phenomena. Such philosophers turn the fact of being minded into a fact about possessing something called 'a mind' itself filled with 'mental entities', 'inner states', 'inner events', and 'mental processes' which one 'owns' and over which one has 'agency'. Once we've developed such an objectivized conception of mind it may seem unproblematic to use it to frame an explanation of how we come to treat our own thoughts as external phenomena. Perhaps, for example, we should just think of a thought as being like a hammer with which at one moment, when we're using it to bang down a nail, we're identified, and with which at another moment, when it looses from our hand or when we're attentively looking for it in the workshop, we're disidentified. Yet, for all this, a thought is not a hammer: it's not an object with which we can identify or disidentify – i.e. it can't become notionally incorporated into or extruded from the body schema. And it's not a phenomenon, since it doesn't appear, but instead occurs, to us.[65] Or, to turn now from thoughts to acts of thinking: might it not be that the inner monologues which normally constitute our thinking have, in the psychopathological case, become disowned and objectified? The difficulty for this suggestion is the absence of any purely psychological criterion to use to determine whether the same monologues are in play in the normal and the psychopathological cases. For sure we could revert to a physical or physiological criterion: the same laryngeal or brain activity is present in both. This, however, is to change the subject, since we don't individuate inner musings by reference to bodily happenings. In short, such approaches only seem to get a thesis about inner objectivization off the ground by themselves relying on an illegitimately objectivized conception of thinking. For sure, and as we'll see in more detail in the next chapter, the schizophrenic may well talk as if (something like) thoughts nevertheless appear, rather than occur, to him; our difficulty, however, is in understanding what that means.

We might describe our problem here thus: that, hoping to improve our understanding of what it means to be in one's own world, we're tempted by philosophical articulations of what it is to be minded which already turn our mindedness into the possession of an inner domain replete with contents with which we're said to enjoy intentional relations or to 'be in touch', and correlatively to construe avowals of thoughts and feelings as reports on inner goings on. Following this assimilation of mind to entity, of the openness of intentionality to the thinghood of phenomenality, we find it natural to describe Barbara as talking of or experiencing objects and events as if she were talking about or experiencing 'inner objects' and or 'inner events'; or alternatively, think of her as somehow experiencing her own mind as if she were encountering a world. Or perhaps we moot that it's the schizophrenic subject, not the psychopathologist, who here assimilates the subjective to the objective order. But the problem remains that it's impossible to positively say what it could mean to actually effect the mooted assimilation. The psychopathologist is simply left without any criterion for saying what it is for the patient to *really* be talking of reality (yet for her talk to logically ape that pertaining to the inner), or to really be experiencing her own thoughts *as if they were objects*, or to really be *experiencing as a thought* one of the denizens of objective reality.

For sure, certain aspects of a patient's psychopathology may be most vividly articulated, by her or by another, as the experience of now objectivized thought. We may even urge that to so much as have these psychopathological experiences just is to have such experience as is spontaneously described by patient or clinician in just these terms. We may notice too that whilst the pre-psychotic patient talks of her own experience as being somehow objectivized, the psychotic patient simply talks of what we (but not she) know to be her own experiences as if she were talking of objective reality. Yet whilst this is all nicely indexed, none of it is explained, by talk of her experience as having become actually objectivized.

An apophatic approach to apophany

Given such failings of intelligibility-recovering approaches, it behoves us to consider what an apophatic answer to the question of what it is for delusional worlds to dawn might look like. For taking an apophatic approach doesn't involve us looking in vain for an unforthcoming criterion in terms of which we establish the validity of some or other positive description of the content of the patient's experience. Instead, it offers us understanding just as it acknowledges how our best efforts to capture it within a meaning-finding scheme are doomed to failure, and how the context presupposed by any successful wielding of our ordinary criteria for assessing meaning is here abrogated. The apophatic theologian takes herself to appreciate the terrible reality of God only as she grasps how even the most superlative forms of description she offers inevitably fail to do justice to their divine object. So too does the apophatic psychopathologist come to appreciate the depth of psychotic disturbance in the same confessional moment as the inexorable inadequacy is acknowledged of attempts to recover rational intelligibility.

If we describe Barbara's experience in terms that are abstract and remote from the lived quality of her experience, such understanding may seem manageable enough. Met with in the flesh, however, and the understanding can be bewildering, despair-engendering, and grievous. When she's lost to her psychosis, the gamut of our living expectations of, and readiness for synchrony with, her are rebutted or disintegrate, rather than received and reciprocated. The other's 'face' – which is to say, her manifestation to me which 'invites me into a relation', whether to understand, flee, or help her – becomes impenetrable.[66] And at this point we have a choice: to cope by switching to a nobody-at-home biomedical mode which thinks in terms of mechanistic malfunction rather than of illness proper; to cope by switching to a business-as-usual, normalizing, psychological mode and thereby falsify her experience; or to do our best to stay faithful to, rather than evade, her actual experience and her brokenness. Such faithfulness involves, in part, quietly taking the measure of – and in this way trying to bear with her in – those painful experiences which, because of her vulnerability, she herself couldn't bear and so which made her ill. As discussed in the penultimate chapter, we find symbolic traces of these intolerable experiences in the content of Barbara's delusion. When sane, Barbara can talk of 'leaving behind a mess of reality with which I was totally incapable of coping'. Yet when she's in her delusional world we find – instead of the real-life assemblage of backstabbing colleagues, and apt emotional responses to that of shock, horror, and anger – a council of Operators who, with voices filled with 'shock, horror, and anger', declare Barbara to be 'a monstrosity and a source of danger, something that has to be put out of the way'. By staying with the fact of her brokenness, rather than turning away from her impenetrable face, we stay alive to what was too disturbing for her. And now we may encounter even her so-called 'negative symptoms' not simply as deficits but as craters constituted by the delusional dismantling of her life's intolerable experiences.

The potent notion of the delusional mind as suffering a 'short-circuit' provides a helpful exemplar of the apophatic approach.[67] Consider that icon of loneliness, the homeless schizophrenic man shuffling past you on the street. He's in 'a world of his own', he's 'talking to himself'. A true address awaits the response of another who, in his hearing of it, gives sense to its making, but this man awaits no answer from any person before continuing his mutterings. The place where the other should be has, in this short-circuit, been taken by himself; the current of his mind no longer flows out into and back from the world beyond. You notice too how his eyes take no part in the normal social dance of 'acknowledge the stranger but avoid intrusion'. The path he treads is similarly unstructured by social conventions governing proximity and distance. He's neither invasive nor ordinarily shy, both such options implying an aliveness to sociality which here is voided. Within his short-circuiting mind, risky alterity gives way to futile solipsism, and needs are pacified with hallucination rather than satisfied or frustrated by reality.[68]

Perhaps at first we're inclined to consider our shuffling man's self-talk his way of 'keeping himself company', but soon we realize the futility of, and evasion perpetrated by, that description, a futility shown by the fact that this self-talk voids the space where both company and an awareness of its absence may be registered. It stops him feeling lonely, but only by dismantling rather than meeting his need for love. Here we meet not with he who imagines himself being measured against another, but with he who 'measures' himself by putting his hand on top of his head, or who 'gives' himself a 'gift' by passing it from one hand to another.[69] The form of such activity carries an echo of the practices of measurement or gift-giving but, since measure and measured, or donor and recipient, are here of a piece, what we meet with is but illusion. To truly live is after all to inhabit a world – to meet with its resistance to one's wish, to register its independence, to experience one's desires and fears being genuinely fulfilled or vanquished or perduring despite their manifest unfulfilment. But this morbid dreamer's longings and needs of sociality are, far from finding registration in his inner life, instead eternally dissolved in the ocean of his autism. They meet not with any real fulfilment but only with that dreamy palliation which obtains when the very distinction between the imaginary and the real is effaced and the mind's capacity to register presence and absence is dismantled.

To truly compete in a race one must, despite the hardships involved, run its gamut; taking a shortcut nullifies your result. In order for a battery to illuminate a bulb, electrons must flow from the battery's cathode to its anode via the bulb, the resistance of which must in the process be overcome. A short-circuit also has the electrons arriving at the 'finishing line' of the anode, but now they bypass the resistance-providing lamp. By analogy: when the mind short-circuits, it does not simply fail to overcome the world's resistance. Its desires, its attempts to gain comprehending mastery of a situation, its attempts to resolve conflicts, aren't merely thwarted. This mind now neither achieves the fulfilment of its desires, nor is left experiencing what has become the world's insurmountable resistance. Instead, a bypass is taken, a bypass taking the shape of delusion or hallucination.

The shuffling man 'palely loiters' his way along the pavement. The current of his mind has met with too much resistance from the world, but rather than develop a way to tolerate experiences of unmet need or of profound anxiety, his mind short-circuits. Now he 'lives in his own world', which is to say, lives but a half life where 'the sedge has withered from the lake', where 'no birds sing'. Now he himself has become one of the 'death-pale' kings or princes, muttering with 'starved lips in the gloam', alone 'on the cold hill's side'. Or, to switch between the above-cited poets, from Keats to Yeats, now he can't hear or miss 'the lowing of the calves on the warm hillside'; the 'kettle on the hob' can't now 'sing peace into his breast'. Or consider again Julie, Laing's above-quoted patient, 'possessed by the phantom of her own being', for whom reality 'did not cast its shadow or its light over any wish or fear' and every 'wish met with instantaneous phantom fulfilment and every dread likewise instantaneously came to pass in a phantom way'. In her own words (when in her psychosis she sometimes speaks of herself in the third person):

> I'm the prairie.
> She's a ruined city....
>
> She's the ghost of the weed garden....
> The pitcher is broken. The well is dry.[70]

Why should this now be her broken, dry, life? Well, we know why. It's because – the world's more full of weeping than she can understand.

5

The Divided Self

Introduction

The psychiatric intuition has always been that the sufferer of madness, especially of such madness as we call 'schizophrenic', is 'breaking down', 'falling apart', 'fragmenting'. She's 'no longer herself'; she's 'out of her mind', 'beside herself', a 'divided self'; she disintegrates. To repurpose Yeats' words: 'Things fall apart; the centre cannot hold.'[1] This sufferer is alienated; certainly, as we've already seen, from others and her milieu; but also, in some sense, and just as paradigmatically, from herself.[2]

Bleuler's concept of 'the schizophrenias' provides us with our prototype mental illness syndrome by consolidating just this intuition of interior division: 'I call dementia praecox "schizophrenia" because ... the "splitting" [*Spaltung*] of the different psychic functions is one of its most important characteristics.'[3] Areas of intolerable emotional conflicts (i.e. complexes) become split off from what's left of the dominant personality; trains of association are blocked.[4] The indefeasible intimacy of interior monologue, the metaphysical unity of person and act, thought or feeling: somehow these all come apart. Unable to achieve an ongoing integration the sufferer takes considerable leave not only of her world but also – and in some sense – of her very self. She now suffers: trains of thoughts which, unbeknownst to her, veer so off course that their meaning crumbles; inner speech which dissociates into 'voices' which she 'hears'; actions, thoughts, and feelings which become somehow impersonal and alienated or, at the delusional extreme, are now experienced as somehow 'belonging to another'; and an 'unlived' body which becomes the site of alien energies, spirits, and mechanical and electrical effects.

We intuit something of this fundamental breakdown, this splitting into pieces of a unity that was more than any mere union, this becoming other/alter of what before was self/ego – but we do not understand it. The ease of our formulations disguises the paradoxical character of the words here reached for by both patient and psychiatrist. For what could it even mean to become alienated from *one's own* mind? Or: isn't *my self* the one thing from which it's impossible for *myself* to become estranged? We can linguistically hive off 'Me's from their 'I's all we like, separate out 'egos' from 'selves' – but such a linguistic proliferation of personae hardly sheds light on the real possibility of radical self-estrangement.[5] If it were a merely contingent fact that we experience our own thoughts and feelings, that we perform our own actions, that it's our own body which furnishes the living substance which we are – just as it's a contingent truth that, say, it's our own car that we normally drive – then we could at least imagine having thoughts that belong to another. Yet our minds and bodies don't belong to us as just so much alienable property. And whilst ordinary speaking is distinct from ordinary hearing, it's surely of the very nature of the inner that such a distinction finds no analogue there – where, inner speaking and inner listening being indissolubly one, we need no inner ear to listen in on our inner soliloquy. Yet then again, whilst I just wrote 'indissolubly', it's seemingly just such a dissolution we seem to meet in the schizophrenic who – again, in *some* sense – now takes his own self-talk for that of another.

The concern of this and the next chapter are those paradigmatically schizophrenic disturbances we call *Ich-Störungen* or disorders of the ego/self/I.[6] The sufferer somehow becomes confused as to which are his own, and which are someone or something else's, properties or qualities, thoughts or feelings, actions or utterances. The present chapter documents how philosophers and psychologists have been tempted to make sense of the psychotic patient in terms of some or other concept of 'self-alienation'. The following chapter considers instead the use of the concept of 'ego boundary disturbances' to theorize the self-disorders. (What distinguishes the two chapters is not so much their subject matter but the theorizations under critical review.) In the hands of theorists of self-alienation, mental faculties proliferate: a new psychology offers us both inner voices and inner ears; inner thoughts or impulses and a now separable inner perception of such thoughts and impulses arrive on the psychological scene – as more generally do a range of theoretical versions of now separated inner 'I's and 'Me's. And such psychologies seem to provide a theoretical framework within which the above-described symptoms may – it's alleged – be rendered intelligible. Rendered intelligible, that is, as the kinds of *mistakes of inner sense* that anyone would surely make should they too be unfortunate enough to fall apart in the ways the theorists propose. In this way is delusion reduced to illusion; in this manner does psychopathological theorizing now aim at dissolving the paradoxes of psychotic self-estrangement, at cataphatically understanding 'how such cases of introspective alienation are possible', at providing 'the key to making sense of such reports, the key to making them coherent', the means of 'rendering the phenomenon more tractable'.[7] Perhaps, it's suggested, the study of schizophrenic splits even gives us insight into such structure within the sane mind as would otherwise remain hidden.[8]

The danger of attempting such cataphatic paths is that we unwittingly lose our bearings both on the intrinsic inalienability of true selfhood and on the inherently paradoxical quality of psychotic self-alienation. The opportunity then becomes lost for appreciating just what it is in the psychotic process that's truly overwhelming of intelligible mindedness. That, at least, is what this chapter shall argue. Tempting as we may find it to 'make coherent' – and in effect thereby evade – the derangements of the psychotic mind, our better aim shall be to acknowledge and stay with that mind in all its brokenness. The path we shall take will then instead be apophatic, which is to say: we shall aim at offering acknowledgment to the depths of psychotic devastation precisely through refining our grasp of the futility of our attempts to dissolve self-alienation's paradoxes.

From automatism to passivity experience

In his *Dementia Praecox or the Group of Schizophrenias*, Bleuler describes for us a range of what he calls 'automatisms'. With automatism proper,

> the entire automatic action is split off from the conscious personality of the patient. The limbs do something, the lips say something, of which the patient is informed by his senses as if he were an observer during his action, as if he were a third person. In particular, writing and speaking often present themselves like this.... [P]atients themselves are surprised by what . . . their tongues have said. They grasp it only by means of their own auditory sense. At times, 'the words are placed on their tongues, so that they must speak it out;' or the 'mouth speaks without the patient willing it.' . . . Willingly or unwillingly the patients direct their attention to external or internal processes; or 'something goes on thinking inside,' 'ideas are made to come to their minds.' Thinking is not experienced as a spontaneous process.[9]

Before pressing on, let's just pause to note that whilst it would take considerable psychopathological tone-deafness to be able to make nothing of Bleuler's talk of 'limbs and lips doing and saying' things, it would also take considerable philosophical tone-deafness to think its meaning straightforward. The ordinary use of such phrases is after all metonymic. When Anglicans engage in the call and response:

> Priest: 'O Lord, open thou our lips'
> People: 'And our mouth shall shew forth thy praise',

they're speaking poetically rather than inviting possession and predicting automatism. Metonymy, however, is precisely not how Bleuler's words are here to be understood. How instead they should be understood is what we shall consider later. For now let's consider patients' descriptions of their own experiences.

Lucinda has a history of indulging dissociation with the aid of a Ouija board. Here she describes what in retrospect she perceives as the origins of her psychotic illness:

> I was sitting in a German lesson, a little bit bored, and all of a sudden my pen started moving, and it was writing to me. And I had this written conversation with the voices from the Ouija board, even without a Ouija board being there. . . . I'd sit there with Ouija boards and move my finger around. And after 6 months I didn't need to move my finger any more, and my eyes would just be drawn to the right letters. . . . And then eventually it didn't need to be a Ouija board, it could even be a keyboard: by looking at the keyboard, my eyes would spell out letters.[10]

The Ouija board phenomenon relies on subtle ideomotor effects whereby the highly responsive planchette on which the participants each have a finger moves in an apparently mysterious way over the board's letters, thereby spelling out words. Such productions are in fact guided by the participants' subconscious expectations; blindfold the participants, turn the board about, and the effect disappears.[11] As expected the intrapsychic and self-world dissociations are most pronounced if the context (low lighting, a passive and submissive stance, uncanny and fearful emotions aroused by the thought of 'communications from the dead', etc.) impairs the normal ways that coherent selfhood and reality contact are co-enacted. Yet as the months go by and Lucinda moves from a sane to a prodromal (pre-psychotic) state, her own boredom provides enough by way of reality detachment to allow the emergence of another automatism: automatic writing.

As the transition to psychosis deepens we typically find a seemingly paradoxical pairing of both heightened and diminished automaticity. The paradox dissolves once we note that the loss of automaticity has to do with what could be called a dis-identification of the self from the body or mind, and the heightened automaticity has to do with that body from which one is disidentified seemingly taking on a life of its own. Sidrah demonstrates the former when she talks of her loss of spontaneous, un-reflective agency when she becomes unwell:

> Simple little things, like making myself something to eat, or showering, become like a huge task. It's like trying to conquer Everest ... It's like, my autopilot that I have when I'm well just malfunctions. I can't switch off; I'm always thinking all the time ... [My] body just doesn't feel my own ... [It's] ... like a layman trying to make a rocket ...[12]

Whereas Anthony, suffering an active schizophrenic psychosis at the time of interview, describes being a body which has become a battleground for autonomous spirits:

> Spirits ... become quite powerful, and they can interact with my body, and it feels like a big war of energy. And they can use your energy against you, and it's a bigger, bigger presence. I feel them wriggling around inside me, like a worm or something. Usually it's only a foot area in my stomach, but sometimes it can be more. I've felt spiritual presences which have filled my entire body up.... [The spirits] took a sword blow to my neck, yeah, and in my opinion they broke it. And there was blood that started rushing through my body, yeah, like in other places that it's never rushed. It was like pressure going round, down my arms and shoulders and other places. Erm, my neck felt different when I was lying down. It felt like it was moving, like it was in movement even though I was still, lying down.[13]

And Kim describes an experience of the return of healthy automaticity and reidentification with his body, an experience he identifies with the remission of psychosis:

> When I was ill, I couldn't trust what I was going to do about something. For example, sometimes there'd be a celebration in the park, with a bouncy castle, and everything else for children. And I have nieces and nephews, and ... they'd go on there. And I'd know that it was dangerous [but] I didn't have the power of thought to think to get them out ... But one time, it just disappeared.... I knew my illness

had disappeared. I was able to think clearly – that 'that's dangerous'. My nephew's crawling so fast, under this car. Just my instinct to grab him, in going there.... And I took him home ... and something gave me a feeling, you know ... that my illness had suddenly gone.[14]

As the transition to frank psychosis deepens, automatisms become experienced in a delusional manner, as the direct intervention of another agency in one's actions, thoughts, and feelings. The psychopathological literature borrows from patients the terms 'passivity' or 'made' experiences to characterize such delusional experiences:[15]

> [Fay, a 33-year-old restaurateur] 'has no longer been able to know herself'. She has felt that 'her thoughts are not hers.' When walking, she feels that it is her legs that carry her, but feels that they are 'moving on their own'. She has the feeling of not being herself, 'as if she had no soul in her body'. On further enquiry, she complained that she felt that her actions did not originate in herself; her thoughts did not come from her. She can no longer recognize herself as being the same person doing her thinking and acting, and yet she does not believe herself to have become another.[16]

> [Katie, a] 23-year-old female patient reported, 'I cry, tears roll down my cheeks and I look unhappy, but inside I have a cold anger because they are using me in this way, and it is not me who is unhappy, but they are projecting unhappiness onto my brain. They project upon me laughter, for no reason, and you have no idea how terrible it is to laugh and look happy and know it is not you, but their emotions.'[17]

Katie doubts that we could form an idea of just how terrible such passivity experience is. What follows will ultimately agree with her, and will suggest that it's only through an understanding of why such an idea can't be formed that we can begin to appreciate the terror she suffers. But first let's consider the views of those who attempt to understand her by forming an idea of what is going on for her.

Cataphatic explanations of passivity phenomena

Anthony, the above-described patient who experiences alien sensations from spirit entities at play in his body, also once – as he put it – found his hands typing numbers into his phone without his bidding. His psychologist suggested to him that such beliefs were produced by attempts to make sense of unusual bodily sensations and movements. This didn't wash with Anthony, whose delusional experience was *ab initio* one of foreign agencies at work within him. And on this matter the classical psychopathologists agree with Anthony; as Jaspers has it, 'the patients are not merely interpreting various abnormal organic sensations in one way or another but have an immediate perception of this "coming from outside"'. Far from us meeting with a rationalization of an abnormal inner experience, 'we are discussing here ... something radically different, an *elementary* experience of *being actually influenced*'.[18] Anthony's psychologist, however, succumbed to the temptation of imposing his own cataphatic scheme (which inexorably sees beliefs as resulting from attempts to make rational sense of experience) on his patient's experience. He thereby failed to pay due phenomenological attention both to the immediacy of Anthony's experience of foreign agency, and – precisely because he renders them in overly tractable, insufficiently *outré*, brushstrokes – to the delusionality, of passivity experiences.

Both Jaspers and Schneider proclaim the 'incomprehensible, difficult to imagine, and not open to empathy' character of passivity phenomena.[19] Yet whilst Jaspers urges that we 'just have to accept these accounts as outsiders',[20] many psychopathologists (including, as we shall see below, Jaspers himself) are tempted to try to render passivity experiences intelligible. That's to say, they're tempted to offer the kind of account which, all going well, would have us exclaim: 'Ah yes, now that you've elucidated what the underlying disturbance of inner experience is, I can see how, were I also to be placed in such experiential circumstances, I too would take the thoughts, feelings, and movements which in some sense are yet mine to nevertheless be under alien control.' Let's now consider some of these attempts at retrieving cataphatic intelligibility.

Such efforts typically begin by inviting us to reflect on what secures our alleged knowledge that our ordinary thoughts and actions are our own. Thus one author suggests that thoughts are 'normally accompanied by a sense of effort and deliberate choice as we move from one thought to the next.' It's on the basis of this sense of effort, then, that we judge them ours. Our actions too are said to be taken for our own because (rightly or wrongly) we experience them as caused by inner acts of will. How does this relate to delusions that one's bodily movements are the work of other agents? Well, with such an understanding of ordinary agency in place, delusions of control can now be considered to result from 'a loss of the feeling of effort or intendedness that is normally associated with willed actions'. And the delusional experience of thought insertion? Well, if 'we found ourselves thinking without any awareness of the sense of effort . . . we might well experience these thoughts as alien and, thus, as being inserted into our minds.'[21]

Such suggestions provide clear evidence of the ascendancy of the cataphatic impulse over the endeavour to attend to the phenomenological details either of ordinary action or of psychopathological experience. For, to start with ordinary action, what we find there is no experience of bodily movement accompanied or preceded by acts of will: 'When I raise my arm I do not usually *try* to raise it.'[22] Instead, we find intention to be fully intrinsic to and immanent within such ordinary movements ('picking up a cup or combing one's hair'[23]) as may be delusionally experienced as influenced. We may note too that the involuntary movements our limbs sometimes make are not typically experienced as caused by another agent. Something similar may be said also of thinking: thought is simply not 'normally associated with a sense of effort and deliberate choice as we move from one thought to the next' – especially if we consider the kinds of thoughts that form the content of reports of thought insertion ('kill God'; 'I will now buy bananas').[24] Furthermore, what are we to make, really, of the idea that ordinary inner cogitation involves 'deliberate choice'? It surely can't be that I choose which thoughts to have next, since then the thoughts which are supposed to be happening next would already have obtained within that choosing. And if deliberate choices are themselves to be counted as mental acts, we should require an infinite regress of such choices to choose to choose to think . . .[25] A similarly futile regress appears to threaten the idea that it's in virtue of our awareness of a sense of effort attending our thoughts that we're inclined to think them our own. For how shall we know in turn that this sense of effort is ours? Or, if the latter knowledge is allowed to be brute, why not the former too? And to turn now to matters psychopathological: if delusions of mental or physical passivity really did result from experiencing an absence of feelings of effort or deliberate choice, then, given the effortlessness and spontaneity of much of our cognitive and agential lives, we should all experience the majority of our thoughts and actions in a psychotic manner.

Another cataphatic approach adverts not to a sense of effort or inner intention but to a putative 'sense of mineness' in ordinary thought and action, a sense which is absent in passivity experience – hence the aberrant experience of certain of one's own thoughts and actions as alien. Taking this tack has been popular from the beginnings of psychopathological thought on automatism. Thus Schneider first offers us the aptly cautious note that:

> Disturbances of identity have received a great deal of description. It is not an easy concept to grasp, in that we cannot say plainly or unequivocally what the criteria for normal self-awareness may be. The literature is often of slight value. There is so much misleading and sometimes artificially inflated self-portraiture, spoiled by sensationalism; there is much hasty theorising of a psychological or physiologic, but nearly always partisan, kind before the phenomena in question are even grasped, and in this field it is a hard enough task to get a grasp at all.

But he too soon goes on to posit an obscure 'sense of mineness' the lack of which is said to underlie the psychopathological phenomena:

> Because this sense of 'me' and 'mine' is so elusive a concept to grasp, its disturbances are ill defined and hard to sample. This particularly applies to thinking and somatic experience . . . Only when the sense of 'me' and 'mine' is encroached on from without can we grasp at the disturbance.[26]

Despite the elusiveness of the concept, Jaspers, like his colleague Schneider, is also confident that there must be some basic 'sense of mineness' present in ordinary experience and absent in passivity experiences

> Self-awareness is present in every psychic event. . . . Every psychic manifestation, whether perception, bodily sensation, memory, idea, thought or feeling carries *this particular aspect of 'being mine'* of having an 'I'-quality, of 'personally belonging', of it being one's own doing. . . . If these psychic manifestations occur with the awareness of their not being mine, of being alien, automatic, independent, arriving from elsewhere, we term them phenomena of *depersonalization*. . . . In the natural course of our activities we do not notice how essential this experience of unified performance is.[27]

The question arises, then, as to what's meant by this 'sense of mineness'. On what basis are the psychopathologists so sure that our ordinary experiences of doing, thinking, and feeling involve such a sense?

The sense of 'sense' here in play has, I take it, to do with experiential judgement: we have senses of outrage, foreboding, injustice, something being not right, someone standing silently behind us, etc. Because they have to do with judgement, it's essential to senses, thus understood, that they can be misleading: it's of their nature to involve us in getting something right or wrong. My outrage may be misplaced; there may be nobody behind me. Yet when I avow my thoughts and feelings, or say what I'm doing, I precisely don't do so on the basis of a sense that such thoughts, feelings, and actions are mine. Rather, it's of the nature of such first-person avowals that neither the attitude nor the subject is in need of identification. (We may call such declarations 'primitive'.) Perhaps I 'tell you what I think': here I no more need become acquainted with who is thinking than with what I think; instead, I simply 'speak my mind'. After all it can't be that all my avowals of psychological facts about myself are based on such alleged senses, since then my avowal that I now have this or that sense would itself require yet another sense to tell me that this sense was mine – and so on ad infinitum.[28] Might we not, then, do better to stop the regress at the very first step, and accept the idea of a primitive capacity to self-ascribe thoughts, feelings, and actions which capacity is not dependent for its proper functioning on a sense of any kind?

Perhaps it's said that all of this makes too heavy conceptual weather of the idea of having a sense of one's thoughts or actions as one's own. For maybe we should think of having such a 'sense of mineness' as instead just like, say, my having a sense that my arm is now outstretched – where the criterion for having that sense is simply that I'm not confused about the matter (as I may be on coming round from anaesthetic). But agreeing to that criterion will also force on us agreement with the assertion that reference to an absence of a sense of mineness is now utterly non-elucidatory when it comes to passivity phenomena. If to enjoy a sense of X simply is to not be in state of confusion about X, then we cannot suppose ourselves to form any clearer an idea of what it is to be in state of confusion about X by adverting to the absence in the confused state of a sense of X.[29]

Or perhaps it's suggested that for me to have a sense of my arm being outstretched is in addition for me to be able to say that my arm is outstretched, when it is outstretched, without having to check or be told. (We might call this a 'non-observational sense'.) Yet whilst there may be room for such a notion of non-observational sense when it comes to knowing where one's limbs are, knowing what one's feeling by way of sensations, knowing what one thinks, etc., it's entirely unclear what it could mean to say that one has a non-observational sense of who it is that's here striking such a pose, feeling this sensation, or thinking that thought. The reason for this is that the identity of the subject of experience isn't here something about which I could meaningfully be thought to be in error – unless by 'being in error' is meant losing control of my words or thought, becoming confused in such a way that no coherent thought as such is being had by me. Furthermore: which poses, sensations, and thoughts does this subject have in mind when he allegedly relies on an inner sense to answer the question of whose is 'this sensation', 'this posture', 'this thought'? He doesn't point to the sensations and thoughts, and it will not do to specify them by their content (many people can after all have a thought with the same content at the same time). The suspicion surely arises that the 'this' here stands for 'the sensation/posture/thought which *I'm* now having/holding/ thinking'.

Two stories bring out the general conceptual point. Consider first William James's anecdote about Baldy:

> In half-stunned states self-consciousness may lapse. A friend writes me: 'We were driving back from —— in a wagonette. The door flew open and X., alias "Baldy," fell out on the road. We pulled up at once, and then he said, "Did anybody fall out?" or "Who fell out?"—I don't exactly remember the words. When told that Baldy fell out, he said, "Did Baldy fall out? Poor Baldy!"'[30]

Baldy's disturbance is manifest not simply in his confusedly calling himself by his own name, as a young child might, but by his falling out of the carriage and knowing that someone had fallen out – but not who![31] Far from Baldy's disturbance showing up a failure to engage in an allegedly normal business of correctly picking himself out as the subject of his own activities, our sense of its absurdity instead shows up the nonsensicality of that very idea.

The idea that being able to express 'I' thoughts ('I've fallen out of the wagonette!') involves correctly identifying oneself is also nicely parodied in the following Sufi tale attributed to Mullah Nasruddin:

> After a long journey, Nasruddin came at night to the marketplace and lay down to sleep. But so many people were there in the hubbub that he feared not knowing which was he on waking. To make himself identifiable, he tied a gourd to his ankle, and then went to sleep. His mischievous neighbour, seeing what the Mullah had done, untied the gourd and affixed it to his own ankle. On waking Nasruddin was mightily disturbed and exclaimed: 'It seems that he is me. But if so, then who now am I?'[32]

Nasruddin's confusion here, we might say, consists not in his actually confusing himself for his neighbour – since it's not clear what that could even mean – but in his confusedly thinking that he so much as needs to identify himself in the first place. In truth neither error nor (guaranteed or fallible) success in picking out the right object – oneself – is here in play, since the having of such 'I' thoughts doesn't involve us in the business of self-identification. We can imagine peculiar cases in which I'm mistaken about whether, say, Richard Gipps is hungry (perhaps in my senility I've forgotten my own name). But what we don't find cogent is the suggestion that I may be mistaken (or correct, for that matter) about whether it's I who is hungry.[33]

It's sometimes suggested that we can draw on a distinction between being the agent and being the subject of one of our own 'mental episodes' (*m*), so that a 'person suffering from introspective alienation with respect to *m*' is properly understood as acknowledging 'that he is the subject in whom *m* occurs, but ... has the sense that somebody else is the agent of *m*'.[34] This is supposed to help us undo the paradox of thought insertion – i.e. of the psychotic experience of my having thoughts in my mind that I nevertheless don't take for my own – by distinguishing two different senses of 'own'. Thus perhaps I own the thoughts in that I experience them as occurring in my mind, but don't own them in the sense that I don't experience myself as their author. Such talk of thoughts occurring in rather than to us, or of our being these thoughts' author or agent, is apt to sound as delusional as the phenomenon here under investigation. But the suggestion is that we can gain our conceptual bearings here by comparing ordinary thought and mental passivity experiences with ordinary action and bodily passivity experiences. Thus: 'Just as I may experience myself as either agent or patient with respect to a particular bodily movement, I may experience myself as actively or merely passively involved in the "movements" of my mind,' and so 'my admitting that thought ... *m* occurs in my mind while denying that I think *m* is like my acknowledging that my arm went up but denying that I raised my arm.'[35]

The distinction between arm raising and arm rising is clear enough.[36] Whether or not we can illuminate it by adverting to distinct experiences of either agency or ownership, we surely do sometimes suffer distinct experiences either of involuntarily moving our arm (twitches, post-anaesthetic phenomena, etc.) or of being acted on. Even so, when passivity experiences obtain, it's often for complex coordinated performances such as talking, and it's not at all clear what it would mean to effect a distinction analogous to that between arm raising and rising in relation to such performances. We can imagine complex performances surprising their agents (to his own surprise a violinist pulls off note-perfectly a fiendish cadenza). But as soon as we get to the idea that a subject is surprised that a complex performance – one which to an observer looks like the subject's own – is obtaining at all, we appear to be approaching the domain of the unintelligible.

The lack of clarity becomes more pronounced still when it's thinking rather than acting that we're considering. It's true that we distinguish between wanted thoughts (e.g. comforting daydreams) and unwanted thoughts (e.g. obsessional doubts, earworms, etc.), and between sudden inspirations and more involved ruminations. It's also true that we deploy a range of idioms for ordinary thoughts which have a surface appearance either of agency ('I think we should ...') or passivity ('It occurred to me that we should ...'). But we don't experience 'passive', out-of-the-blue, inspirations as ego-alien, and it's not clear what it would mean to talk of mistaking an active consideration for a passive inspiration. We understand too what someone who says her thoughts are in truth those of another might be getting at; perhaps she's finally acknowledging either a post-hypnotic suggestion or that the thoughts she previously voiced as her own thoughts were in truth plagiarized. Yet none of this amounts to her denying that it's she who's thinking her thoughts, since what she'd be denying if she denied that would be not an empirical, but rather a conceptual, truth. (How do I know my thoughts and actions are my own? Or, for that matter: How do I know that my eye colour is mine? ... Because I know how to use the word 'my'?) Or to put it otherwise: her 'denial' would amount to nothing but nonsense.

In short, the psychopathologist borrows a distinction between activity and passivity derived from certain bodily contexts, and attempts to render passivity experiences more tractable by applying this distinction to cases of complex coordinated action and thought. What is prima facie more plausible, however, is that it's instead by understanding precisely the inapplicability of the distinction between doing and undergoing to thinking and to actions such as talking that we enhance our reflective understanding of agency and thought. Or even if we did find ourselves wanting to describe certain unusual complex bodily performances as somehow not being done by us – a kind of Tourette's syndrome for whole sentences, say – the step to their being another's is still a leap across a conceptual chasm. And turning now to thought rather than action: to invoke the distinction between agency and passivity in an explanation of what it means to suffer thought insertion is to attempt to explain a mystery by invoking a mystification. To suggest that we should, say, simply make *the same* distinction in the mental (thinking) case as in the physical (arm raising/arm rising) case helps us not at all, since the very thing we don't understand is what that would be. We might as well be invited to understand a toothache transplant on the model of a tooth transplant.

A more plausible approach to rendering passivity experience intelligible takes a lead from considering the possible responses that may be had to electrical stimulation of the cortex. We can imagine that when a neurologist directly innervates some part of it in an experiment or surgical procedure, thereby causing a bodily movement or vocalization, the patient may sometimes experience the results as involuntary. Such movement would be akin to automatism; we might also imagine a seizure or some other disturbance of cortical interactivity giving rise to such experience. Perhaps, then, there is some or other failure of connectivity – of feedback or feedforward perhaps – in the schizophrenic brain which gives rise to such experience?[37] And perhaps, then, reference to a disconnection at the neurological level could here explain the kind of self-alienation we find at the psychological level?

Yet to be able to provide a neurological, causal, explanation of delusional automatisms is not to make such experience itself more intelligible. Or, at least, is not to make it more intelligible if what we're after, when we seek intelligibility, are the sufferer's reasons for thinking that someone's moving his arm 'from the inside'. We may well imagine that we too, on suffering a particular brain dysfunction, would suffer the same delusional experience as does the passivity experience sufferer. We may understand – in the sense of knowing what the cause is of – why this would happen. But what we don't thereby understand is why – in the sense of having any kind of reason – we should think what the delusional subject thinks. Which, to restate the Jasperian claim, is just what we should expect when what we're dealing with is truly delusional experience.

Herein too lies a key difference between our understanding of delusional and illusory/hallucinatory experience. Were a neurologically caused auditory hallucination of, say, a choir to arise in someone, we can well understand why she might actually believe a choir was singing or a record playing. And we may well understand why someone with a passivity experience of being controlled by alien forces has a delusional belief with the same content as the experience. In both cases a failure to challenge the reality of the experience leaves the subject with the belief in question. But whereas a failure to challenge illusion results in the bedding in of intelligible error, a failure to recover enough reality contact to challenge delusional experience results in the bedding in of rationally unintelligible confusion. We understand *that* the delusion arises from the delusional experience, but we don't understand *it* – perhaps because, the Jasperian thought goes, it's not an intelligible item.

The final cataphatic understanding of passivity experience to be considered here is owed to the phenomenological psychopathologists.[38] We can, they suggest, understand the passivity experiences of the schizophrenic subject if we see how he has become inwardly withdrawn from his own body and ultimately even from his own mind. Any of us may become de-immersed from that environment with which we previously enjoyed a participatory engagement, now becoming its static alienated onlooker. The schizophrenic, so the suggestion goes, takes this retreat further. Now he no longer inhabits, but instead somehow merely encounters, his own body; his body is no longer 'lived', is no longer the transparent medium of his intentional relations to a world, but instead is an opaque object of his experience. And, retreating now to an even greater remove, thoughts and experiences themselves now become not the transparent medium of his intentional relatedness to the world, but the opaque objects of an inner sense.

This phenomenological proposal may be read in two different ways; I shall call these the 'expressive' and the 'explanatory' readings. On the expressive reading, which shall be pursued in the chapter's final section, the proposal consists in an evocative collocation of expressions of psychotic experiences of automatism and passivity. The accuracy of the account is measured in terms of the justice it does to the gamut of psychotic subjects' delusional and non-delusional expressive articulations of their inner experience. By contrast, on what I'm calling an 'explanatory' reading, the accuracy of the phenomenological account is instead thought to be a function of its doing justice to something which allegedly transcends such first-person expressive articulation – namely, 'the actual structure of consciousness' itself. On this reading the 'because' in 'he speaks of thoughts in his mind which are not his own *because* he has become alienated from them' is supposed to be an explanatory 'because'. The thought continues: 'And if you'd experienced such a misidentification from your own thought or action or feeling, so that they now appear as but ego-alien objects of inward encounters, then you'd also be inclined to say that your experiences are "made", and your body "lived", by another.' The self, as envisaged by the explanatory account, actually lives out, one could say, the dismal world- and body-alienated predicament that Cartesians, empiricists, solipsists, etc. misguidedly paint as the ordinary human mind's existential condition.

The difficulty with such a reading is that we don't understand it. We no more know what's meant by a thought or feeling becoming an entity, something inwardly perceived rather than lived, than we know what's meant by the idea of a number becoming a shed. To think a thought is after all not to have an entity or process present to the mind, but instead to silently invent or rehearse a conversational move, to make an as-yet-unvocalized decision, to ponder or consider something, to have something to say in response to 'what were you thinking?', etc. We understand neither what it could mean for the more active forms of thought to become mere occurrences, nor what it could mean for either such active thoughts, or for such thoughts that pop into our heads, to appear to become objects of an inner sense. If, *per impossibile*, thoughts were initially tethered yet ultimately detachable entities floating within the mind then, we might imagine, we should know what to do with the notion of now experiencing ourselves as such thoughts' alienated inner observers. At that point we could also take ourselves to have a reason-providing understanding of why the subject believes she has thoughts in her mind that she doesn't recognize for her own. But since we can't make sense of this explanatory conception of the psychotic subject's inner predicament, we also can't make sense of her delusional beliefs as what anyone with such a predicament would think.[39]

Passivity phenomena: An apophatic understanding

Whilst cataphatic approaches to passivity experiences tend to invoke the category of the 'acted *upon*', what actually defines automatisms, especially in their delusional elaboration, is their embodying an experience of being 'acted *through*'. 'Possession' – with the kind of meaning the term enjoys in 'spirit possession' – is the relevant category here, and it's precisely by way of their contrast with, rather than instantiation of, the category of the 'acted upon' that passivity phenomena are understood. The categories of 'done by' and 'done to', as manifest in the distinction between (say) raising your arm and having it hoist by another, place an experience in a recognizable humanly intelligible domain. By contrast the category of 'acted through', whether applied to action or thought, carries with it the sense that human intelligibility has here been abrogated just as the constituting unity of the human subject is eroded.[40] Cataphatic attempts at understanding psychosis effectively aim to preserve, rather than acknowledge the defining loss of, the essential intelligibility-conferring unity of the human subject. They do so, in effect, by tacitly locating a sane and unified human subject as a remote interior occupant of the body or mind. That unity of intention and action which is lost in the psychotic subject is now preserved in the retreated subject's 'inner acts of will' – acts which then have an effect on the body and ultimately the world. Or it's preserved in the retreated subject's 'introspections' of her own thoughts and feelings. Even if these thoughts or feelings have, within the cataphatic psychopathologist's theorizing, become mere objects of a retreated subject's purview, the unity of thought and thinker is now preserved in those thoughts, newly invented by the theorist, which constitute the 'introspective acts' themselves. It's by empathically grasping these acts of will and baffling introspections that we're invited to understand, in the sense of 'make sense of', the psychotic subject. Yet in truth all such attempts to preserve unity and hence intelligibility fail to help us understand the nature of psychotic thought whilst also cheating the psychotic subject of his brokenness.

The patient who experiences non-delusional automatisms will typically relate his experience with phrases like 'as if': 'It is for me as if the thoughts in my mind were put there by someone else.' The phrase 'as if' is often used to make comparisons such as: 'The dinner was so exquisite it was as if Heston Blumenthal himself had prepared it.' The intelligibility of such a sentence is a function of the manifest intelligibility of the suggestion that one really could eat a dinner prepared by Blumenthal. If that were the logic of 'as if' at play in the suggestion that 'It's as if the thoughts in my mind were placed there by another', then our understanding of that phrase would depend upon the intelligibility of the suggestion that one really could have thoughts in one's mind placed there by another. But we don't really know what that means, so it's as yet equally unclear what it means for an experience to be 'as if' that were the case.

There is, however, another significant use of 'as if' which is not to make comparison with something already understood, but to individuate an experience by reference to something that one's simply moved to say of it. The modifier 'somehow' makes this clearer: 'It's as if, at this point in the symphony, the music is somehow freezing over'; 'It's for me somehow as if someone's putting his thoughts into my mind.' To understand these sentences we don't need to know what it would really mean for music to freeze over or for someone to have thoughts inserted into their mind. What instead we need is access to experiences which inspire a similar verbal reaction from us. Perhaps we've suffered anarchic hand syndrome, have had strange hypnagogic, hypnopompic, post-hypnotic, post-anaesthetic, or epileptic experiences, or used a Ouija board, and thereby experienced part of our body, or something we're touching, moving as if 'with a mind of its own'.

Such a use of 'as if' helps explicate what in the previous section I called the 'expressive' reading of the phenomenological psychopathologist's thesis regarding psychotic experience. Thus perhaps we talk of 'introspective alienation' or even 'loss of mineness' not because we have any sense that ordinary thinking involves either introspection or a sense of mineness, but simply because the psychotic subject, and we who listen to his self-expressions, are moved to articulate his experience thus. Consider again what was discussed in the previous chapter – the significance of staring in the engendering of certain illusions of philosophical sense and for our comprehension of psychopathology.[41] Lie face up, static and alone, on the ground, with limbs and digits splayed, and stare straight up into the slowly moving clouds. Are you not now more inclined than normal to articulate your experience as one of looking at a film which somehow lifts off of reality? Or to think yourself somehow at the centre of the world, to feel yourself discarnate, to think your present experience to be all that's real, to think everything obtains only in relation to your own experiencing mind? Such solipsistic doctrines, Wittgenstein suggests, are (nonsensical and so) not even false; even so we may be far more tempted to entertain them, far more gulled by the illusions of sense they proffer, when passively staring than when actively engaged with our worlds.[42] And so too for prodromal (pre-psychotic) experience: are there not states of mind, underpinned by a partial disintegration of reality contact, wherein the world may appear somehow 'unreal', somehow as if it were a mere representation or stage set?[43] Yet what makes 'unreal' the right word here? Nothing; but it's the word for which we spontaneously reach, and the experience is itself individuated by just this reaching. Other phrases and sayings may well now come along on its coat tails, phrases such as 'I feel I wouldn't be surprised if those trees slowly fell backwards like a two-dimensional stage prop.' Similarly for automatisms: there are states of mind wherein the subject spontaneously reaches for words such as 'it's as if someone were putting thoughts into my mind'. Nothing in the experience itself, independent of the inclination it induces in us to proffer these words, makes these the right words to use to describe it. Our language here functions purely expressively.

Turning now from automatisms to passivity experiences proper, we find reality testing to be lost. As a result, not only is there now no work for the simile indicator (e.g.

'as if') to do, but there's also now no fact of the matter as to whether one's words are intended in a metaphoric or literal sense.[44] Herein lies the delusionality of the passivity experience: such experiences are now individuated by words which are not intelligible other than metaphorically, and which yet express a thought the form of which no longer embeds a distinction between appearance (metaphoric truth) and reality (literal truth). An experience which, before the psychotic collapse of reality testing, might have been expressively articulated with words such as 'it's for me somehow as if someone's projecting unhappiness onto my brain …' now becomes 'it is not me who is unhappy, but they are projecting unhappiness onto my brain. They project upon me laughter … and you have no idea how terrible it is to laugh and look happy and know it is not you, but their emotions.'[45]

To understand what it is to suffer passivity experiences without attempting to provide a reading of them which reconstructs their thought's rationality – or, as we could also put it, without attempting to make sense of them by making them make sense – it's helpful to think first on automatisms and passivity experiences of movement. Recall Fay, the 33-year-old restaurateur who was 'no longer … able to know herself. … When walking, she feels that it is her legs that carry her, but feels that they are "moving on their own". She … felt that her actions did not originate in herself; her thoughts did not come from her.'[46] On the one hand her actions (like walking) appear intentional: they're coherent and manifest goal-directedness. On the other hand she's moved to disavow such attributions. If we were to succumb to cataphatic temptation we'd try to decide between these two options. We might, for example, suggest that her actions actually are intended, but that she can no longer recognize her own intentions.[47] Yet put aside the confused idea that we're in the business of recognizing our own intentions, and we can instead acknowledge that the criteria for the intendedness of action are dual, and involve both what's said ('I'm walking') and what's done (walking). In the normal run of things these criteria are either both met, or both not met – and herein the unity of intention, both of the concept and of the phenomenon. Such unity of utterance and act is, however, contingent: in certain twilight states we temporarily experience their disunity, and in schizophrenic breakdown we encounter their more prolonged, and sometimes non-reversing, fracture.[48]

The same disjunct of criteria is found in she who voices certain thoughts but denies that they're her own. But what of she who reports having thoughts in her head that are yet not hers? Looked at historically we can think of thinking *in foro interno* as the result of a developmental sequence: first the child learns to converse; then to talk out loud when others are absent; then to 'keep her thoughts to herself' by 'talking in her head'. (The schizophrenic who mumbles to himself as he shuffles along the pavement struggles with the last stage, and the voice hearer can sometimes be found to be unconsciously subvocalizing.) And this might incline us to seek a similar disunity of criteria when thinking of thought insertion. But here matters are less straightforward, since the only criterion for ascribing thought insertion is what the patient avows. The disintegration of the psyche doesn't here take the direct shape of a dissociation of criteria. Instead, it takes the form of a contradictory report of a thought, which report rather invites us to understand it as a report of a 'made' act – i.e. of an act which is marked by such a dissociation of criteria.

It's essential to the ongoing enaction of coherent selfhood and thought that we're naturally moved to avow intention in conjunction with expressively manifesting it in our acts. Yet we should consider too that it's not only in the conjunction, but also in a certain disjunction, of our ascriptions of mental states that our and their intelligibility-conferring unity is preserved. That is, it's also essential to our sanity that we're naturally moved to ascribe thoughts to others on the basis of our observations of their actions and utterances, yet to ourselves on primarily non-observational bases. This disjunction is essential to healthy individuality and autonomy, but it too is radically compromised in the psychotic subject who now talks as if it were intelligible to ascribe thoughts to others – to the alleged originators of his inserted thoughts – on non-observational bases.

In a move proving influential on the twentieth-century's construction of psychopathology, Schneider offered passivity experiences as 'first rank' symptoms of the schizophrenias – which is to say, he suggested they be taken as highly pathognomonic of such conditions. Their specificity to the schizophrenias has since been questioned, although it's true that reliable inference to a schizophrenia diagnosis can often be achieved by diagnosing passivity experiences, and true that they occur far less frequently in other conditions.[49] Such empirical matters are of course not our concern, but they reside in close proximity to another matter, both conceptual and phenomenological, which has to do with the quality of distinctly schizophrenic experience. The concluding suggestion of this chapter is, accordingly, that the deep kind of fragmentation we find in passivity experiences clues us into the real meaning of that 'splitting of the different psychic functions' which caused Bleuler to rename dementia praecox 'schizophrenia'.

As we've seen, those hoping to recover speaker's meaning in sufferers' articulations of their central symptoms are naturally tempted to offer psychological reductions of them. In Bleuler's terms, 'different psychic functions' are still ascribed to patients, and dissociations are posited between what are supposed to be in-principle separable functions. Separate functions of producing and introspecting thoughts and intentions are invoked, for example, and disparities between their results are offered as the cause of delusional passivity experiences. Delusion thereby collapses into illusion – i.e. collapses into the making of mistaken judgement caused by the malfunctioning of a putative psychic function – and in this way delusional experience is considered to embody the kind of empathically intelligible mistake of a sort we could imagine anyone making who was in that predicament. But when we consider the dissociation of intention and thought in the passivity experience sufferer, we find a 'splitting' far more profound than can be captured by the notion of a dissociation of functions. The concept of 'splitting' we're instead here after is one which acknowledges a splitting within the very constitution of functions themselves.

The schizophrenic subject disintegrates, falls apart, is a 'divided self' for whom 'the centre cannot hold'. What we find in prototypically schizophrenic experiences is a dissociation of the diverse criteria which, when conjointly met, underpin our ascription to the subject of particular and determinate thoughts and experiences. It's not only the schizophrenic subject who is split thus. Derivatively, empathic observers are too when they try to predicate humanly intelligible thought or experience of their interlocutor.

We want to say one thing but also the opposite. 'It's as if he really thinks what he's saying is true, or yet again as if he's rather exercising imagination, or somehow both at the same time.' 'It's somehow as if he's expressing a thought but also ascribing a thought to someone else at the same time.' 'It's as if he's truly to be thought of as speaking – since nobody else is, but then again, given that he sincerely disavows agency, we also aren't really meeting him in the words coming from his mouth.' We're naturally drawn to approach him as we approach people every day, by making positive sense of what he's saying and doing – but now the jigsaw pieces of our concepts no longer fit together. Still reluctant to relinquish the comforting ambition of positive sense-making, we invent new mental functions and senses which allegedly mediate the relation between ourselves and our very own thoughts and experiences: 'He has somehow become alienated from his own thoughts, thoughts which no longer have that feeling of familiarity which normally marks them as one's own.'

It should be noted that what makes such illusions of sense problematic is not the above-offered descriptions themselves. Understood apophatically they can be acknowledged as illusory at the very same time that they're offered or apprehended. The fact that the sense of these careful articulations of psychotic experience breaks down, the fact that their paradoxes cannot be ironed out, itself registers the depth of psychotic breakdown. An expressive, as opposed to explanatory, phenomenological psychopathology can acknowledge this. But if instead we indulge such illusions of sense as are conjured up by our own words without acknowledging their illusory character, too confident in our own positive contribution to understanding psychotic experience, we stave off the experience of disintegration that attends meeting the other in his truly terrible disintegration. And in this way we turn our face against him and his real need: the need to be tolerated, borne with, and accepted in his brokenness.

6

Self and Other

Introduction

Sufferers of schizophrenic psychosis have long been said to show 'disturbances of the ego boundary'. Along with 'disturbances to self-consciousness' (Chapter 5), references to disturbed boundaries offer the principal psychological understandings we have of such self-disturbances (*Ich-Störungen*) as are at least somewhat pathognomonic of the schizophrenias.

Talk of disturbed self-consciousness, and talk of becoming inadequately demarcated from others, may appear to reference different pathologies. But often enough the principal difference lies in the form of our representation and the theoretical allegiances we enjoy – phenomenological (disturbances of self-consciousness) or psychoanalytical (disturbances to ego boundaries). I somehow experience the thoughts in my mind as belonging to you: we may chalk this up either to a disturbance of 'self-consciousness' such that my own thought now appears alien, or to my 'ego boundary' being drawn too near, so that some of what are actually my own thoughts now appear to lie outwith it. Even so, to suffer a damaged ego boundary has been proffered – principally by psychoanalytically-minded but also by otherwise-inclined psychiatrists[1] – as 'the basic disturbance in schizophrenia', and the patient's 'confusion regarding his own identity' held up as its most direct manifestation.[2] But what is this 'ego boundary', and what is meant by its disturbance?

As we saw in the previous chapter, confusional phenomena invite confused theorizations; and as can be seen from the literature discussed below, this remains the case when they're theorized in terms of ego boundary disturbance. Yet it's not only confusional phenomena, but also the very idioms with which we characterize psychotic experience, that invite confused theorizing – unless, that is, we stay alert to their idiomatic character. Thus it's not clear that idioms designating an intrapsychic disturbance (Chapter 5) are always more than rhetorically differentiated from idioms designating interpersonal breakdowns (this chapter). But consider too what earlier in the book was described as losing contact with reality (Chapter 3), and what it means to instead live in a delusional world of one's own (Chapter 4). If we rested content with considering the superficial form of such locutions, we might struggle to understand how someone utterly in his own world could yet be suffering that indistinction from the world characteristic of ego boundary loss. Yet when we recall that to be 'in one's own world' (or for 'reality testing' to fail) is for the form of one's thought to no longer instantiate the distinction between the imagined and the truly judged, the appearance of contradiction between 'being in one's own world' (schizophrenic autism) and 'becoming fused with the world around one' (schizophrenic ego boundary loss) ought to evaporate. Furthermore, being clearly distinguished from reality and yet enjoying reality contact are so far from contradicting one another that they're better considered conditions of each other's possibility.

Victor Tausk, who seems to have invented the term 'ego boundary', originally gave us the symptom of thought broadcast as its paradigm disturbance:

> This symptom is the complaint that 'everyone' knows the patient's thoughts, that his thoughts are not enclosed in his own head, but are spread throughout the world and occur simultaneously in the heads of other people. The patient seems no longer to realise that he is a separate psychical entity, an ego with individual boundaries. A sixteen-year-old patient in the Wagner-Jauregg Clinic indulged in gay laughter whenever she was asked for her thoughts. Catamnesis revealed that for a long time while being questioned she had believed I had been jesting; she knew that I must be familiar with her thoughts, since they occurred at the same time in my own head.[3]

Over time, however, the term's meaning has spread out to designate a larger range of identity confusions of the sort found especially in the schizophrenias. In fact, before Tausk wrote specifically of *ego* boundaries, Bleuler was already writing of how the schizophrenic subject 'loses his boundaries in time and space' such that they 'identify themselves with some other person, even with inanimate objects, with a chair, with Switzerland':[4]

> A patient often claimed that she had holes in her hands and was half-blind; now she maintains the attendant also has holes in her hands and is half-blind. Many patients believe that their relatives are mentally ill; or, even, more frequently, they believe them at last to have been committed to the mental institution; or these relatives are receiving electro-therapy like themselves. A patient strikes himself twenty times, thinking that he is striking his enemies. Another patient screams, but thinks that it is his neighbour who is screaming. A third one speaks in a confused way but accuses the doctor of being unable to express himself clearly; her eye glasses do not fit, so she says to him: 'What awfully silly glasses you are wearing!' . . . A patient hits the attendant on the head and screams, 'Oh, my poor little head!' Another seeing the attendant, calls out, 'There goes the maid with the lantern. I am the maid with the lantern.' . . . A patient's neighbour died; the patient thinks that he himself has died and covers his face with the sheet. . . . Things seen may likewise be appersonated: the chief attendant holds a black-bordered letter in his hands, hence the patient's hands become completely black.[5]

We already met Laing's tragic patient Julie – the 'ghost in the weed garden' – in Chapter 4. Here, to supplement Bleuler's offering, is an extract from Laing's description of Julie's ego boundary loss:

Together with the tendency to perceive aspects of her own being as not-her, was the failure to discriminate between what 'objectively' was not-her and what was her. . . . She might for instance feel that rain on her cheek was her tears. . . . William Blake in his description of split states of being in his Prophetic Books describes a tendency to *become what one perceives*. In Julie all perception seemed to threaten confusion with the object. She spent much of her time exercising herself with this difficulty. 'That's the rain. I could be the rain.' 'That chair . . . that wall. I could be that wall. It's a terrible thing for a girl to be a wall.'⁶

Before turning to consider what's meant by this 'ego boundary', let's first clarify some of the terminology for confusional experience. Thus, first, when speaking of 'confusion', or of the 'suffering' of ego boundary disturbance, we may have in mind either a subject's own self-acknowledged confusion regarding, and distress about, his identity, or the unacknowledged confusion he suffers such as is characteristic of delusional states. The more a patient is delusionally sunk into his confusional experience, the less he experiences himself as confused; that designation is then instead left for us to apply to him. At times, we may imagine, Julie delusionally mistakes herself for the chair; at other times, as in the extract Laing offers, she is reflectively puzzling this over. It's worth noting, however, that profound confusions such as these are not easily pacified by delusion-formation; they manifest no mere muddle-headedness, instead often evincing terror. A chronic patient declared: 'I have lived with these other people (patients) for so long and we have eaten and drunk together. Now they are all part of me and I am part of them. I'm frightened – I only want to be myself.'⁷ A 27-year-old schizophrenic woman sought a consultation because of:

her fear that her husband 'might have to commit suicide' should she desert him, as she was planning to do. . . . In the course of my talk with her, the girl – a pathetic, beautiful Ophelia clad only in a torn nightgown – pulled me down to the couch where she had seated herself. 'Let us be close,' she said. 'I have made a great philosophical discovery. Do you know the difference between closeness, likeness, sameness, and oneness? Close is close, as with you; when you are like somebody, you are only *like* the other; sameness – you are the same as the other, but he is still *he* and you are *you*; but oneness is not two – it is one, that's horrible – horrible,' she repeated, jumping up in sudden panic: 'don't get too close, get away from the couch, I don't want to become one with you,' and she pushed me away very aggressively.⁸

Second, what also marks such confusion as psychotic is its occurring in what psychiatry calls 'clear consciousness'. (Contrast Baldy from Chapter 5: Baldy fell out of a wagonette, bumped his head, asked if someone fell out and, when told that Baldy fell out, said 'Poor Baldy!' Baldy's confusion isn't to be taken as psychotic because it occurred not in 'clear' but in 'clouded' consciousness – i.e. when he was concussed.⁹)

Finally, a little nomenclature will be helpful for articulating the different forms of ego boundary confusion. Thus *transitivism* will, in what follows, be restricted to designating the experiencing of aspects of one's psychological or bodily self as belonging to others. By contrast, *appersonation* will be the term used to describe the thought and experience of the patient who in some sense assimilates the characteristics of others to herself.[10] (Confusingly, these may occur together, as when a patient thinks whatever he does (e.g. scratching himself) is done to him by another who he also feels to be himself.) Self-object fusion or indistinction, the sheer loss of ego boundaries, will be styled *dedifferentiation*; this may take predominantly transitivistic, appersonative, or indeterminate forms.[11]

Projection and introjection

As reported above, the concept of the 'ego boundary' is, whilst not exclusive to psychoanalytic psychology, rather more prominent within it than within general psychiatry. Psychoanalysis has also provided its own explanation of ego boundary disturbance. It behoves us then to first consider whether this explanation sheds light on what it means to suffer such pathology.

The explanation offered by psychoanalytic psychology offers us *splitting, projection,* and *introjection* (and their conceptual cousins *projective* and *introjective identification*) as ways to make sense of the coming about of a variety of healthy and pathological states of mind, experiences, capacities, and incapacities.[12] Appersonation is taken to result from introjective identification: the incorporation of elements of the other within one's own self-understanding and self-experience. Transitivism is taken to result from projective identification: the splitting off from aspects of the self and their projection into the other as one experiences him. Deployments of these mechanisms with psychotic results are often distinguished from neurotic uses through the adjective 'massive' (i.e. 'massive projective identification'). The term looks quantitative but, I suggest, instead indexes that we're here talking about an enduring projection of one's essential rather than accidental properties.[13] It has been suggested that dedifferentiation results from a regressive desire to secure for oneself, by (as it were) becoming, that on which one both depended yet also experienced as painfully unavailable. (In psychoanalytic terminology, we find here an 'omnipotent' identification with the 'good breast'.) This is a defence which is backfiring to the extent that it also prompts catastrophic fears or actual experience of loss of the self.[14]

A first question to ask is: what makes such a theory more than a congeries of pleonastic neologisms? Is 'introjective identification', say, not in truth just another term for 'appersonation'? The answer lies in psychoanalytic theory's invocation of motivation: projection, introjection, splitting of the self, and identification with the other, are here conceived as essentially deployed to a defensive (hence motivated) end. In this way the theory not only redescribes the appersonative, transitivistic, or dedifferentiated fate, but also articulates the alleged activity and ends, of the psychotic subject. The defensive end of splitting off from certain of one's attributes and then projecting them into another may, for example, be to rid the experience of the self of intolerable qualities. Bleuler's above-mentioned patient speaks in a confused way – *so* she accuses him of being unable to express himself; her glasses don't fit – *so* she tells him he was wearing silly glasses. To read these as expressive of projection is to understand them as motivated by a wish to avoid intolerable shame, this motivation being registered by the 'so's in the preceding sentence.

Another of Bleuler's above-referenced patients 'hits the attendant on the head and screams, "Oh, my poor little head!"' Here perhaps we find an aggressive, envious attack combined with a projective, blaming defence against guilt. It has the superficial form of ordinary projection: you and I have an argument but, unable or unwilling to own my part in its arising, I blame you for it. And yet the projection is 'massive', inviting description as involving a real confusion of identity. A clearer example of such projective identification is manifest in the following:

> We're near the end of the evening of an open mic night, and Karl, a young schizophrenic man, now has his slot. He brings his guitar on stage and sings what is in effect a bizarre parody of the last two performances, a parody that appears to simultaneously evince both envy and scorn. The audience finds this deeply uncomfortable and disturbing, and so offers only the requisite minimal polite applause. Karl is, it seems, dissatisfied with this; at any rate he refuses to leave the stage. Eventually the next act, a talented singer-songwriter duo, is forced to start up with him still standing there. At their act's end the audience applauds and Karl now takes a bow along with the performers, leaving the stage with them.[15]

Here Karl radically conflates himself with those whose performance comes after his own. The identification not only undoes what otherwise would be the too-painful contrast between his own poor offering and that of others, but also allows him to take for himself the praise offered them.

Psychoanalytic theory is sometimes talked of, by both pundits and critics, as if it offered merely an abstract set of posits which 'explain' the behaviour in question by 'telling a story' about it – one that can be hard, or perhaps impossible, to assess for truth – in which case, critics suspect, we have nothing more than a 'just so story'.[16] But whether or not this is, in any particular instance, the case depends on whether we can justify the claim on the table. True, one has no right to go about simply saying that, say, Bleuler's patient was projecting her shame. But if, when she recovers her sanity, she owns shame about her confusion and ill-fitting glasses; if she generally becomes transitivistic only when the properties in question are galling to her; if the transitivism clears up when the glasses are fixed or when therapeutic work helps soften her self-critical attitude (which in turn reduces her projection of self-criticism into Bleuler) – then we have good grounds for the motivational claim. What wouldn't here count as valid critique would be a request for further evidence that, in all the situations just envisaged, the transitivism is truly caused by a mechanism of projective displacement. That request is invalid because to project simply is, in those circumstances, to react in the way envisaged.

This clarifies what the particular circumstances are in which we should want to say that transitivism is a function of projection, or appersonation a function of introjection. But what if it be asked whether projection explains transitivism in general? Must Julie's confusion of herself with the rain, or Bleuler's patient's experience of himself having black hands after seeing the attendant holding a black-bordered letter, really be considered a result of defensively motivated introjection? This is surely unlikely. As (say) with eating, which may be done for reasons other than hunger (greed, habit, politeness, self-soothing, etc.) without this impugning the claim that it often truly is inspired by hunger, we needn't expect psychological understanding to have, nor impugn it for not having, a law-citing structure. And so sometimes we may find a particular transitivistic experience to be not itself the end of projection but instead one of its effects – as when massive projective identification unwittingly hoovers up innocuous properties of the self in its efforts to project those which are unwanted. And sometimes, it's surely at least imaginable, it may arise for no motivationally explicable reason at all – as a manifestation not of a self-stabilizing strategy of an overwhelmed mind but, instead, of mere confusional breakdown.

A more perspicuous objection to the psychoanalytic theory points out that it doesn't by itself show how massive projection is possible. Talk of 'defence mechanisms' and 'intrapsychic processes' may for a while distract us from this unmet need – since we do after all enjoy an understanding of how references to mechanisms and processes do their explanatory work in straightforwardly mechanical and material contexts. In truth, however, the psychoanalyst's talk of defence mechanisms doesn't so much reference separately identifiable pieces of psychological machinery underlying the alterations in psychological state which they explain, as provide a way of bringing these alterations under motivation-citing descriptions.[17] And regardless of the emotional gain which a psychoanalytic psychology shows projective transitivism to achieve, what this doesn't yet tell us is how such transitivism is possible – or, to put it differently, what it is for someone to so much as: mistake himself for his own mirror image, confuse the death of a neighbour for the death of herself, or not know whether one is sitting in an armchair watching and listening to the TV or whether it's the voice in the TV which is one's own. Talk of someone 'using massive projective identification' keeps us attuned to the relevant phenomena under a potentially relevant description, but by itself sheds no light on the distinctive form of confusion here encountered. The same may in fact be said of talk of 'ego boundaries': psychoanalytic psychology freely deploys the term but typically fails to elucidate its meaning.

The ego boundary: Cataphatic attempts

So what is this 'ego boundary', and how does reference to its abrogation or faulty registration help make sense of transitivism, appersonation, and dedifferentiation? Freud provides an early, oft-cited contribution:

> Pathology has made us acquainted with a great number of states in which the boundary lines between the ego and external world become uncertain or in which they are actually drawn incorrectly. There are cases in which parts of a person's own body, even portions of his own mental life – his perceptions, thoughts and feelings –, appear alien to him and as not belonging to his ego; there are other cases in which he ascribes to the external world things that clearly originate in his own ego and that ought to be acknowledged by it.[18]

Unfortunately, however, he provides no further clarification, nor more detailed examples, of the notions of uncertain or incorrectly drawn ego boundaries, of what it is for something to appear to not belong to one's ego, and of what it is for something to originate in a particular ego. Looking for clarity, then, we naturally turn to the principal architect of a revised 'ego boundary' concept – Paul Federn – who tells us that:

> Whenever an impression impinges, be it somatic or psychic, it strikes a boundary of the ego normally invested with ego feeling. *If no ego feeling sets in at this boundary, we sense the impression in question as alien.*[19]

Federn consistently writes about this boundary as if reference to it will aid in the explanation of the disturbances which concern us in this chapter. Other authors repeat his principal claims and take forward his explanatory ambition:

> The ego cathexis [i.e. charge of psychical energy] invests the periphery of the ego, the ego boundaries. . . . The ego boundary takes on the function of a sensory organ in order to become aware of everything that goes on outside the ego. What is sensed as thought is a process occurring within the mental and physical ego boundary, what is sensed as real lies outside the body. . . . The . . . deterioration of the ego boundary results in a failure to differentiate the self from the outside world . . .
>
> It is this . . . ability to differentiate the self from the environment, that we regard as being damaged in chronic schizophrenia. . . . We believe that, once this basic disturbance is appreciated, all other schizophrenic manifestations can be viewed as necessary elaborations of it.[20]

Such talk has the form of a psychological or psychophysical explanation, one which aims at making sense of that kind of 'failure to differentiate the self from the outside world' which concerns us here. The suggestion is that dedifferentiation experiences and beliefs obtain *because*, or *as a result*, of the deterioration of ego boundaries. That which normally marks for someone the boundary between self and other has deteriorated *and so* he can no longer readily distinguish himself from the other. Other authors influenced by Federn write in a similar manner: 'A . . . clear differentiation of the self from the rest of the world . . . *is largely predicated upon* good "ego boundaries."'[21] This all gives us hope of arriving at an explanation with the form: 'Julie takes the rain on her cheek to be her own tears *because* she's suffered deterioration of her ego boundaries.' But how shall we understand this 'because'?

One use of 'because' is to signal which of several possibilities is met with on a given occasion. Consider Anne who is sitting in the rain, deeply distressed and preoccupied by news of her aunt's death. Standing up and pulling out her handkerchief to dry her face, she mistakes the moisture on her cheeks for tears – when, truth be told, her tears had long since been washed away by the rain. Anne's confusion is not due to psychopathology; she suffers no disturbance of ego boundaries. Now consider instead Julie who, when utterly lost to her delusional experience, suffered a true transitivistic catastrophe, now taking the rain for her tears even when she has no reason to think that she's been crying other than, say, experiencing a general feeling of sadness. If someone, not knowing of Julie's schizophrenia, and hearing of her symptom only under the description 'mistaking the rain for her tears', asks us 'why does she do that?', we may helpfully reply that 'it's because she's suffered a disturbance of ego boundaries'. We thereby rule out possibilities such as Julie here being confused in the way Anne is confused. The question which concerns us here, however, is whether someone who already knows full well that Julie's experiences are appersonative is learning anything new when, on asking 'but why does she delusionally perceive the rain on her cheeks as her own tears?', he is told 'it's because she's suffered a deterioration of the ego boundary'. Is reference to ego boundaries explanatory of transitivistic and appersonative phenomena which have already been apprehended as such?

One reason why someone might take reference to ego boundaries to explain dedifferentiation phenomena is because they've been misled by talk of 'boundaries', taking it too literally. Imagine that the fence marking the boundary between your own and your neighbour's property had fallen down. It now becomes rationally intelligible – 'empathically understandable' in Jaspers' idiom – why you mistake some of his garden for your own. We have a clear and distinct idea (from the property deeds) of where the boundary lies, a clear and distinct idea of what the visible marker of it is (the fence), and a clear and distinct idea of what it is for someone to make an error about what belongs to whom. Or imagine, alternatively, the case of the cell membrane.[22] Here – by contrast with the fence – the position of the physical membrane itself determines the boundary's location. We can clearly imagine it taking an unexpected shape; we can clearly imagine it rupturing; and we can clearly imagine a microscope-wielding scientist making an intelligible mistake about whether a particular organelle belongs within that cell or within another.

If ego boundaries were akin to property or cell boundaries, then we could readily understand how appealing to disturbances in them, or in our perception of them (if that be a different matter), could explain Julie's delusional experience. And yet we find nothing in our experience corresponding to the perception of a boundary of this kind. Or, at least, nothing aside from our skin.[23] Yet whilst the boundary provided by the skin might be said to help individuate us in our physical being, we don't determine whether attitudes, characters, identities, thoughts, and feelings – properties which, along with body parts, are mislocated in ego boundary disturbances – belong to ourselves or to another on the basis of whether we perceive them within or without it. It's unclear, then, that reference to the ego boundary has any power to make further sense of such disturbances as are already understood as forms of delusional dedifferentiation. It seems more likely, that is, that the term 'ego boundary disturbance' simply collocates, rather than explicates, the phenomena of transitivism and appersonation – and that the psychoanalytic psychiatrists' explanatory ambitions have here got the better of their phenomenological sobriety.

At this point we do well to note that Federn himself often warns us against reifying the ego boundary into a literal membrane:

A highly esteemed discussant of this theory refused to accept the idea that the ego has a distinct boundary because he felt that this term would indicate a strict linear, ribbonlike, or ditchlike circumference of a territory. It seems to me that this discussant is not quite free of a static conception of the mental processes.... The use of the words 'boundary' or 'periphery' is necessary to express the fact that the ego is actually felt to extend as far as the feeling of the unity of the ego contents reaches. This feeling sharply distinguishes everything that belongs to the ego in an actual moment of life from all the other mental elements and complexes not actually included in the ego. Because the feeling of a unit exists, there is also a boundary or a limit of the unit. This is mere phenomenological fact finding.[24]

Yet here and elsewhere, despite his welcome denial that ego boundaries have a quasi-physical character,[25] Federn's arguments in fact lead us into further confusion. For the more important issue which underlies the complaint of those who protest that no ribbon or ditch circumscribes the ego, is not whether ego boundaries have a process-like as opposed to a state-like character, but whether the 'boundary deterioration' concept is able to play an explanatory role *vis-à-vis* such phenomena as are already understood as instances of transitivism or appersonation. If we're unwittingly held captive by the picture of a literal boundary, we might take ourselves to be dealing with a phenomenon which could enter into explanations in the way in which reference to a section of missing fence can enter into explanations of why you mistook your neighbour's plants for your own. But if the ego boundary's solidity and location is not a separate matter from the subject's degree of sanity-constituting self-possession or proneness to suffer sanity-abrogating dedifferentiation experiences, it can't sensibly be considered explanatory of such phenomena as are already apprehended under such descriptions as 'transitivism' or 'appersonation'. No more do we explain why Ronnie is a never-married man by adverting to his bachelor status. The story's moral, then, is that we must not only cancel the misleading impression of a literal ditch-like or ribbon-like boundary, but also remember to simultaneously void the expectation of explanatory prowess that the appeal to such boundaries produces.

Federn's own positive suggestion is that talk of the 'ego boundary' is nothing but a way of talking about the extent of the 'ego feeling' or of the 'feeling of the unity of the ego'. He doesn't tell us what this means, and our concern must surely be that it amounts to little more than that spurious 'sense of mineness' – critique of which was offered in Chapter 5 – allegedly accompanying everything physical, behavioural, and mental which belongs to the ego. The curiously schizoid picture suggesting itself to us here is, to recall, one of parts of ourselves as so many 'free-standing' particulars – thoughts, feelings, sensations, bodies, body parts, actions, perceptions, etc. – which we inwardly apprehend and then, based on the presence or absence of the ego 'feeling', know either for our own or to belong to another.[26] Yet whilst Federn describes the positing of this 'ego feeling' or 'feeling of a unit' as 'mere phenomenological fact finding', it's not at all clear on phenomenological grounds that we do normally enjoy any such feeling. Rather than saying that we normally enjoy a feeling of being all of a piece, it would be far more accurate to say simply that normally we don't suffer feelings of not being so. Why, then, does the theorist still propose the feeling? One possibility is that they've already committed to making dedifferentiation experiences rationally intelligible as forms of error. Another is that they've been misled by the psychopathologists' descriptions of dedifferentiation experiences as involving 'pathological *error*'.[27] (Describing the pathology as involving 'error' runs the risk of encouraging the unhelpful thought that the non-pathological state involves getting something 'right'. And from there we may imagine further that there must be some *means* – such as noting the presence of a feeling – by which we normally achieve this right result. This, however, all rather ignores the clinical use of the term 'pathological error', which is typically to designate something like an unwitting and enduring breakdown in intelligibility occurring in the midst of an otherwise intelligible mental life.)

On the ego

A question we've not yet considered is what it is for something to be of the ego. Neither Freud nor Federn tell us what their talk of the 'ego' (*das 'Ich'*) means; they instead assume we already know this and move straight on to describe its 'functions'. Yet whilst Freud's use of the term has it referring to a part of the 'psychic apparatus' (in his tripartite structural model he talks of the ego alongside the superego and id), Federn's use of it is more in line with our more ordinary talk of 'selfhood'.[28]

The clarificatory prescription I offer here is that what it is for something to belong to the 'I' or 'ego' is for it to be something (sensation, emotion, thought, position, utterance, or movement) that may be 'immediately' or 'directly' avowed or known. Such sensations, emotions, and movements 'belong to my ego' as I may self-ascribe without relying on observation.[29] My knowledge of the sensations of others is mediated by observation of their behaviour, but I need deploy no such observation when I 'immediately' (non-mediatedly) ascribe them to myself.[30]

This proposal brings the ego in its bodily aspect in direct line with an aspect of what phenomenologists describe as the 'lived body':[31] the body which I may immediately move, the positions of which I immediately know, sensations in which I can feel, and the orientation of which affects which environmental features perceptually show up for me. These four features occasionally dissociate, but their interlocking manifests in the guidance of movement by proprioception, and in the effects of movement on sensation and perception. (If we wished to interpretatively rescue the concept of 'ego feelings', we might say that the 'ego boundary' is 'felt' whenever one presses on something in which one does not experience pressure sensations (contrast pressing one hand on the other with pressing one's hand against the wall), or when movement of a sense organ (including movement of the body or body part to which it's attached) enables the perceptual determination of what does and what doesn't lie outwith the self.) Notable too is that it's a fact determinative of our concept of a 'person' that lived bodies don't overlap between individuals: the body which I can control, in which I can feel sensations, from whose vantage I perceive, and whose positions and movements I immediately know, is not the same as yours.

The above description of what makes it apt to talk of something 'belonging to the ego' provides us with a means to understand what ego boundary disorders amount to. On this understanding we shan't be said to suffer boundary disturbance if one of our limbs becomes truly insubordinate to our will, or insensate, or void of proprioception.

Instead, that appellation shall be reserved for cases in which we take ourselves to be able to feel sensations, directly move, or immediately judge movement and orientation where we cannot possibly.[32] (By extension we may also wish to refer to ego boundary disorders when someone takes another person to be able to immediately move and enjoy proprioceptive knowledge of his body, or to avow what in truth are thoughts and feelings which, being his own, can only be avowed by himself.) The ego boundary is not, then, to be understood as corresponding to something experienced, such as a sensation or something perceived. Like, say, the edge of the visual field, the ego boundary neither shows up within experience (as something perceived) nor constitutes a type of experience (like a sensation). Reference to it provides but a formal characterization of the categorical division of what one can immediately avow from what one cannot.

Consider Bryan who's standing by the window, looking out at the setting sun, performing Tai-Chi-style movements, talking with his psychologist. Bryan spontaneously reports that with these movements he's 'setting the sun'.[33] He doesn't so much take his actions as somehow eventually effecting a distal causal impact on the sun as instead experience them as coextensive with that sun's setting. His belief about what he's doing ('setting the sun') is immediate in the way that our knowledge of what movements we're currently making is immediate. It's in virtue of the collapse for Bryan of the differentiation of himself from the sun, such that his own movements themselves become for him the inner impetus of the sun's setting, that we say he's suffering an ego boundary disturbance. Or consider Karl – we already met him above – who remains silently standing on the stage whilst others play and sing alongside him. His ego boundary disturbance consists in his not differentiating these others' actions (playing and singing) and perceptions (of the praise they receive) from his own. Or consider again Laing's patient Julie who sometimes experiences herself as the wall or chair, and at other times shows a more conscious confusion about this experience. Her saying, just by itself, 'I am the chair' will not by itself count as an ego boundary disturbance. Instead, it's when this goes along with various expectations – e.g. of feeling sensations in the chair or wall when they're touched – that it becomes natural to describe it as a boundary disturbance.

Now that we have a determinate conception of the ego and its differentiation we may ask what explanatory power – *vis-à-vis* the kinds of pathologies described above – is enjoyed by references to it. What I propose is that its positive explanatory power is exhausted by its alerting us to certain further claims that the sufferer of ego boundary disturbance shall be inclined to make. Julie tells us that she and the chair are one. If this manifests an ego boundary disturbance, rather than a passing moment of delirium, then we should expect her to answer 'yes' to at least one of our inquiries into whether, say, she expects to feel sensations in it, or expects to know without observation where it is or that it has moved. The use of a psychopathological concept to generate such further expectations of the behaviour of the person described by means of it provides an important sense in which it can be said to illuminate, explain, or generate understanding of that person's experience.[34] Aside from this, the only further rational expectation aroused by talk of someone's utterance manifesting an 'ego boundary disturbance' is of her suffering other related disturbances. Thus Julie sometimes conflates herself with the chair or wall, yet she also sometimes takes the rain on her cheeks to be her own tears.

None of this, however, is to say that reference to the concept of 'ego boundary disturbance' helps make that behaviour which evinces it empathically intelligible in Jaspers' sense. That is, whilst we can understand that someone who thinks herself the wall may also expect to feel sensations in it, we have no good idea of what it means to truly expect that. We can understand why someone who somehow thinks $5 + 3 = 10$ may also think $5 + 4 = 11$, but we don't on that basis understand how anyone knowing these terms' meanings could really take the sum of $5 + 3$ to be 10. And if *per impossibile* we did understand this, or understand why Julie thinks herself the wall, then the beliefs in question should not properly be treated as delusional.

Perhaps we might try to understand boundary disturbances by analogy with our experience of illusory phenomena such as the 'rubber hand illusion'.[35] (To create the rubber hand illusion: rest both arms on the table in front of you. Occlude your right arm, place a visible rubber arm next to it, and have someone repeatedly brush both arms at the same time and place. After a while it's likely that you'll find yourself wanting to say that you feel the tickle from the brush in the rubber hand which you can see being brushed. Here, we might say, our brain's impetus to integrate tactile and visual stimulation results in its incorporation of the rubber arm in the body schema, despite our knowledge that the arm is rubber and not attached to our person.) The analogy is surely plausible. Yet whilst we find ourselves wanting to say that we 'somehow' feel tickle sensations in the rubber hand, what makes the scenario illusory rather than delusional is our simultaneous acknowledgement that what we're inclined to avow is impossible. We register this by the use of statements like 'I *can't help but imagine* that I'm now feeling sensations in that rubber hand' or 'I'm now *impossibly* feeling sensations in the rubber hand'. The delusional subject, however, 'believes the impossible' - an achievement not helpfully unpacked by saying that she somehow manages to genuinely believe what the rest of us can only imagine, but instead by noting that her thought is not helpfully characterized as an instance of belief *as opposed to* imagination.[36]

The upshot of all of this is that to talk of 'ego boundary disturbance' is to say no more than that someone suffers a delusional form of dedifferentiation. Bleuler's above-cited inpatient cried out 'There goes the maid with the lantern. I am the maid with the lantern.' To chalk this up to a loss of ego boundaries is to imply that the patient: is delusional, is not joking or simply delirious, may well also delusionally take herself to be responsible for performing the maid's duties, etc. In this way it doesn't do more than describe her as suffering appersonation; it doesn't provide any kind of explanation which helps us understand, by the provision of a reason, why she takes herself to be the maid with the lantern. It doesn't help us find a way to make that belief humanly intelligible; instead, it leaves us with the fact of someone 'believing the impossible'. It's true that by bringing the loss of ego boundaries under a further motivational scheme – i.e. by describing, when it's appropriate to do so, the delusional experience as rooted in, say, the patient's wish to enjoy the relatively greater prestige of the nurse – we do something to make it psychologically intelligible. Yet even here we're providing not her reasons but her motivations. We understand that a nurse may well enjoy more occupational pride and status than a chronic schizophrenic, and can therefore understand why Bleuler's patient might wish that she was the former rather than the latter. In this way we understand why she's unconsciously motivated to develop the delusion that she is indeed the maid. But what we don't thereby make into an intelligible thought is her belief that she (who is watching the maid with the lantern walk past) is in fact herself that very maid.

Conclusions

Reference to disturbed ego boundaries looks as if it offers an explanation as to why someone suffers transitivistic or appersonative experiences and beliefs. Yet in truth it merely redescribes these phenomena. Articulating these phenomena in terms of projective or introjective identification is, however, less tautologous: here – so long as the situation warrants it – we add to our understanding by bringing the patient's thought under a motivation-referencing description, thereby providing a psychological understanding of it. Such an understanding is not, however, the same as a rational or (in Jaspers' terms) 'empathic' understanding: seeing why someone's emotionally motivated to form a delusion is not the same as understanding why it makes rational sense for him to think that thought.

The suggestion of this chapter has been that the appeal to ego boundaries often seems explanatory simply because of the way it invokes a picture of a visible boundary to the ego which may become less visible and hence lead to intelligible error. When, however, we remind ourselves of the merely metaphoric character of such boundaries we also need to cancel our expectations of being provided with a sense-making form of explanation. Federn's suggestion that the ego boundary is but the outer limit of the 'ego feeling' also appears to offer a sense-making explanation (Julie mistakes herself for the wall because she's misled by an ego feeling that has spread out to include it). This loss of 'ego feeling', however, appears to be but a mythical posit; and, as with the 'ego boundary' disturbance itself, reference to it collapses straight back into a non-explanatory redescription of the psychopathological phenomena.

At this point one may be left thinking the results of our investigation to have been purely negative – that whilst we may have better understood the ego boundary theory, what we haven't better understood is the patient and her experience. This, I suggest, would be a mistake. For what we've come to see, when reflecting on the failure of psychopathologists' best efforts to empathically comprehend the thought of the dedifferentiated subject, is something about the depth of the disturbance itself. It is, I suggest, precisely in acknowledging the impotence of such sense-making schemes that we're most forcefully brought face to face with the dementing loss of selfhood suffered by the patient. When this loss is non-motivated we encounter her directly in her brokenness. Our best theoretical efforts can't force her mind back into the kind of shape which makes comfortable sense to us. And when it is dynamically motivated we bear witness not only to that underlying fragility in her which makes possible the use of such radical defences, but also to the depth of mental suffering prompting such a catastrophic 'solution'. Bleuler's patient is so ashamed by such a small matter as her ill-fitting glasses that she is compelled to berate his own. Karl utterly fell apart in the spotlight of the open mic and, wanting to belong but lacking the resource, delusionally merged with the other performers. In these ways we see once again with Schopenhauer how:

> if such a sorrow, such painful knowledge or reflection, is so harrowing that it becomes positively unbearable, and the individual would succumb to it, then nature, alarmed in this way, seizes upon [massive projective or introjective identification] as the last means of saving life. The mind, tormented so greatly, destroys, as it were, [its own identity] and thus seeks refuge in madness from the mental suffering that exceeds its strength . . .[37]

7

Hallucination

Introduction

Ask someone on the street what they take for a quintessential sign of madness and they'll speak to you of hallucination, in particular of auditory verbal hallucination. They'll make mention, that is, of schizophrenic subjects 'hearing voices' which, amongst other things, berate or otherwise comment on them. In this they're on track, yet we also know full well that hallucinations may be experienced by those who, not being deluded about their hallucinations' veridicality, will properly be counted sane. The questions arise, then, not only of what it is to hallucinate, but also of what the connection is between hallucination and insanity, and why hallucinations in the mentally ill have the character and content they often do. This chapter's aim is to see how far we can get with these questions, having first made adequate acquaintance with the real phenomenon, yet whilst refusing to budge from the reflective armchair.

What kinds of hallucination are met with in psychotic mental illnesses? On this topic Eugen Bleuler's writings are amongst the most evocative. Consider this from his treatise on the schizophrenias:

> The patients hear blowing, rustling, humming, rattling, shooting, thundering, music, crying, laughing, whispering, talking.... They feel things, animals, and people, and are struck by rain-drops, fire, sticks. They experience all tortures, as well as every pleasurable sensation which the sense organs can transmit ....
>
> The usual occurrence is that the 'voices' threaten, curse, criticize and console in short sentences or abrupt words; that the persecutor or heavenly figures, certain kinds of animals, fire or water and also some desired or hoped for situation are hallucinated: paradise, hell, a castle, a robber's cave is seen; that ambrosia or some frequently mentioned poison or a vile substance is tasted in food; that a poisonous vapour or a wonderfully glorious perfume surrounds the patient. They feel the passion of love or all kinds of torture that can be effected by physical means on their abused bodies.
>
> ... The 'voices' are the means by which the megalomaniac realizes his wishes, the religiously preoccupied achieves his communion with God and the Angels; the depressed are threatened with every kind of catastrophe; the persecuted cursed night and day.... The voices not only speak to the patient, but they pass electricity through his body, beat him, paralyze him, take his thoughts away ...

. . . While the patient is eating, he hears a voice saying, 'Each mouthful is stolen.'' If he drops something, he hears "If only your foot had been chopped off."[1]

For a more personal take, one revealing something of how hallucinating can be situated in the living of a life, consider the following testimony from Peter Reynolds, a 52-year-old married father of two who works as a mental health advocate:

I hear voices behind me and I also hear them in my ears. . . . When I was psychotic, I believed that I was being talked to by aliens. . . . Now I feel that my voices come from me. They are clouded memories of things that have gone on in my past.

I hear six voices: I have *Socrates*, and he comes along when he fancies. I can't conjure him up but when he comes, he talks of philosophy and psychology and medicine, all sorts of brilliant things. On the bad side, one is my *father*. It is not his voice but it is what he would say. He ridicules me and makes fun of me, just generally taking the piss out of me like my father did. His voice tells me that he never did anything to upset me, which just isn't true. I have the *blasphemer* and he just swears all the time, along with *profanities*, another voice that curses me. There is another one called *dangerous*. He tells me to walk in front of buses and cars all the time . . . He's a bastard. He wants me dead, very much like my father did when I was younger. One of the voices is *the man my mother had an affair with*. He talks to me about my mother sometimes. What he says is crude and horrible. . . .

It didn't start off with voices; it started with noises when I was about 9 years old. I could hear whistling noises coming from behind me. . . . They had always been in the background as noises I could hear – schoolyards in my head, children shouting and screaming. I think the voices were provoked by my mum and dad's relationship. My mother and father were always accusing each other of sleeping with other people; my father hit me once and said, 'I don't know if you are even fucking mine' – so if that isn't stress for a child then I don't know what is. . . . I was trying to deal with puberty as well. A lot was said about sex. Shouting and screaming: 'You took him up your Nan's and fucked him on the settee', and it left me with a sexual problem. I started self-harming; I'd pour surgical spirits and bleach on my genitals; I thought I was diseased; I wouldn't eat or drink in the house because I believed I was being poisoned.

When I was 13, my mum died . . . I had all these unresolved problems, and then I was seduced by my sister-in-law . . .[2]

We shall return to Peter later. But, our exposure to the phenomenon now in place, let's return to our first question: what is it to hallucinate?

Hallucination as percept

Before 1817 'hallucination' was used either to refer to the entertaining of unfounded notions or to signify visual disturbance; Esquirol then finessed the term's scope – 'If a man has the inner conviction of truly experiencing a sensation for which there is no external object, he is in a hallucinated state, he is a visionary' – and ever since we've used the term somewhat in his way.[3]

To many the ('what is it to hallucinate?') question has seemed readily answerable, hallucinations being 'perceptions without objects', 'false perceptions that spring up by themselves', 'percepts experienced in the absence of external stimuli', 'percepts lacking the objective bases which they suggest', and instances of 'seeing, hearing, smelling, tasting or feeling things that don't exist outside their mind'.[4] Some such talk may be thought paradoxical insofar as, in their primary senses, terms like 'perceive', 'see', 'hear', etc. are what we call 'success' verbs. That is, talk of my truly perceiving a cat typically implies both that there's a cat there to be seen and that I succeed in making its visual acquaintance. And yet, in a separate sense of 'perceive', the term does indeed properly extend to cover hallucinatory episodes. In this latter sense, if we want to know whether and what someone sees or hears, we need only ask him – and now whatever he sincerely offers by way of answer, regardless of whether what's referred to also exists 'outside his mind', shall count as telling of perception. To speak with the philosophers we might say that, whilst only real cats afford the possibility of such perception as necessarily meets with 'material' objects, the very same 'intentional' objects (i.e. cats) can obtain both for hallucination and for such perception as would be undone by a lack of success.[5]

So far so anodyne; the use of a single word – 'perception' – to cover both cases presents neither conceptual illumination nor theoretical challenge. And yet difficulties arise early in the theory of hallucination when it's further assumed, as it often is, that perception's intentional objects enjoy a kind of existence akin to that of material objects – except 'in the mind', as it were, rather than in the world about us. In this conception, what gets called 'percepts' are the alleged inner objects of inner analogues of perceptual faculties – percepts being encountered with the 'mind's eye' (or heard with the mind's ear ... or, presumably, smelled with the mind's nose). In effect, this conceptual picture takes what is merely a philosophical grammarian's construction – the 'intentional object' – and turns it into a ghostly copy of its material cousin. Thus, it seems, are born the psychologists' 'percepts', 'phantasms', 'sensory traces', 'ideas of sensation', 'sense data', and 'sensory representations'. Just to complicate matters we have, running unhelpfully close to this misleading picture, such otherwise innocuous idioms from everyday psychopathological discourse as 'hearing voices', 'seeing things', or 'sensing presences' – idioms which obtain their evocative power precisely by paradoxically deploying what are typically success verbs in situations where no actual voices, things, or presences are on the cards. Given such abundant invitations to confusion we oughtn't be surprised when they're sometimes taken up, in relation both to perception and to hallucination. Thus as regards the former, it's urged that 'instead of calling hallucination a false external perception, we must call external perception a true [or 'controlled'] hallucination.'[6] (As if perception's world-disclosing function had now somehow become a merely accidental property of it; as if someone who didn't know what it is to perceive could somehow yet know what it is to hallucinate.) And, as regards the latter, we're offered – by way of alleged conceptual analysis – the notion that hallucinations involve such 'percepts' as obtain in ordinary, veridical, perception except in the absence of their typical outer causes. The result is that 'percept' now slips from representing an ambiguous disjunct of success-apt perception and hallucination to referencing a putative psychologically real common element of both.[7] (As if it were enough, for providing an explanation of what it is to hallucinate, to reference a hypothetical entity or process which obtains in the absence of what's alleged to be its typical cause.)

Another misleading implication of the suggestion that hallucinations are 'percepts' without their typical worldly causes is that the hallucinator experiences his hallucinations rather as the veridical perceiver experiences her perceptions. No doubt this is sometimes the case but it remains empirically true that it often isn't – not only for the sane but also for the psychotically unwell.[8] Both the extraordinary content and the atypical form of the hallucination can mark them apart from ordinary perception. Hypnagogic hallucinations, for example – as of seemingly hearing someone calling your name when you're half-asleep – may be experienced as somehow sounding 'in the head' rather than as environmentally located. And the schizophrenic symptom of 'hearing voices' is not always clearly distinguishable from the experience of having thoughts inserted into one's mind or hearing one's own thoughts spoken aloud, and there need be no fact of the matter as to whether a hallucinated voice is loud or soft, male or female, harsh or gentle.[9] Furthermore, even when a sufferer doesn't distinguish hallucination from veridical perception, this needn't mean that his hallucinations have taken on all the phenomenal properties of ordinary perceptual experiences – for perhaps his actual world-engagements have themselves become dreamy and subjectivized.[10]

Implicit presences, inadvertent actions

Among the more popular conceptions of hallucination are the 'inner image' and 'inadvertent imagining' theories of hallucinatory visions and the 'talking to yourself without realizing it' theory of hallucinated voices. All can be formulated as no more than truistic, in which case they're as unobjectionable as they are empty. Yet all are sometimes formulated as would-be genuine psychological theories which attempt to offer positive explanatory accounts of something called 'what hallucination consists in'. Behind these would-be explanations appears to be a tempting idea that may be put like this: when you hallucinate, 'an externally irreal but internally real stimulus is present to the mind'. In short, intentional objects are now described as if, like perception's material objects, they too are encountered by or presented to the subject, as if they were stimuli or perceptibilia of some sort. What follows argues not only the misguidedness of such a conception, but also that it positively impedes our understanding of what it means to hallucinate. To put it in what, until we elucidate it later, must remain an admittedly elliptical idiom, we might say that it encourages us to think positively about hallucination in terms of presence precisely when we'd often do rather better to instead think negatively about it in terms of absence.

Talk of 'inner images' is par for the course when voicing both hallucination and vivid imagining. After suffering a heart attack, Carl Gustav Jung enjoyed an out-of-body experience in which he surveyed the whole globe: 'From ... the direction of Europe, an image floated up. ... I knew at once: "Aha, this is my doctor, ... coming in his primal form."'[11] To speak here of an image floating before Jung's mind is to say nothing other than that he was having a visual hallucination: it doesn't tell us in what such an hallucination 'consists'. But why talk of 'images' at all here? Well, we know what it is to see physical images – to look, for example, at photos of friends in an album or at portraits on the wall. We can make visual sense of such images because we've hitherto experientially engaged with what they're of – i.e. with people.[12] And we know something of their impoverishment relative to what they represent – i.e. that they only represent certain aspects of depth, that what is perceptible of the represented object doesn't alter when we change our line of sight, that this object can be seen but not heard. We know too that we can be tricked by *trompe l'oeil* images, mistaking them for what they represent. It is, I suggest, such similarities between our perception of ordinary images and our experience of hallucinations which makes talk of 'inner images' natural when describing hallucination. Talk of an image 'floating before' the mind also makes vivid the way in which hallucinations are unlike imaginings in that, like physical images, they typically enjoy an independence from the wills of those who experience them. (We can choose to look away from, or shut our eyes on, a physical image.) Even so, the images that constitute hallucinations are unlike physical images in that they enjoy no existence independent of our experience of them.

To speak of hallucinated images is, then, to do nothing other than speak of visually hallucinating. In particular, such talk references no object of any kind – no experiential object for an inner sense, for example. For the only 'object' to be met with in hallucination is of a logical sort – namely an intentional object, and this object is not the mental image itself but is rather what the image is of. You may, if you insist, say that in hallucination a merely intentional object is 'presented to the mind'. But once we've cancelled the tacit implication that talk of such presentation normally brings with it – the implication of one thing, an object, being brought before another separate thing, a subject – we see what an empty formulation this is. Act and object are here one, and talk of mental images provides nothing but an evocative yet non-illuminating re-description of the fact of visual hallucination.

Perhaps it be suggested that hallucination involves unwitting imagining. If this amounts to the claim that some of the same brain regions are involved in hallucinating as in imagining, then it seems we have but a neurological hypothesis misleadingly dressed up in psychological garb. Or perhaps it's a reminder that, amongst the various different uses of 'imagine' – such as: (i) as a synonym for 'assume' or 'believe' ('I just can't imagine that you love me, After all is said and done') and (ii) as a term for such inner picturing or envisaging as is distinguished from daydreaming by its self-consciousness and commandability ('Imagine all the people, Sharing all the world') – is (iii) as a synonym for 'hallucinate' ('Is that shining in the distance I see, Real or just imagined?'). If so, the suggestion hardly provides insight into the nature of hallucination: we already need to know what it is to hallucinate before we can successfully disambiguate the term 'imagine'.

Or perhaps the real intent of the 'hallucination as unwitting imagining' pundit is to suggest that hallucination is an inadvertent version of (ii): the subject of visual hallucinations, say, is 'unknowingly picturing'. So far, however, that suggestion appears to be but a seemingly paradoxical invitation to consider hallucination a *passive activity*. And yet there *are* contexts where we talk quite properly of unconscious action and activity – so might not hallucination be considered such an activity too? (To borrow from Freud: a doctor puts his umbrella in the corner of the room, hypnotizes a patient, and says to him, 'I'm going out now. When I come in again, you will come to meet me with my umbrella open and hold it over my head.' The hypnotic session ends, the doctor leaves and later returns, the man then doing as asked. When the doctor questions what he's doing, the patient confabulates ('I only thought, doctor, as it's raining outside you'd open your umbrella in the room before you went out').[13] Here, despite the real reason and intention being unconscious, we still talk of action.) Might not hallucination also then be considered an activity of unconscious imagining? And yet it's the difference between the cases that's more telling than the similarity. With the hypnotic action there's the visible behaviour which, in its structure and in its relation to the hypnotic instruction, makes it at least somewhat natural to talk here – despite the lack of self-consciousness – of a form of intention. With typical hallucination, however, we find no such markers of unconscious agency. And when it comes to imagining *qua* inner envisagement, the only criterion for its obtaining is the subject's avowal that this is what she's doing – which avowal is of course precisely what we don't have with hallucination.

Similar difficulties attend the suggestion that the hallucination of voices amounts to 'talking to oneself without realizing it'. The theory has a long history; one recent incarnation suggests that 'If hallucinations are caused by inner speech, then the problem is not that inner speech is occurring, but that patients must be failing to recognise that this activity is self-initiated. The patients misattribute self-generated actions to an external agent. I have called this a defect of "self-monitoring".'[14]

At least here we seem at first to find a use for the notion of a 'passive activity', since it's well-known that voice hearers sometimes do unwittingly make subvocalizations corresponding to the content of their voices.[15] (Whilst the idea of unwitting activity lacks meaning when the only criterion for their being any activity per se is the subject's say-so – which here is, *ex hypothesi*, unforthcoming – at least with subvocalization the activity may be detected by others. We may hear the hallucinator faintly muttering, or quieter mutterings still may be picked up by a microphone near the larynx.) And yet theorists, aware that not all auditory verbal hallucinations are accompanied by subvocalizations, are apt to instead insist that hallucination is unwittingly engaged in purely inner speech – i.e. is fully 'in the head'. Now, however, we are back to the paradoxicality of the 'inadvertent imagining' theory – since the only criterion for someone engaging in such inner speech is their sincere say-so – which say-so is precisely what the hallucinator will not offer.

Or perhaps it be suggested that the inner speech theory be tested by investigating whether people still hear voices when engaging in tasks that normally suppress inner speech (opening the mouth wide, humming, etc.), or if their Broca's area (involved in the production of normal and inner speech) is knocked out by transcranial magnetic stimulation. The results of such experiments are, as it happens, mixed.[16] But regardless of the results, what such experiments presuppose is that the 'inner speech' theory has a content in the first place. One way to save it from emptiness would of course be to cash it out neurologically. But then we no longer have a psychological theory, but instead just the neurological hypothesis – that the material basis of voice hearing involves activity in (say) Broca's area. That is not nothing, but finding it to be true would not be to confirm, but merely to give (an albeit metaphorical) meaning to, the otherwise empty idea that voice hearers are 'talking to themselves without realizing it'.

Projections and anticipations

Hallucinations are commonly described as 'projections'. Four different senses of 'projection' can be distinguished in the literature.

The first is exemplified by Wilhelm Griesinger who understood hallucinations as 'subjective images that are projected externally and acquire an apparent objectivity and reality'.[17] More recently Oliver Sacks wrote: 'To the hallucinator ... hallucinations seem very real; they can mimic perception in every respect, starting with the way they are projected into the external world'.[18] Such uses appear to offer non-elucidatory re-descriptions. To have a 'subjective image' presumably means either to imagine or to hallucinate. How now shall we understand 'projected into the external world'? One, phenomenological, option has us 'projecting' just so long as we lack self-consciousness regarding the image's origination with ourselves; this now collapses the 'projection' view into the 'inadvertent imagining' formulation discussed above. The other, metaphysical, option construes perceptions, imaginings, and hallucinations as 'inner' phenomena, and now – worrying about incompatibility with the phenomenological fact that perception truly, and hallucination seemingly, put us in touch with an 'outer' world - looks for a mechanism to explain the phenomenology (voila: 'projection'). Perhaps this is but a modern expression of the seventeenth-century idea that in perception we're somehow most proximally in contact with 'ideas in the mind' (or 'inner representations') only through which do we gain a merely distal contact with a world about us.[19] If so, then we'd do well to recall the myriad objections against such conceptions.[20] The principal one, perhaps, is that it's hard to grasp how we could have ever so much as come by the idea of an 'external world', or for that matter of other people to talk to about it, if it was never something we actually encountered. It's also worth recalling that using the cinematic 'projection' metaphor to characterize both vision and hallucination risks undermining itself, since we understand what it is to see a projected image only by contrast with what it is to see non-projected phenomena (such as the canvas onto which the image is projected). How, then, could we honestly invoke the former in explanation of the latter? Considering now the use of 'projection' to characterize only hallucination (rather than perception as well), there's perhaps nothing, aside from a taste for perspicuity, that should stop us speaking thus. At the same time, however, we must acknowledge that all we're thereby doing is providing a non-elucidatory re-description of the fact that the intentional objects of hallucination can sometimes be characterized in terms like 'distance from us', 'shape', 'depth', 'over there', etc.

A second sense of 'projection' references the seeming displacement of the perceiver rather than of the experience, especially in 'out of body' (autoscopic) experiences.[21] Here it seems to the hallucinator as if what she takes for her perception of the world is from a vantage (e.g. from the room's ceiling) other than that which her bodily location (e.g. on the bed) could afford. And here such talk of the hallucinator's 'projection into space' again offers nothing more than non-elucidatory re-description.

A third use also involves the projection of a perceiver but now the projection contributes not to the vantage but to the content of the hallucinatory experience. The hypnopompic hallucination, typically with accompanying sleep paralysis, of night-time intruders (space aliens, succubi, etc.) standing at the end of the bed is one such example of the 'projection of one's own body image'.[22] What this use of 'projection' really amounts to has not yet been made clear in the literature, although it gestures towards the hypothesis that the properties of the hallucinated image are a function of the neural dynamics underlying the body schema. In any case, such phenomena are but a small subset of hallucinations, and don't inform the wider discussion, so we may leave them aside.

A final use of the term 'projection' is provided by psychoanalytic psychiatry, and refers to a defence mechanism. Freud and Lacan described hallucination as itself a distinct defence mechanism from projection.[23] Nevertheless, psychoanalysis has often explicated hallucination in terms of projection; for example, a 'patient's auditory hallucinations might be full of vile and cruel comments and instructions. Here there is splitting and then projection of the unacceptable from self to other'.[24] Such talk of hallucination as being 'formed by' projection (or projective identification), and description of projection as a 'mechanism of' defence, may sound like the provision of a causal account of the steps underlying hallucination's genesis. What such dynamic notions instead achieve, though, is the bringing of a symptom under a motivational description. That we should wish to rid ourselves of intolerable thoughts and feelings, and experience them instead in the external world, is readily intelligible. But reference to projection doesn't explain how – by what means – it should happen that an intolerable self-critical thought becomes experienced instead as an external critical voice. Nor does talk of such projection (or projective identification) as results in hallucination explain why, say, a self-critical thought should still, post-projection, appear to relate to oneself, rather than to the irreal speaker. That object-relativity is, after all, what we do sometimes find in neurotic projection: it's not I who am disappointed in myself, but rather you who are disappointed in yourself. Or perhaps it be said that reference to 'massive projective identification' rather than to ordinary 'projection', explains this: it's not just that a current feeling, but that the self's very capacity to feel that feeling, is projected. Yet whilst the terminological distinction is apt, it doesn't so much explain, as instead simply honour, the psychopathological difference.

Let's turn now from attempts to understand hallucination as projection to efforts at understanding it in terms of anticipation. So: you're approaching the escalator, and perfectly well see that it's broken. Mounting it, you imagine, should therefore be just like walking up a normal staircase. But as you take the first step, you stumble forward a little; it seems to you as if the escalator lurched backwards under your feet.

Or, to move from illusion to hallucination proper: you wear a chunky wristwatch yet, unless telling the time with it, barely notice it there on your wrist; in particular, you're no longer aware of the extra weight it adds to your arm or of the pressure the strap exerts upon your wrist. Your body schema incorporates the watch within itself: you habituate to the sensations it causes in your wrist, and you automatically compensate, when making arm movements, for the weight and bulk it adds. But one day the battery runs out, so you take it off. And now – well, what shall we say? – you seem to positively feel its absence; the unusual lightness of your arm and the decompression of your wrist have resulted in an experience there of an 'anti-watch', a 'ghost watch'.

Here now is an example of a hallucination you can readily induce at home. Stare unblinkingly at the dead centre of a negative image of a young woman for thirty seconds (follow the link in the reference for the image[25]). Now look up at the ceiling and blink. There you'll find a ghostly positive afterimage of her appear: black skin and teeth become white; light hair, irises, and lips become dark.

Or consider the following: experimenters have been able to induce auditory hallucinations of tones by first repeatedly pairing the presentation of a chequerboard with a tone and then displaying the chequerboard alone.[26] (Those who frequently 'hear voices' are the most susceptible to this conditioned hallucination, but it affects all of us.)

Common to such hallucinations is the carrying forward in time of a non-conscious sensory readiness. These hallucinations reveal how structured our everyday experience is by such readiness: whether we're listening to a tune, watching a bird fly through the air, or reading a text, new sensory readinesses as to what shall come next are enlivened and quelled in us at every moment, structuring our living experiential comprehension of that which confronts us.[27] Often such readinesses will correlate with what we we'd avow if asked about what we expect, but the above examples clearly show that they've a life of their own. They primarily show themselves not in avowal but in our increased competency in experientially dealing with the familiar, in the overall coherence of our moment-to-moment experience, in our blindnesses, and, through their absence, in our stumblings. But as the above-reported hallucinations reveal, we can be spuriously readied for, or ongoingly habituated to, what is in fact now absent. And when such a readiness or habituation persists despite its current irrelevance, illusions or hallucinations can result.

So far so empirical, but might there not here also be enough to warrant risking a metaphysical claim? Thus one suggestion has it that to hallucinate is to have specific sensory readinesses persist uncancelled despite one simultaneously registering the absence of the actual experience for which they ready us.[28] Despite the fact that you can see that it's static, past experience of mounting the escalator still readies you for an upwards pull; that pull is unforthcoming; the combined effect of the unrelinquished anticipation of movement and the actual stasis *is* an illusory experience of downwards movement which persists until the readinesses are relinquished. Or to turn again to hallucination proper: when the habituation of the experience of the watch on your wrist persists despite the watch's removal, you experience a haptic hallucination of a watch on your wrist.[29] And so too with the afterimage: the habituation to the negative image persists despite the image's removal; you now 'see' its inverse on the ceiling.

A clear difficulty for this answer to the 'what is hallucination?' question is generalizing it beyond such cases as introduce it. Consider voice hearing. Peter is lying on his bed, and hallucinates a voice saying 'you're a worthless wretch'. Perhaps we can understand why, given his history and his psychology, he might anticipate hearing that, and we can also understand why, once he's heard 'you', he's primed to hear 'are', 'a', etc. But acknowledging that is not enough to get the anticipation account off the ground, for what that account still owes us are the criteria whereby these anticipations are properly ascribed to Peter at the time of hallucinating. So far as he was concerned, the voice came out of the blue, and so we can't ascribe the anticipation to him on the basis of his avowals. Furthermore, we have here the difficult business of understanding what the 'negative' of an expectation of hearing 'you', 'are', 'a', etc. is. We can see why the result of, say, spinning round on the spot and suddenly stopping should lead to an illusory experience of the world now appearing to turn in the opposite direction (think too of the escalator, the 'ghost' watch, and the tone-reversed afterimage). But it's not at all clear what's meant by hallucinating the inverse of an auditory expectation. What instead we find is a hallucination with the same, rather than with some kind of inverse, content of the sensory anticipation.

Despite such failings in generalizability, the notion of hallucination as anomalously uncancelled sensory readiness may yet serve to help undo the widespread notion that hallucinations involve the positive presence to the mind of some kind of inner stimulus. For with, say, the case of the ghostly wristwatch, what we intuitively understand is that here we have no actual stimulus but rather simply the failure of the readiness for such a stimulus to be cancelled, or of a habituation to wear off, despite our knowledge of the stimulus's absence. We intuitively understand, that is, that a hallucination of a watch is, in the absence of any actual stimulation from a watch, just what we should expect were we to fail to relinquish our sensory readinesses whilst also registering the absence of that for which they ready us. By generalizing from the watch case to that of the inverted afterimage we can see here too how hallucination may be reflectively understood in terms of absence rather than in terms of the positive presence to the mind of some kind of inner version of an outer stimulus.

A related suggestion, albeit one with a neuropsychological twist, has it that hallucination be accounted for in terms of 'prediction error'.[30] Rather than understand perception as resulting simply from the brain's processing of sensory stimuli, the 'prediction error' theorist invites us to see our experience as constituted by what sensory stimuli the brain predicts. These predictions are generated by prior experience, and (amongst other things) facilitate the disambiguation of otherwise 'noisy' (i.e. ambiguous) sensory data – with the erroneous result that what in a quiet room might have been accurately heard as the curious 'oh no, the beard police' is in the noisy pub confidently misheard as 'another beer please'. In effect, this predictive brain 'constantly hallucinates at the world ... thereby generating the content of phenomenal experience', and the task is to generate 'hallucinations' as accurate as possible.[31] This is all achieved by the brain's minimization of 'prediction error' – that is, by its minimizing the difference between what's predicted and what stimuli are actually encountered. Mistaken predictions occur if the neural instantiations of such predictions start to trigger themselves, or if there's a failure in their calibration by prediction error information.

The question naturally arises as to what's left of this theory once we strip it of its metaphor. For literally speaking the brain of course makes no predictions (it's people, not their organs, that do that); veridical perceptual experiences can't possibly be hallucinations or predictions; and hallucinations can't possibly be predictions (the criteria for ascribing each are utterly different). A promising way to preserve its sense would be to render it fully neurological: 'prediction', etc. now becomes a picturesque way of talking about certain prefrontal activations. The now merely biological story might have it that a creature's tight perceptual grip on the world is maintained when sense-organ-derived activation in lower sensory cortical regions is ongoingly balanced by activations generated by higher prefrontal cortical regions. And a neurobiological understanding of hallucination might have it resulting when, say, prefrontal activations obtain excessive dominance over sensory signals.[32]

As an empirical theory of hallucinations' neurological causes, the predictive processing account clearly lies outside of this conceptual investigation. I mention it here though because it's sometimes presented as an account of what hallucinations are – i.e. as the suggestion that hallucinations are constituted by 'predictions' in the brain. In this it's akin to the other above-described theories (of hallucination as: percepts without objects, projected inner images, unwitting imaginings, unwitting self-talk, unchecked protentions or predictions) in that it's an attempt to answer the question of what hallucinations consist in. But is this even a good question?

On hallucination's alleged constitution

Our original question, to recall, was 'What is it to hallucinate?' The above-canvassed answers are to what may appear its equivalents, namely: 'what's an hallucination?' or 'in what does hallucination consist?' These latter questions, however, already seem to presuppose either that hallucination is an entity, process or action, or that, whatever it is for something to consist in something, hallucination may sensibly be said to do just that. Such presuppositions are questionable. Let's consider them in turn.

Questions with a 'what's an x?' form find particularly ready application when 'x' refers to an objective phenomenon. You ask me 'what's a coelacanth?' and I know just what to do. Depending on the context, saying 'a fish', speaking of a large size, lobed fins, and particular prehistory, or giving its genus and species, will be acceptable responses to the latter question. By contrast it's no more clear, right off the bat, what someone asking 'what's a hallucination?' is really after than it is when she asks 'what's an anticipation?' or 'what's time?' Of course it's not that we can't, in particular contexts of enquiry, imagine anything sensibly being offered by way of response to such questions. But we might rather suspect that our questioner is here suffering a conceptual illusion, and find that the response which best clears things up for her is 'Ah, "hallucination" isn't actually the name of a thing', perhaps followed by an explication of what's essentially true of she who hallucinates (for which, see below).

Perhaps it be said that 'hallucination' is the name not of a thing but of a process – and we surely know how to answer questions about processes. Such questions naturally take a 'what is x?', rather than a 'what is a y?', shape ('what is metabolism?', not 'what is a metabolism?'), and gerunds formed from psychological verbs ('thinking', 'hallucinating', 'hoping', 'hearing', 'feeling', etc.) function like process terms in so far as they more naturally replace 'x' than 'y'. Yet the concept of a 'process' has to do with a happening in stages, each stage causally depending on that which precedes it, and the typical point of asking the 'what is x?' question of a process is to elicit informative talk about its constituting stages and (if relevant) its purpose. But when we ask, say, 'what is thought/ thinking?' or 'what is hallucination/hallucinating?', we aren't enquiring into something that always has stages or a purpose. We shall therefore once again be forgiven for still not knowing here what this questioner is after, and so needn't think poorly of ourselves for coming up short.

As noted above, sometimes when we ask 'What is x?' what we're interested in is what x consists in. Various of the above-proffered answers (in terms of inner images, projections, anomalously un-cancelled anticipations, etc.) took this tack with the 'what is it to hallucinate?' question. Such answers may fail, but isn't it at least clear what the question thus understood means?

Well, what is it for x to consist in z? Note that we aren't, with this talk of x and z, talking about two different particulars or sets thereof. Some or other book consists (inter alia) in such-and-such pages glued together, but these pages aren't helpfully described as 'something other than' that book of which they're part. In talking of its 'constitution' we're rather talking of what Aristotle meant by its *material* causes. For the book these include paper, glue, and ink – whereas its *formal* causes (which determine its identity as a book) include its legible and portable nature and authorial origin; its *efficient* causes (that bring it into being) include the motions of the printing press; and its *final* causes (its purposes) include being read, entertaining, imparting information. The question on our table, then, is whether every x – and whether hallucination in particular – enjoys a constitution or material cause.

If someone were to insist that everything must enjoy every form of Aristotelian cause, we moderns should quickly accuse him of an *a priori* prejudice. It is, for example, surely very doubtful, at least to secularists, that every phenomenon enjoys a final cause. (Consider the salt in the sea, or the stars in the night sky.) But must everything have a material cause? Especially when we turn to non-entitative (abstract) phenomena, the claim is hard to make out. Thus consider Usain Bolt's acceleration at the start of a race. Its formal cause is his increasing speed; its efficient causes include the egg sandwich he had for breakfast; its final cause is winning the race. But material cause? Nothing comes to mind.[33] And the suggestion I now offer is that psychological phenomena quite generally, and hallucinations in particular, typically provide no more surface for questions about constitution to grip onto than does Bolt's acceleration.

We can see this by focusing on what's required of us, by way of demonstration or investigation, if we're to adequately answer questions about that in which something consists. Asked by a language teacher what a particular book is made up of, we reach for 'printed pieces of paper', 'covers', 'glue', etc. Asked instead by the biology teacher, and we talk of the pulped wood of coniferous trees. Asked by an antiquarian bibliophile, we might investigate whether the paper has a watermark. Or, to take a different kind of example, if we're asked what a particular non-entitative phenomenon – a ritual such as a marriage ceremony, say – is, we refer to the marriage vows, to a priest or registrar's performative pronouncement of the marriage, the signing of a licence, exchange of rings, etc. Our knowing what to do is here of a piece with our grasp of the sense of the question. But when asked what a toothache or thought or hallucination consists in, no obvious routes of enquiry or demonstration open up. Again, this isn't to say that a route couldn't be contrived; we might, for example, decide that Peter's hallucination of a derogatory voice saying 'You're pathetic' shall be said to be constituted by its most proximal causes, and so make elucidatory reference to various aspects of his psychology, particular cortical activations, and so on. Or perhaps we decide to restrict answers that shall count as proper to such causally necessary conditions as obtain in his cortex – or restrict it further still by ignoring all such conditions as would have anyway been necessary for him to remain alive and awake. The point being made here, though, is that such decisions are no more mandated by the mere asking of 'what is hallucination's constitution?' than they are when we're asked about the constitution of Bolt's acceleration. It's only if we ignore just how much stipulation has here been engaged in, so as to provide an initially opaque question with a sense, that we shall consider hallucination to enjoy the same manner of existence as is had by such phenomena as are more naturally enquired about with such questions. To refuse to provide an answer of a similar sort to those canvassed above to a question about hallucination's constitution need not, then, be seen as a reluctance to set out on any clearly envisaged quest. Instead, it can be seen as of a piece with a deeper insight into the kind of existence hallucination enjoys: that it no more has a constitution than numbers have durability or economies a sense of humour, and that the suggestion that it does stems merely from that misplaced reification which turns hallucinations into 'inner stimuli', 'percepts', or 'appearances'.

What it is to hallucinate

Let's regroup. Our original question asked 'what is it to hallucinate?' The psychologists' talk of 'percepts', 'phantasms', and 'mental process' conjures an illusion of sense that beguiles us into attempting to answer this question in such terms as are apt for entities, processes, and other such phenomena. But if hallucination doesn't enjoy the kind of reality enjoyed by entities or processes, what shall we say about its form of existence?

By way of answer I suggest that it enjoys that kind of existential form which itself is fully elucidated by apt answers to questions about its ascription conditions. To questions, that is, which ask 'what's essentially true of he who hallucinates?', or 'when's it proper to say of someone that she's hallucinating?' In this it's similar to Bolt's acceleration: we understand what it is for him to accelerate when we understand what makes it true to say that he's accelerating: namely that his velocity is increasing over time. So, what does make it true to say of Peter that he's hallucinating a male voice saying 'you're pathetic'? It's in part that Peter would sincerely say, whether asked or unprompted, something like 'I just heard someone say "you're pathetic"', or 'It somehow seems to me that a man was just telling me "you're pathetic"'. But more than that, it must also be the case that Peter neither actually heard (in that sense of 'hear' which is success-evaluable) nor imagined (in that sense of 'imagine' which involves direction by the will) what he here reports. Or, to finesse this a little: we may properly be said to hallucinate what we also perceive or imagine, but in order for such hallucination

ascriptions to be sustained there must be some difference in their intentional objects
– i.e. in the content, character, timing, etc. of a hallucination and what's actually heard
or imagined. If someone, either standing eyes open before a Friesian cow, or avowedly
imagining doing just that, tells us 'I seem to be hallucinating a Friesian cow right in
front of me', we shall struggle to find a meaning for her words. Only if she tells us
something to distinguish the seeing from the hallucinating (perhaps the hallucinated
cow is a little to the left) shall her hallucination report remain credible.

Whilst such avowals – either of hallucination or, wrongly, of perception – provide
the surest criteria for hallucination, we also properly ascribe hallucination on the basis
of other verbal and non-verbal behaviour. That dishevelled old man we pass on the
street – the one with staring eyes and startled mien: sometimes he seems to be
answering questions put to him by no mortal soul. Or consider the dog staring into the
room's empty corner, barking fiercely exactly as she does when strangers enter the
house. Sometimes the hallucination ascriptions we make here are defeasible: the old
man is reciting lines for an amateur dramatics production; an ultrasonic sound has
disturbed the dog. It's important to note that, whilst we may feel less secure in making
hallucination ascriptions in the absence of perceptual avowals, our lack of certainty
here need reflect no lack of informedness on our part. Little Renée has recently made
an 'imaginary friend' to whom she talks whilst playing in the garden. Shall we say of her
either that she's hallucinating or that she's imagining this companion's voice? Various
factors may push us one way or the other – for example, does Renée happily acknowledge
the friend's non-reality? But the idea that there *must* be a right answer to our question
is merely an unwarranted stipulation. The further we are from such paradigm
hallucination as is straightforwardly ascribed on the basis of avowals of perceiving or
hallucinating, the further we are from making determinate hallucination ascriptions.
Rather than always presume that difficult cases involve a fact of the matter beyond
our ken, we do better in such cases to reconsider our confidence that there is any such
fact.

To summarize: the principal criteria for the meaningful ascription of hallucinations
are someone's sincere say-so either that it's for them somehow as if they're perceiving
even though they aren't, or that they're perceiving something which we know to not
obtain. Less paradigmatic, but still conceptually relevant, is their other possible
behaviour: we sometimes ascribe hallucination to a strangely barking dog or to
someone utterly lost in an unreal conversation. And the suggestion that reference to
these indices of hallucination still doesn't tell us what hallucination itself is can now be
rejected – not because we're compelled to consider that question aptly answered by
reference to the aforementioned criteria, but because without some such reworking the
question's sense remains unclear. We could of course invent a method for answering it,
and in doing so provide it with a sense. Perhaps that method would have us look to
certain brain processes in the hallucinator: Peter's hallucination of a hostile voice
'consists in' or 'is', we now say, such and such an activation of his superior temporal
gyrus. To turn an empirical truth (the hallucination *requires* the activation) into a
conceptual truism (the activation *is* the hallucination) in this way might be useful if, for
example, we're wanting to achieve economy of expression in a neuroscience laboratory.
Yet the cost of such decisions should also be borne in mind – the principal one being

the invitation they extend to become confused about the form of existence enjoyed by hallucination.

Hallucination and lost reality contact

Investigations of hallucination's causes tend to be empirical in character, aiming as they do to arrive at new knowledge through scientific enquiry. This of course is not here our method or concern, focused as we are on developing instead our reflective understanding of what's already known. So when what follows addresses the questions of what hallucination's connection is to lost reality contact, how it arises in mental illness, and how it bespeaks – when it does so bespeak – as-yet-unprocessed emotional disturbance, our concern shall not be with the proffering of novel causal hypotheses, but rather with showing how what at first may appear quite diverse phenomena can be brought under a unifying description. Our concern, that is, is with what's been called 'genetic phenomenology' – i.e. with revealing the continuity of form enjoyed by otherwise diverse-seeming experiences and thoughts over time. It's one thing to believe, on the basis of good evidence, that mental illness and unprocessed emotional overwhelm can result in voice hearing, but another thing to understand why this should be the case – and it's with this understanding that we're here concerned.

Hallucinations can – yet need not – be symptoms of mental illness. In understanding why they often are, it's important to first acknowledge that what's in common to hallucination's causes is a diminishing of reality contact. All going well, our sensorimotor lives remain tightly looped in with our surroundings: we spontaneously track environmental changes; sensory stimulation caused by our own activity and that caused externally are not as it were conflated; goal attainment results nicely in the cessation of strivings; and sensory readinesses are either fulfilled in experience or cancelled when no longer apt. In such ways is a unified self enacted in relation to a self-independent world. If, however, the opportunity for this fine-tuned self/world differentiation is reduced, reality contact is impaired, and the soil in which hallucinations can quickly grow is thereby prepared. We don't see the loss of reality contact as indicative of mental illness unless it also precipitates a loss of reality testing (i.e. unless delusion supervenes).

In various situations, reality contact may flicker in and out. Thus as twilight turns into the witching hour, 'creatures from inner space' temporarily manifest on our experiential horizons. Darkened rooms – or, even better, sensory deprivation chambers – are their preferred abode.[34] An absence of afferent stimulation from lost body parts leads to phantom sensations in phantom limbs.[35] Deafferentiation (the loss – due, for example, to retinal degradation – of input to sensory cortices) also explains the visual hallucinations in sufferers of Charles Bonnet syndrome.[36] Children, who have yet to develop a tight sensorimotor coupling with their environments, are more likely to hallucinate than adults.[37] Drug intoxication diminishes reality contact and induces hallucination. Visions – but also auditory, olfactory, and somatosensory hallucinations – are common in hypnagogic (between wake and sleep) states.[38] And the near total loss of reality contact during sleep is a condition of ordinary dreams' possibility.

Two metaphors from the literature stand out as making evocatively real for us the relation of hallucination to this lost reality contact. These are the notions of hallucinations' 'release' and the 'short-circuiting' of the hallucinating mind.

We owe the 'release' concept to pioneering neurologist John Hughlings Jackson who suggested that aberrant behavioural and cognitive activity can be 'released' when the top-down inhibiting control of lower (subcortical) activity by higher (cortical) centres dissolves.[39] Louis Jolyon West later redeployed it in offering a neurological theory of hallucination: a hypothesized mechanism of 'scanning and screening' normally excludes irrelevant neural trace activations from reaching consciousness but, in conditions of reduced sensory input and increased cortical arousal, disinhibited 'perceptual traces may be "released" and re-experienced, either in familiar or new – even bizarre – combinations'.[40] Yet well before West's scientific use of the concept, others had used it to characterize hallucination's onset.[41] The possibility canvassed here, then, is that the concept's value isn't exhausted by its role in empirical theorizing, but that something in it corresponds to what we intuitively understand regarding hallucination. For what such talk of 'release' intuitively evokes is the idea of a hallucination that's waiting to happen once freed from the bounds of reality contact and repression. A butterfly released from its cocoon now enjoys a new form of existence; someone released from the prison of low self-esteem now draws on previously dormant resources to live a flourishing life. The question arising, then, is: what do we intuitively understand to have been lying dormant within and to be released when reality contact is diminished? And one answer to this, canvassed already above, is that it's sensory anticipations which are released and which, like anticipatory caterpillars turning into hallucinatory butterflies, metamorphose from mere sensory readinesses into ersatz perceptions as they take flight. Compare: (i) I apply a strong upwards force to hold the heavy suitcase perpendicular to my body and steady in the air – but it breaks away at the handle, suddenly releasing my arm's sudden upward movement. And: (ii) I have, especially when anxious about my obligations, a residing readiness for being urgently addressed; as reality contact is lost, the readiness is released, thereby transforming into a hallucination of my name being called.

Our second metaphor has it that, in the absence of the world's resistance, the mind is prone to short-circuit.[42] Reality contact requires us to be both ongoingly differentiated from, yet also constitutively bound up with, the world about us. Our constant and consistent readiness that part-constitutes our fluid sensorimotor engagements ensures that we neither merge into, nor lose our experiential grip on, our surroundings.[43] Yet when reality contact is lost, the 'anode' of sensory readiness and the 'cathode' of sensory experience suddenly come into direct contact without their normal worldly mediation, resulting in a hallucinatory spark.

Essential to both the 'release' and the 'short-circuit' metaphors is the devolution of something with a place in the order of reason to something obtaining without it. Actions (of lifting suitcases) become mere movements (of arms into the air); well-placed or misplaced sensory readinesses that part-constitute reality contact become hallucinations that manifest its absence. The true value of the 'release' metaphor in particular is not to be met with in the idea of an ontologically self-same 'perceptual trace' registered, stored up, and released within and from the brain. It works instead by reminding us of the understanding we already enjoy of all such instances of causal continuity combined with ontological transformation.

Hallucination, suffering, and mental illness

Our concept 'mental illness' implicitly references not only a loss of reality contact but often also the intolerable suffering which can occasion it. Reading the literature one often gets the impression that the only relevant suffering here is that which madness throws up – rather than that which inspires it and remains mutely skeined in its flesh. Our final question regarding hallucination, then, concerns its relation to such suffering. How may hallucination itself evade yet encode what for the psychotic subject are the unmanageable pains of life?

As a way in, consider first the hallucinations of the bereaved. Perhaps a third of us hallucinate our dearly departeds; a half 'feel their presence'.[44] Here Marion C. describes to Oliver Sacks her experience of 'seeing' and 'hearing' her recently deceased husband:

> One evening I came home from work as always to our big empty house. Usually at that hour Paul would have been at his electronic chessboard playing over the game in the New York Times. His table was out of sight of the foyer, but he greeted me in his familiar way: 'Hello! You're back! Hi!' . . . His voice was clear and strong and true; just the way it was when he was well. I 'heard' it. It was as if he were actually at his chess table and actually greeting me once more. The other part was that, as I said, I couldn't see him from the foyer, yet I did. I 'saw' him, I 'saw' the expression on his face, I 'saw' how he moved the pieces, I 'saw' him greet me. That part was like one sees in a dream: as if I were seeing a picture or a movie of an event. But the speech was live and real.[45]

How shall we understand this? Why should it be that it's only after his death that Marion's anticipations of seeing and hearing Paul should, when he's not there, bleed through into ersatz experiences of him? Well, consider that Marion's task in mourning is to relinquish such readinesses for shared experience as form part of her marriage's living structure. This is no easy task: they've become wired into the existential fabric, into the deep habit structure, of her body. The tearing wrenches of grief index the relinquishing of those bodily readinesses as the fact of his death gradually becomes registered within her body's anticipatory and intentional fabric. And this painful task requires ongoing reality contact since otherwise Paul's real loss from the world can't be registered. When he was alive, but out for the evening, there was no difficulty in relinquishing for a while the anticipation of his presence. Now, however, that task is associated with a greater one: relinquishing the expectation of ever seeing him again. And so it's no surprise that, especially when tired after a day's work, less tightly bound now to the world, and less resistant to the faerie call to evade the world's pains, her living readinesses are not cancelled but instead short-circuit, collapsing into ersatz perception. Marion 'encounters' Paul's 'ghost', a spectral 'presence' which is really the inverse of what can't currently be tolerated – i.e. his absence. Such 'ghosts' can even start to 'haunt' the bereaved; they won't leave us alone; they have something to tell us before they can move on from this life to another world. In reality, however, it's we who still wish to say something to them before we shall let them go; we who beckon to, and vainly reach out toward, them from this world, not they to us from the 'other world'. It is then not the 'ghost', but we ourselves, who are trapped between the worlds, ghosts being – in the terms of an above-discussed illusion – in truth but our own lurches on the escalators of our animal souls, absences in the guise of presences.

Now mourning is, all being well, not psychosis: we typically find here no truly enduring consolidation of defence, or no utter breakdown, which prevents sensorimotor reality contact's reestablishment. No delusion sets in. Even so, it provides us with a model for understanding such hallucination as manifests mental illness: here too hallucination may express such intolerable pain as would have been felt had reality contact remained secure. By way of analogy consider how defensive denials express that which they deny: it's precisely in the agitated and clipped manner in which Amy denies that her ex meant anything that we see just how painful is this loss to her. Or consider the old shuffling man talking to himself on the street: the sensitive observer can't but be struck by that loneliness in him of which he himself, so deeply lost to or merged with it as he is, is largely unaware. The pain's full force can't here be avowed or straightforwardly witnessed.

To make ready sense of psychotic hallucination, however, we require one further concept – I shall call it 'crystallization' but we might also talk of 'concretization' or 'symbolization'. This has to do with a relieving crystallizing out, from a pervasive moody solution, of a specific and momentary ersatz perception. In this respect, we may compare hallucination's formation with the unconscious way in which children develop themes for their play, or with automatic (trance) writing, or the formation of night-time dreams, or the emergence of paranoid delusion out of a diffuse and awful state of 'trema' ('*something* is going on').[46] The relief comes precisely because the unthinkable and unformed has now become an ersatz thinkable form. Bringing these lines of thought together now, we can understand such hallucination as expresses the pain that breaks the mentally ill as the crystallizing out, whilst reality contact is compromised, of discrete ersatz perceptions. And what they crystallize out from is an intolerable longing and dread which the hallucinator, like the shuffling man, is more merged with than alive to. In such ways hallucination's formation may mirror that of delusion: maintaining a structured reality contact is simply too undoing; a diffuse unstructured confusion is also unbearable; a discrete hallucination or delusion which enjoys an ersatz thinkability is, by contrast, more tolerable. And as also with delusion, at no point should we think of hallucination's motivated formation as rooted in a literal choice of symptoms. The hallucinator no more chooses his experiences than a reservoir chooses to discharge through the sluice gates which offer least resistance.

Most schizophrenic hallucinations are distressing – and we shall turn to them shortly. Yet Bleuler, with whose examples of hallucination the chapter began, talked also of voices that 'are the means by which the megalomaniac realizes his wishes' and 'the religiously preoccupied achieves his communion with God and the Angels'; of voices that 'console'; and of hallucinations of 'every pleasurable sensation which the sense organs can transmit'. And Peter Reynolds, whose voices were also reported at the chapter's head, mentioned one 'Socrates' who 'talks of philosophy and psychology and medicine, all sorts of brilliant things'. These are not obviously distressing experiences, and so it's natural to question their relationship with such pain as breaks the mentally ill. Now we are of course not obliged to consider all the hallucinations of those who are sometimes mentally ill as directly expressive of that pain which elicits the illness: sometimes they may express quite different, even healthy, aspects of a mind which has nevertheless originally been thrown out of orbit by mental pain. Even so it's not implausible to see various benign voices as sometimes also testifying to intolerable predicament. We obviously can't know this to be so in Peter's case, and we shouldn't indulge armchair empirical theorizing – but we can nevertheless offer a hypothetical formulation to show the intelligibility of a possibility. Thus we can imagine that it mightn't have been safe for Peter to enjoy his own philosophical thoughts, so quickly would they have been snuffed out by real or internal critics, thereby leaving him brokenly demoralized; instead, these would-be thoughts now safely crystallize out as ego-alien voices. In this way the pain that elicits the illness is manifest not in the hallucinatory content per se, but in the need for such thought as the hallucinator enjoys to take an hallucinatory form. Or consider the case of a young woman whose thwarted longing for intimacy devolves into an hallucinatory experience of genital stimulation. There is, we intuitively sense, something tragic here afoot. By attending to the collapse of unintegrated and intolerable – hence also unsatisfiable – longing into its own hallucinatory pseudo-satisfaction, the sense of pathos which attends such cases should now make ready sense.

Let's return now to the more explicitly dismal hallucinations. Peter, you will recall, hears not only Socrates but five other voices:

> *father* . . . ridicules me and makes fun of me, just generally taking the piss out of me like my father did. His voice tells me that he never did anything to upset me, which just isn't true. . . . the *blasphemer* . . . just swears all the time, along with *profanities*, another voice that curses me. . . . *dangerous* . . . tells me to walk in front of buses and cars all the time . . . He's a bastard. He wants me dead, very much like my father did when I was younger. . . . *the man my mother had an affair with* . . . talks to me about my mother sometimes. What he says is crude and horrible . . . .

Whilst he has in the past been psychotic when hearing voices – at which time he believed aliens were speaking to him – his temporary losses of reality contact now no longer provoke a loss of reality testing. Now Peter is mentally stronger he takes his voices for aspects of his own psychology, and reasonably contends that they, along with his prior sexual problems and paranoid beliefs about being diseased and poisoned, were provoked by his parents' highly dysfunctional and aggressive relationship, his mother's death, and his teenage seduction by his sister-in-law.

So how are we to understand the relationship between traumatic early experiences and later hallucination? We may take our lead from Peter's claim that his voices are 'clouded memories' of his past trauma. If he'd enjoyed a preternatural degree of self-possession as a child, then Peter could have clearly experienced and comprehended the abuse he suffered. He would have known 'this isn't me; it's not my just desert; this isn't how a father should act'. To have arrived at such thoughts would, however, have itself been destabilizing: children are helpless and the thought that one is living amidst ego-destructive forces is itself terrifying. It is, then, both because they naturally lack ego strength, and because they're motivated to not recognize parental abuse, that children instead 'introject' or 'internalize' such destructive forces into the fabric of their psyche. This renders them blind to the external trauma; it numbs them and 'clouds' the trauma. In psychoanalytic language: the 'introjection of the bad object' (or 'identification with the aggressor') leads to a 'scotomization' of the actual experience of a bad parent.[47] The child now swims in dismal inchoate traumatic seas: the trauma becomes not a thinkable moment of reality contact but instead the mind's very fabric or form.

To be left swimming endlessly in such seas is, however, unendurable. For quasi-thinkable content to emerge back out of diffuse unthinkable form, crystallization must take place. Voices precipitate out of the inky solution: thinkable droplets of experience condense out of the dark clouds. It might be asked: how can this be understood as a motivated, pain-relieving, function since the voices – *father*, *dangerous*, *profanities*, etc. – too are clearly terrible? But to ask such a question is to misunderstand the toll that such internalization of serial abuse takes, and to misunderstand the relief that ersatz thinkable form has compared with an unthinkable atmosphere, at least when the terrors of an abusive situation are no longer externally present. Peter is still fated to swim in these bitter seas, but at least now their toxic saturation is reduced as accusatory and hateful voices crystallize out of them. And so what might, in happier circumstances, have bodied forth as a cogent feeling of hurt or anger instead now takes the shape of a voice. Peter may not be able to own, and curse in, anger – but the *blasphemer* can shout abuse at the world. The hatred that was directed to him but which couldn't be consciously experienced is now released in the voices of *father* and *dangerous*. And once the crystallization begins, the anticipatory dynamics of hallucination take over. Just as a dream unfolds as each successive moment associatively inspires the next, or just as the first words of the Ouija board inspire those that come next, so too do hallucinated voices auto-construct moment to moment.

How may such voices abate or at least be managed? Peter finds respite and solidarity by joining the Hearing Voices Network. He developed much by way of ego structure, holds down a job, remains in touch with reality, and knows such voices as do remain for unresolved aspects of his own traumatized inner life. This transition from intolerable, unthinkable, pain and hallucination to acceptance and reality testing is well-illustrated by the Grimm fairy tale *The Shroud*:

> A mother had a little boy of seven years who was so attractive and good natured that no one could look at him without liking him, and he was dearer to her than anything else in the world. He suddenly died, and the mother could find no solace. She cried day and night. However, soon after his burial, the child began to appear every night at those places where he had sat and played while still alive. When the mother cried, he cried as well, but when morning came he had disappeared. The mother did not cease crying, and one night he appeared with the white shirt in which he had been laid into his coffin, and with the little wreath on his head. He sat down on the bed at her feet and said, 'Oh, mother, please stop crying, or I will not

be able to fall asleep in my coffin, because my burial shirt will not dry out from your tears that keep falling on it.' This startled the mother, and she stopped crying. The next night the child came once again. He had a little light in his hand and said, 'See, my shirt is almost dry, and I will be able to rest in my grave.' Then the mother surrendered her grief to God and bore it with patience and peace, and the child did not come again, but slept in his little bed beneath the earth.[48]

8

Disordered Thought

Introduction

Such discourse as manifests *formal thought disorder* is variously: circumstantial, tangential (marked by 'knight's moves'), dominated by irrelevant associations, readily derailed, populated repeatedly and without acknowledgement by invented and misused terms (neologisms and 'stock' words), forgetful of its goal, over-inclusive, stilted, governed by sound rather than meaning ('clanging'), suddenly interpenetrated by unrelated themes ('inspirations'), mimicking of the interlocutor ('echolalia'), unspecifying of the referents of the pronouns within it, self-interrupting and halting ('blocked'), and confused (people and places condense into single objects; self and other change place). Some of these features also characterize our dream thoughts; they're another aspect of that to which the conception of psychosis as *waking dream* draws our attention. Alongside lost reality testing, disorders of thought's form provide the clearest exemplification of what it is to 'lose your mind'.

An example: the year is 1887 and Babette Straub – a 42-year-old seamstress, 'brought up under sad domestic conditions, amid distress and hard labour', sister of a prostitute – is admitted to in Zurich's Burghölzli asylum where she's to live out her days.[1] Before admission she hears accusatory voices and wants to drown herself. Soon after admission she begins to write such letters as:

> 5 July
>
> Dear Superintendent:
> With these lines I request you once more to instantly discharge me. My head, as I already remarked to you in my last letter, is clearer than ever. What I have to suffer secretly on account of novelties in all domains is unfortunately known to me alone, and is too smashing for my health as well as for my mind. Unfortunately they have gone so far as to torture to death poor victims by secret cruelties, for I suffer more than you can imagine and in this manner fully expect my end, which sadly touches me more and more. I hope you will act in your capacity as physician and will have no need of any further reflection.
> Yours faithfully, etc.[2]

These missives are delivered in a completely unemotional manner. Babette maintains that she has a fortune of millions, that her bed is full of needles or snakes, that she hears voices over invisible telephones. Over time her discourse becomes increasingly incoherent and perseverative: by the following year she frequently becomes 'the monopoly'; 'Rubinstein from Petersburg' sends her money 'by the wagonload'; her 'spinal marrow is torn out at night'; back pains which 'do not stick in the body and do not fly about in the air' are 'caused by substances going through the walls covered with magnetism'; 'extracts' are made by 'inhalations of chemistry'; 'Station for station must keep its proper governmental position so that existence-questions of the ward cannot be chosen to hide themselves behind, all things can be chosen.'

By 1892 the situation arises that Babette and 'Naples ... must supply the whole world with macaroni'. Three years later she's the owner of 'a seven-floored note factory with coal-raven-black windows, which signifies paralysis and starvation'. In 1896 Babette becomes 'Germania and Helvetia of exclusively sweet butter', 'but now I have no more butter-content than a fly would leave behind – hm-hm-hm – that is starvation – hm-hm'. Before long she also becomes Socrates, the Lorelei, and 'Noah's Ark, the boat of salvation and respect, Mary Stuart, Empress Alexander'. In 1897 'Dr D. recently came out of her mouth ... the little tiny D., the son of the Emperor Barbarossa'. By the turn of the century she repeatedly whispers mantric 'power words' to herself whilst at work on her sewing, words that crop up in phrases such as 'Yesterday evening I sat in the night train for Nice, had to go through a triumphal arch there – we have established all that already as a *threefold world proprietress* – we are also the *lilac-new-red-sea wonder*.'

As the years pass Babette remains able to talk with lucidity on various everyday matters, but at other times slips into a thought-disordered mode, as when she repeats that – for example – she's 'the double polytechnic irreplaceable', 'I am the master-key ... the house belongs to me', 'I am triple owner of the world', 'I affirm the asylum', 'I am a Switzerland', 'on a Monday between eleven and twelve o'clock I slept and established a million Hufeland to the left on the last splinter of earth up on the hill'. Or she 'suffers hieroglyphical', 'I was shut up fourteen years so that my breath could not come out anywhere', 'then the poisoning, it is invisible – it is shot in through the window ... as if you were in ice ... this also belonged to the monopoly. . . . Forel should have paid me 80,000 francs nine years ago, because I had to endure such pains'. Or 'The hedgehog is *so* long [she indicates about a foot] and on Sunday morning it crawled as far as the well – yes, Mr Zuppinger, it was through pork sausages. Mr Zuppinger has eaten pork sausages'; 'Once when I affirmed my 1000 millions in a dream, a little green snake came up to my mouth – it had the finest, loveliest feeling ... just as if it wanted to kiss me.'

Such discourse is expressive both of delusions and of formally disordered thought. But how are we to tell these apart? Psychiatry typically uses a form/content distinction to this end: delusion involves a disturbance to thought's content, formal thought disorder a disturbance to its form. But this may seem doubtful, since the delusionality of delusion is more helpfully understood in terms of a disturbance to the form of a subject's reality relation rather than in terms of a false or exceptional content (see Chapter 3). We can move past this apparent impasse by noting that the use and therefore the sense of the form/content distinction differs in the two contexts. In relation to thought disorder its deployment aims to register the fact that, whilst in delusional discourse it's clear *what* the person thinks, in the sense that we can at least readily give a value to 'x' in 'he delusionally believes that x', it's far harder to identify particular 'x's in thought-disordered discourse. Despite being rationally unintelligible, *delusional* thoughts may still be said to admit of paraphrase, to recur over time, and to provide the basis for certain inferences and the content of certain explanations. ('James believes he can set the sun with his arm movements.' Paraphrase: 'James thinks that, by moving his arms, he can set the sun.' Inference: 'James thinks that, if he doesn't move his arms thus, the sun shall not set.' Explanation: 'James moves his arms like that because he believes that, by so doing, he shall set the sun.') That the same possibilities of paraphrase, inference, and explanation are not so available for *formally disordered* thought tells us something essential about what it means to suffer it. The thought-disordered subject's discourse may, for example, at first appear to be setting off in one direction – the direction perhaps being set by a situation, a memory, or a question put to her. Very quickly, however, she becomes derailed by associations not pertinent to what we might have assumed was going to be her theme. In paradigmatic cases the result is that the presumption that she truly has a particular direction or theme itself becomes unsustainable, it becoming clear that the theme in question was itself only a product of a projection of our own, one rooted in a misplaced presumption of her sanity.

Notwithstanding this conceptual differentiation of delusion and thought disorder it's important to note that there's not always a fact of the matter as to whether a certain stretch of talk should be deemed expressive of a short-lived delusion or be seen as formally disordered. We might sometimes be able to answer a question about this by putting to the psychotic subject questions such as: 'did you mean to say what you just did say?', 'do you consider the following paraphrase apt? . . .', etc. Nevertheless, actively psychotic subjects may respond with silence or with rationalizing, evasive, or nonsensical answers. It's then hard to see what could rationally motivate the claim that there must here be a fact of the matter to be determined. If, however, particular bizarre claims are repeated at other times, if recognizable paraphrases of them are repeated, and if their negations are denied, then we shall be more likely to diagnose delusion. Delusion's diagnosis requires a certain constancy, hence it cannot go ahead when peculiar claims are quickly acknowledged to be awry or are abandoned for no discernible reason.

What follows attempts a closer understanding of what it is to suffer formal thought disorder. First, we shall consider the intrinsic pitfalls of following either those psychologists who would explicate the thought that's therein disturbed in terms of alleged inner processes of thinking, or those linguists who would direct our attention instead only to outwardly demonstrable grammatical or syntactical disturbances. But also notable about such purely dysfunction-based approaches is that they fail to relate the having of disordered thought to the struggles encountered in the living of a human life – or, at least, they only show how such struggles result from, rather than manifest in, the disordered thought. The rest of the chapter will then consider just how it is that formal thought disorder manifests and expresses what the mentally ill subject experiences as life's intolerable pains.

Thought disorder and discourse

Whilst poorly put together thought may be found in various psychotic conditions, formal thought disorder has traditionally been most closely associated with a schizophrenia diagnosis.[3] (A talent for milder versions of anomalously structured discourse in which thought disorder manifests has been found not only in schizophrenic subjects – whether or not currently unwell – but also in their first degree biological relatives; it appears to be under partial genetic control.[4]) Along with a disposition to self-other and imagination-reality indistinction, a disposition to associative dreaminess has long featured in psychopathologists' theories of the key determinants of the schizophrenia diathesis. Bleuler, our inventor of 'the schizophrenias', suggests that the only feature which is both 'fundamental' (i.e. essential) and (causally) 'primary' to schizophrenic illnesses is a 'disturbance of associations', a disturbance not limited to, but showing itself most clearly in, formally disordered thought.[5] The disturbance of associations he noted most frequently was that of their 'loosening'. Such a focus on association is of a piece with his longstanding adherence to an associationist psychology – i.e. to a psychology which hopes to capture important truths about apt and disturbed thinking, understanding, and recollection by focusing on the causal and contiguous relations between separable ideas.

To investigate thought disorder Bleuler would sometimes invite his patients to repeat back to him stories such as this Aesop's fable:

A donkey loaded with bags of salt had to wade across a river. He slipped and fell and remained lying comfortably in the cool water for a few moments. Standing up, he noticed how much lighter his load had become because the salt had dissolved in the water. Long-ears [i.e. the donkey] registered this advantage and decided to use it the following day when he was carrying a load of sponges across the same river. This time, he fell deliberately but was badly disappointed. The sponges had soaked up a great deal of water and were far heavier than before. Indeed, the load was so heavy that it drowned him.[6]

Seven decades later two psychologists repeated this investigation and received the following from a schizophrenic subject:

A donkey was carrying salt and he went through a river ... and he decided to go for a swim ... and his salt started dissolving off him into the water ... and it did ... it left him hanging there ... so he crawled out on the other side and became a mastodon ... it gets unfrozen ... it's up in the Arctic right now ... it's a block of ice ... and a block of ice gets planted in ... it's forced into a square, right? ... ever studied that sort of a formation, block of ice in the ground? ... well, it fights the permafrost ... it pushes it away ... and lets things go up around it ... you can see they're like, they're almost like a pattern with a flower ... they start from the middle ... and it's like a submerged ice cube ... that's frozen into the soil afterwards ...[7]

We readily see how the subject's recollection is derailed by such dreamlike associations as are extrinsic to the story but nevertheless arise along the way in the subject's mind.

A donkey, on climbing out of water, becomes first a mastodon (perhaps a woolly mammoth, of which frozen specimens have been reported) and then a block of ice; the sorry episode of the water-logged sponges and the dismal finale are thereby altogether avoided.[8] Other thought-disordered features are evident too: we lose a sense of what the pronouns refer to; something is both unfrozen and a block of ice; and the pervasive un-self-consciousness about the failure to keep track – and to notice the communicative inadequacy – of what's been said bespeaks a loss of reality testing.

Let's accept that thought-disordered discourse is permeated by diffuse, interrupted, and adventitious associations. The question remains as to whether we can specify what it is for such thought to be formally disordered by referring to a disturbance of associative processes. Consider that when – in his *Essay Concerning Human Understanding* – John Locke first introduced to us the notion of 'the association of ideas' he was referring to an intrinsically pathological process.[9] In the normally healthy run of things our ideas enjoy not an 'associative', but instead what he called a 'natural', connection – i.e. a connection that may be grasped by 'reason'. Sometimes, however, the mind may – through either 'chance or custom' – become governed by mere 'association', and this creates in us a 'degree of madness' (as when, say, a phobia of horses is acquired after suffering food poisoning whilst watching harmless galloping horses). Locke's model, that is, makes no claim that we can articulate in merely associationist terms (i.e. in terms of causality and contiguity – rather than in terms of intrinsic rationality) what the pattern is that constitutes sane thought; 'association' properly remains the name of the problem rather than of that which thought disorder problematizes. To put it otherwise: the thought-disordered patient associates *rather than* remains on rational thought-constituting track. Later associationist models, taking their lead instead from David Hume, attempt to articulate disturbances of thought in terms of disturbances of putative associative processes of thinking. Yet it remains unclear how rational and meaningful relations between thought contents could plausibly be explicated in terms of non-rational relations between thought's instances, since no examination of the contiguity or causation of ideas will by itself tell us which are related rationally and which not.[10]

The idea that 'thought' or 'understanding' are names of an associative process is but one version of a more general claim, quite standard in the psychological literature, that it names some kind of 'inner – or psychic –process', a process that's disrupted in thought disorder. It has, for example, proved tempting to many to imagine that thinking and understanding are both inner processes which as such hopefully inspire our utterances but which may also go on by themselves. Various other gerunds ('oxidizing', 'photosynthesizing', 'dying', etc.) are after all names of processes, so why not 'thinking' too? And since we *can* readily imagine speaking occurring without thought or understanding – as when we speak mindlessly, or in a trance, or repeat the words of someone talking in a language unknown to us – it's tempting to think that thinking and understanding must be inner processes, processes quiescent in us when we're merely parroting, but alive in him who speaks with understanding.

Despite these temptations, nothing in either our ordinary ascription of thoughts, or in our psychopathological ascription of disordered thought, really suggests that thought is helpfully considered an inner accompaniment of such speech as expresses it.

If I ask you to repeat the sentence 'A donkey loaded with bags of salt had to wade across a river' first with, and then without, thought, it isn't clear what you're to do.[11] Perhaps we mobilize more mental imagery in the former case, or furrow our brow a little more, but since such images and furrowings may themselves occur with or without thought, and are themselves hardly self-interpreting, this helps not at all. Or perhaps the thought is supposed to consist in a sentence 'spoken in the mind'? Yet when we express thought out loud we aren't aware of pronouncing any such parallel sentences *in foro interno*. And in any case, inner utterances may themselves be undertaken with or without understanding.

Bleuler may tell his attendants 'The proper functioning of the asylum depends on everyone playing their part, attending thoughtfully to their duties, and trying carefully to understand their patients' unique personalities.' Babette, however, tells us that 'Station for station must keep its proper governmental position so that existence-questions of the ward cannot be chosen to hide themselves behind, all things can be chosen.' To understand Bleuler's utterance as expressing the thought it does, we're not required to infer any particular process going on in him either before or whilst he speaks. It expresses clear thought, but such expression isn't helpfully compared to the way in which, say, a translation does justice to what it translates, or a picture to what it depicts. His thought is not simply identical with his discourse, but neither is it some other thing separable from it in the way texts are from their translations or scenes are from their pictorial representations. For, far from it naming an inner state or process, talk of Bleuler's 'clear thought' references his talking intelligibly (we know what to do with what he says, how to respond to it, how to paraphrase it, etc.), his uttering assertions with clear implications and negations, etc. The thought characterizes his discourse; it's not something separate the occurrence of which we infer on being presented with an as-it-were intrinsically thought-less utterance. In this respect it stands to his talk rather as his taking care does to his driving (when what he's driving with is care), or as his tone of voice does to his speaking.[12] Babette's discourse, by contrast, fails to express clear thought. And here too this isn't something we infer on the basis of her unclear utterance.[13] Instead, her thought disorder is to be met with right there, in her discourse itself. We don't know what to do with her talk, can't really see what it entails, wouldn't know how to paraphrase it, and whilst (as we shall see later in this chapter, and in Chapter 9) it may reveal much by way of Babette's psychology, it doesn't convey much by way of speaker's meaning. Her discourse is accordingly to be counted thought-disordered not because of a disruption of putative thinking processes somehow behind it, but rather because it doesn't itself conform to the pattern of true thought – much as moving the rook diagonally in chess is to be counted a failure not because of what causes it but rather because it doesn't conform to the rules of the game.

Because both pundits and critics often take for granted that what's disordered in thought disorder is an inner process, complaints are often lodged against the very notion of 'thought disorder'. Thus talk of 'thought disorder' allegedly: invites us to make unsafe inferences from what's observable to what lies within;[14] imposes a spurious unity upon what truly are diverse phenomena;[15] frames mere pseudo-explanations of the cause of overtly disordered discourse;[16] and encourages us, in talking of 'thought', to deploy 'a philosophical term' which is to 'be avoided in scientific writing'.[17] The response to such objections has hitherto either been to attempt a defence of the concept of thought disorder[18] or to replace it with allegedly more precise and safer notions (dyslogia, dysphasia, disorders of thinking and language and communication, and speech dysfunction).[19]

Against such complaints and responses we may note that we shall only be talking here of, say, dysphasic speech (i.e. speech with abnormalities in flow, syntax, semantics, and pragmatics) if what's said fails to readily convey cogent thought, and that in studying the linguistic aberrance we shall ipso facto be studying deformations of the subject's thought. The kinds of speech and writing disturbances that inspire a diagnosis of thought disorder are not of a sort that can be investigated in abstraction from the meaningfulness of what's said or written. Yet to talk of meaning is already – in the sense of 'thought' that's relevant here – to talk of thought, just as describing lapses into meaninglessness is to describe someone's failings as a thinker. We may insist, too, that 'thought' is not primarily 'a philosophical term' but rather a perfectly everyday one (a child who sulks 'but I thought we were getting ice-cream!' betrays thereby no philosophical tendencies). Furthermore, we may register that 'thought disorder' was never intended as an efficient cause-citing explanation (and hence is not well considered a circular explanation), but only as a characterization, of disordered discourse: the discourse being that which can no longer be brought under such descriptions as ascribe cogent and reality-oriented thoughts to the speaking or writing subject. This thwarting of our standing ambition to find meaningful what we humanly encounter also explains the unity of the concept, which accordingly has nothing to do with the kind of unity enjoyed by such phenomena as spring from a singular process.[20] Primarily, however, we may insist that nobody here was thinking in terms of inner processes, or any other inner phenomena at all, until the psychologists came along. For such thoughts as are expressed by speech are not aptly portrayed as inner phenomena inferred to obtain on the basis of that speech; instead, they're *abstracta* ascribed to individuals on the basis of what they say and do in particular contexts, how they disambiguate and paraphrase themselves, what they take to be entailed by what they say, etc.[21] And nothing in such diverse ascription conditions suggests that thoughts are well taken to enjoy the kind of reality enjoyed by phenomena. Instead, thought is a good example of an x the nature of which is simply not well approached by asking 'what is an x?' but instead is much better got at through questions like 'what is true of someone if he "is xing"? / if he "has an x"?'[22] Rather than hunt about, then, for the inner process to which 'thinking' (or 'remembering', 'perceiving', etc.) allegedly refers, we instead do better to get at such terms' meanings by considering their apt (non-object-indexing) use.[23]

None of this means that we never do well to predicate cogent thought of he whose discourse is confused. (Perhaps, for example, someone who's had a particular kind of stroke struggles, to his own great annoyance, to convey clear ideas in speech, but can readily write them down.) Even so, far from it being an unargued assumption of the psychiatrist that disorders of communication in schizophrenia manifest disordered thought, the burden of proof instead surely lies on the psychologist or linguist to demonstrate that such communication difficulties are not expressive of disordered thought. What makes it right to say, of she who avows that she's having thoughts that she yet can't voice, that genuine thoughts really are here being had? The answer is that she can write them down or otherwise demonstrate them. At times we might also take her affirmation that a sentence we present to her expresses her thought as enough to forestall our negative judgement as to her having bona fide thoughts. There are, however, important limits to such conceptual largesse: we need to leave room for distinguishing between the person who all along had the thought expressed by that sentence and the person who was previously muddled but became clear on being offered it. (It's not humanly unheard of for someone to claim merely expressive difficulties whilst in truth being quite confused.)[24] In general our rule is that someone who utters confused talk is properly to be considered a confused thinker unless the difficulties can be proved to be merely expressive.

A particularly misleading picture, when used to develop our understanding of formal thought disorder, is that of a thinking subject whose thought may be plotted along two dimensions: the first dimension concerns its 'vertical' fit with the world – the truth or falsity of thoughts; the second – 'horizontal' – dimension concerns how thoughts or their discursive expressions fit rationally one with another. With that picture in place it may be supposed that delusion belongs to the vertical, and thought disorder to the horizontal, dimension. The failings of this (representational) conception of delusion have been canvassed in Chapter 3. But we may also question the value of conceptions of formal thought disorder which characterize it merely in terms of the rational coherence or grammaticality of thought and its expressions. For what such conceptions miss is the *loss of reality contact* of the truly thought-disordered subject. This too is what differentiates thought disorder from aphasia: the aphasic subject's discourse may also be in utter disarray, but nothing in this leads us to diagnose, in the aphasic subject, a loss of reality contact, disturbed reality testing, or a tendency to live in a world of one's own.

The question arises as to why researchers have sometimes tended, despite not having determined it empirically, to moot the possibility of cogent thought underlying schizophrenic discourse. One answer may be the sheer intellectual temptation of the above-described dualistic construals of mind and expression that appear to leave hanging, on some kind of potentially unsafe inference from 'outer' to 'inner', the ascription of disordered thought to him whose discourse is disordered. Another may be that a lack of clinical experience leaves a residual unbelief in the depths of psychotic dislocation. A final answer is that the researchers are motivated by a wish to avoid encountering the terrifying depths of psychotic fragmentation. These last two answers are suggested by the final paragraph of Harold Searles' paper on schizophrenic communication:

> Eight years ago in a research seminar led by Frieda Fromm-Reichmann the question early arose, concerning schizophrenic patients' distorted verbal communications, whether such communications are to be regarded as only a manner of speaking, or whether these are to be heard as reasonably accurate representations of a subjective experience which is actually distorted to such a degree.... [O]ne reason why the therapy of schizophrenia is so complex is that, in the instance of any one patient ... his communications are at one moment toward one end of a scale in this regard, and at another moment, toward the other end....

I have seldom found that a communication initially hard to locate on such a scale proved eventually to have been only a manner of *speaking*; recurrently, instead, I have discovered with awe that the patient's subjective experience is, in a high proportion of instances, as genuinely and terribly distorted – as chaotically fragmented, or rudimentarily differentiated, or bleak, or what-not – as his words suggest.... Becoming able to deal skilfully with schizophrenic communication requires, more than anything else, that one become able to endure seeing, and at least momentarily sharing at a feeling level, the world in which the schizophrenic individual lives.[25]

Yet the truth of this matter cannot be pronounced on in the abstract, for all people and all time, but instead is something to be individually confessed by those who've found themselves tempted in one or another such way.

Thought disorder and sociality

A deep psychiatric intuition has it that thought disorder somehow reflects a disturbed ability to relate – to be truly encountered by other people and to truly encounter them in their otherness. Thought disorder – at least as it obtains in schizophrenia – is, thus understood, another manifestation of that autism which has its sufferer residing in a world of his own, failing to make meaningful contact with his fellow humans.[26]

One (cataphatic) formulation of this intuition makes the problem one of presentation: Babette's thoughts may be coherent in themselves, but she's struggling to package them in a manner suitable for uptake by her interlocutors.[27] If, for example, she misjudges what Jung or Bleuler could realistically be expected to already know about that which she's discussing, then she may fail to provide them with adequate antecedents for her pronouns and adverbs, or fail to tell them the meaning of such words as are her own coinages. (Perhaps she says 'we went to buy by there and the stockingstockers were all closed so we got then a train to the centre to find one open', failing to grasp that they couldn't be expected to already know that she's talking about a hunt for an open hosiery first near the station and then on the high street.)

A difficulty for this formulation, however, is that it isn't mindful of the above-described requirement that criteria must be demonstrably met before we can reasonably say, of some stretch of incomprehensible discourse, that it's an inadequate expression of what nevertheless are cogent thoughts.[28] The disturbance we meet in the thought-disordered subject is, however, no mere mistake or failure of judgement. This subject is not one who says 'Oh silly me, I didn't realize you'd only walked in mid-conversation', or 'Oh, I'd forgotten you weren't there at the time', or 'Oh I was sure I'd already told you my silly name for a hosier's shop.' Far from it being apt to describe her as making faulty assumptions about what her listener understands, what we find instead is someone whose form of mindedness rather precludes the very idea of having a listener at all. In short, the (apophatic) suggestion now on the table is that our sociality – i.e. our capacity for interpersonal engagement, or ability to meet others as others, including our capacity to respect one another's semantic needs in conversation – is, just like our discourse itself, similarly to be understood as essential to thought, and is not merely a mediating factor in discourse's production.

This can be harder to grasp than the consideration that thought is co-constitutive of, rather than antecedent and external to, discourse. But just as that latter consideration is best appreciated by thinking on such thought as is immanent within everyday speech, so too do we best grasp the significance of sociality to thought by thinking on our spontaneous meaningful social interaction. So here I am, rather unreflectively chatting with my neighbour, talking over the events of the day. We've updated one another about the antics of the bats roosting in his chimney, and now are negotiating our different takes on what's to be done about the haphazard refuse collection. Scarcely ever, in the course of this conversational drift, have I cause to ponder on what he means by what he says or on how I must phrase what I say so as to best enable his comprehension of it. And when occasionally I do have cause thus to ponder, the questions I raise within myself are themselves framed in terms provided by the deeper certainties of our connection (just as, say, my wondering where I put my shoes is predicated on my certainty that I have some). An individualistic conception of the self and its cognition may inspire a conception of us as first and foremost enjoying go-it-alone cogitations, yet lucky or inferentially diligent enough to enjoy sufficient correlation in these with those of others for the achievement of mutual comprehension. Yet nothing in the actual individuation of ordinary thoughts – those that are properly ascribed to both my neighbour and I in our bat chat, for example – warrants such a picture's application. Using, as a model for the having of thought, the rarefied and solitary experience of, say, reading or writing an academic text on psychopathology, proves utterly misleading to the extent that the umbilical connection of such thought to the prior participatory contexts of our lives remains obscured. But what consideration of the originary situations in which thought obtains instead shows is that thought's flesh is discourse, that the originary home of discourse is the conversation, and that conversations are had between those in such communion as is itself thought's condition of possibility.[29]

When thinking philosophically about thought's preconditions, it's natural and proper to emphasize those quite general matters wherein we commune: an environment, a language, traditions and customs – along with what we have in common, albeit not conjointly: bodies, instincts, sensorimotor capacities, etc. What, however, is here at issue is that which is always particular, namely my constantly updated attunement right now to my neighbour, at this – and then this – point in this conversation, a conversation arising at this point in our shared history of conversations. My capacity for conversation-sustaining synchrony manifests in my non-reflective grip: on who I am and who he is, on who's to speak now, on who just said what, on what is and isn't now pertinent to say, on what may now be taken for granted, etc.[30] Yet such a grip shows itself not primarily as a content of my thought (it would be but an absurdity, itself inviting psychiatric diagnosis, if I were to go about thinking 'I'm this one here, he's that one over there; he just spoke so it's now my turn; etc.'[31]) but in what I say and more generally in the weft of my discourse. This grip shows up, that is, in the constancy and integration of my responses, in my consistent readiness for certain responses from him, in my apt turn-taking, in my deploying words already in common usage (i.e. not using neologisms), in my deploying words in accordance with their common meaning (i.e. not using 'stock' words), and in general by conforming to such norms of correct usage as render my linguistic impulses meaningfully accountable. In fact my grip on who's who is here nothing distinct from my being a distinct self, such distinctness itself being achieved through a lifetime of enactive interactions with others who share enough by way of a common culture and language to make such enactions possible. In such interactions self and other receive their definition, and the interactions themselves receive corollary definition as moments of thought-replete conversation.

Consider the following, from Harry Stack Sullivan's *Clinical Studies in Psychiatry*:

> [S]ince the referential processes [in schizophrenia] are of a distinctly less focused, less precise character, meaning spreads widely [in] the ... universe of the schizophrenic. Correspondingly, because there is not the neat but often treacherous distinction between *thee* and *me* ..., the boundary between the patient and the universe, particularly the personal universe, undergoes the same diffusion.... If all of us were not able to achieve this very diffusion, this loss of boundaries, in our states of reverie or brown study, we would not get some of our sudden, wonderfully useful hunches. But the point is that the schizophrenic tries to communicate in these terms, while most of us never even know that we sometimes think in them. And when the schizophrenic tries to communicate in this way, it sounds as if he has become involved in the whole universe ...[32]

One of the reasons we might struggle to accept Sullivan's conclusion is our cleaving to the idea that conversation inexorably results from already having something to say. Like the above-critiqued notion of thought as inner phenomenon, this idea can suggest to us that talk is the causal product of thought, and so would cease if thought ceased. But we have only to encounter a fluent aphasic (who, because of acquired brain damage, cheerfully talks unwitting gibberish) or someone high on crystal meth, or for that matter simply to eavesdrop on various conversations down the pub, to know that this truly isn't the case. Much talk is, after all, a product of associations to interlocutors' utterances, which associations are at best subject to the inhibition of embarrassing content before being socially unleashed.[33] Meaningful thought requires that one be able to pay attention to the conversation and its context – to what has already been said by whom, to what the topic is, etc. – and is essential before one can graduate from *homo loquens* to *homo sapiens*.[34] And one of the functions of such attention is to continually differentiate oneself as attender from that to which one attends – namely to other people, objects, and situations. Lose what it provides by way of perceptual and cognitive structuration, and one's selfhood (and correlatively one's discourse) begins to disintegrate – which is why it starts to sound as if the schizophrenic subject 'has become involved in the whole universe'.

Consider again that response to Aesop's fable about the donkey and the sponges provided by the above-quoted schizophrenic subject:

> A donkey was carrying salt and he went through a river ... so he crawled out on the other side and became a mastodon ... it gets unfrozen ... it's up in the Arctic right now ... it's a block of ice ... ever studied that sort of a formation, block of ice

in the ground? ... well, it fights the permafrost ... it pushes it away ... and lets
things go up around it ... you can see they're like, they're almost like a pattern with
a flower ... they start from the middle ...[35]

About this one commentator writes: 'The speaker provides no antecedent for 'they'.
Apparently, he assumes that the listener already knows who or what they are. Possibly
he had snowflakes in mind.'[36] It's by way of contrast with this proposal that the
contention now on the table may be understood. The failure in the patient's sense of
what 'the listener already knows' is not a cause of his failing to adequately articulate
something (a definite thought about snowflakes) that he has in mind, but is rather
partly constitutive of his failing to have a coherent thought in mind in the first place.
Furthermore, the failure of interpersonal understanding here encountered amounts
not so much to a faulty assumption as to a disruption of that unreflective social
attunement necessary for entering into the space of conversation (i.e. into language-in-
use) and thereby into the space of thought itself. Or call it 'faulty assumption' if you
must. But don't let that prevent you from keeping alive the distinction between i) failing
to appreciate that someone else has a different perspective than you do on something
and ii) failing to so much as bring this someone else into view – and thereby also to
constitute oneself, as such, in contradistinction to this someone else – in the first place.

In sum: considered simply by themselves the utterances of he who makes mere
mistakes about what another knows, and the utterances of she who fails to even engage
with another as an other, may sometimes look remarkably similar. It's no doubt just this
similarity that can tempt the (cataphatically minded) psychologist or linguist into
proposing that thought-disordered discourse results from a failure to grasp what an
interlocutor does and doesn't already know and understand.[37] The effect of this,
however, is to assimilate a disturbance that truly bespeaks a catastrophic disintegration
of thought and subjectivity to something like an everyday form of obtuseness. It's by
instead holding true to an apophatic line – i.e. to a line which doesn't envisage the
continued applicability of such schemes of explanation as presuppose the intactness of
subject-hood and meaning, but which instead grasps that such schemes are here
precisely what have been rendered inapplicable – that we do the better justice to the
depths of psychotic fragmentation in the thought-disordered subject. And it's thereby
that we stand the chance of offering her a more genuine recognition in her brokenness.

Thought disorder and emotion

The communicative chaos we meet with in thought-disordered discourse thwarts such
of our empathic endeavours as aim to retrieve rationally intelligible content from it. It
prevents, that is, our predicating of it that kind of intelligibility sought by (but denied
to) Jaspers in the discursive products of an overtly psychotic subject.[38] Yet far from
stymieing the pursuit of other forms of understanding, such a disruption of discourse's
rational intelligibility can even provide a logical precondition for the meaningful
application of such forms of understanding, since a mind in good rational order simply
repels attempts to explain its functioning in what might be called 'psychological' rather

than 'rational' terms. I'm going to the shop. Why? Well, we've run out of milk. My reasons for so acting may of course be several (perhaps I'm also seeking respite from my vexatious housemate). But the action they make rationally intelligible can't also be explained by reference to an unconscious emotion or motive (my unconscious attraction to the shopkeeper, say) unless that explanation also shows up what I offer for reasons as unconvincing rationalizations. Absent such a disturbance of rationality, and such psychological explanations have their permit revoked.[39] What they reference (my unconscious attraction) may be perfectly apt, but without the failure of reason we shall find it hard to bring them into a truly explanatory relation to the action. It is, then, precisely when we do meet with disturbances of rational intelligibility that the search for psychological rather than rational understanding may proceed.

In a brief commentary on such approaches to thought disorder as would make of it merely a neurocognitive dysfunction, Manfred Bleuler rehearses the

> old clinical observation that schizophrenic language (just like schizophrenic thinking and behavior) is not stable. In many patients it undergoes astonishing changes. One patient may speak in a very dissociated way that is difficult to understand, but the same patient may write letters as good as those of a healthy person. Another schizophrenic may speak in a clear and coherent way to me but in a very incoherent and peculiar way to his relatives.... The inconstancy of schizophrenic symptoms is hard to observe if one only deals with schizophrenics for a restricted number of hours during psychopathological research. It is easy to observe, however, when one lives under the same roof with schizophrenics for decades.[40]

The question then arises as to why the thought-disordered subject sometimes ends up in her distinctive state of cognitive disarray. Two answers to this may be distinguished in the psychological literature on thought disorder's relation to emotional distress. The first of these has it that the psychotic subject's thought sometimes *falls* apart under the impact of disruptive emotion. The second has it that the psychotic subject *takes* apart her thought – i.e. that thought disorder is sometimes motivated by a wish to avoid unbearable emotion. The second answer will be considered in the following section, but it's worth mentioning here that these answers are not mutually exclusive. And in fact what I will call these 'causal' and 'motivational' relations between emotion and thought disorder obtain not only together, but also alongside the 'symbolic' relation (see Chapter 9). It's by way of attending to these three dimensions of psychotic thought that the psychiatrist becomes able to tune into what has been dubbed the 'psychotic wavelength'.[41]

To begin to understand the first – causal – answer we may consider our everyday experience of thinking difficulties. For who hasn't had the experience of struggling to think and speak clearly, or even at all, when under extreme pressure, highly anxious, or otherwise out of sorts? We call this being 'discombobulated' or 'lost for words', and by bringing both our cognitive disarray and moments of mental paralysis under such descriptions we elevate the causal relations between them and our emotional disquiet into conceptual relations.

Let's consider this in relation to Babette Straub. This institutionalized seamstress, with whom we introduced this chapter, was in fact one of the earliest patients of the newly qualified Dr Carl Jung who joined her at the Burghölzli asylum in the early twentieth century. At that time Jung was so reclusive, and so maniacal in his studies, that his colleagues assumed he was himself either psychotic or melancholic.[42] What he was busy developing, however, was a psychological understanding of schizophrenic thought, one that applied the principles of Freud's new psychoanalytic theories of hysteria and dreaming to Bleuler's schizophrenic patients. His first (1907) monograph – *On the Psychology of Dementia Praecox*, the fifth chapter of which is devoted to Babette – was the result.

Babette, Jung tells us, usually speaks in a normal manner: 'Her speech is changed only in the spheres of her delusions . . . She repeats what she reads and defines ideas in a clear manner, insofar as they do not touch her complex.' But when her complexes are activated, Babette experiences thought blockage (long pauses in speech which she articulates as 'thought deprivations') and her discourse loses its rational form (whenever 'the relations between emotional life and ideation are disturbed . . . a thought-process akin to flight of ideas is bound to develop').[43] Jung's findings have been echoed by more recent studies showing schizophrenic subjects to manifest a far greater degree of disordered thought when asked to talk about emotionally distressing matters than when invited to discourse on pleasant, unstressful topics.[44]

Unlike the ordinarily discombobulated speaker, however, the thought-disordered subject may manifest her incoherence in the absence of other straightforward indices of emotional disturbance. In such cases she neither avows distress nor straightforwardly betrays it with her tone; as Jung says of Babette, her delusional and disordered thought is presented 'with marked want of emotion', and is more affected than affective. The question arises then as to what the criteria are which govern the judgement that Babette is in some sense yet emotionally disturbed. By way of answer we may cite not only her topic-relative incoherence and thought blocking, but also her apparent lack of emotional reaction itself. Such an answer might at first seem tendentious, but when what we're encountering is a topically incongruous affective display, alongside signs of discombobulation or being lost for words, the matter can be seen in a different light. The situation is, after all, not one in which Babette displays merely less emotion than expected, but rather one in which she evinces no affect, or speaks in an incongruously affected manner one in which she displays either no or a 'fresh' affect. In and of itself such incongruity can reasonably be taken to indicate something 'being up with' her, and especially when we consider it alongside topic-relative incoherence and blocking it's hard to see it as other than an index of emotional disturbance.[45] And such an index, it should be noted, is not something we merely correlate with an independently assayable reading of emotional experience; it instead is that emotion's expression. For this reason the first thing we notice when we've tuned into the psychotic wavelength is the emotional pain that can now be seen in disturbed utterance or writing.[46]

In the previous section we looked at such disturbed social relatedness in schizophrenics as is evident to others. But the key human drama for the schizophrenic subject himself is often articulated as having to do with the tension between his desire for companionable closeness, belonging, and recognition on the one hand and his desire for the safety of distance, eccentricity, and undecipherability on the other – or his giving up on the former to opt for the latter.[47] What remains of this chapter shall therefore consider the extent to which the form of thought-disordered talk may be considered motivated by the subject's concerns about being met with for who he is.

A suggestion encountered in the phenomenological literature has it that thought disorder is a function of the psychotic subject's quite general motivation to avoid human connection.[48] This literature also suggests that sometimes thought-disordered discourse reflects indifference to the semantic needs of listeners. Yet it also qualifies both suggestions: both wilfulness and indifference may be at least partly feigned: if my capacity to remain self-same and rational whilst relating to others is compromised – perhaps on account of endogenous (maturational) factors – then I shall be ongoingly motivated to avoid or attempt control of such encounters. (Thus does biology segue into biography.) Or I may conveniently re-describe my fear-based failures in social relating as a wish-based rejection of a way of life that I now disparage (i.e. I may deploy the defence Nietzsche called 'ressentiment').[49] Language itself may now appear to me as an oppressive conformist system which I'd do well to resist. And just as patterns of defence settle over time into reflexive and enduring aspects of normal/neurotic character, so too may defensive instincts to beat an autistic retreat settle over time into irretrievable aspects of a chronic schizophrenic state. (Thus does biography sediment into biology.)

When we turn to the psychoanalytical literature we find not so much a focus on the general character of the thought-disordered subject's linguistic relations with others, but instead a focus on particular emotionally significant thoughts. And here the thought-disordered subject is sometimes presented as attacking his own extant capacity to represent (attend to, judge, think about) what to him is emotionally intolerable.[50]

As an example of how an idiosyncratic way with words can subserve the thought-disordered subject's self-protective ends, consider Christine's response, during an inpatient group meeting, when the diagnosis of schizophrenia – her own diagnosis – came up for discussion. Until this point her speech had been clearly intelligible and relevant, but at the mention of 'schizophrenia' she related, in a manner that seemed forceful, cheerful, and brittle all at the same time, that she knew perfectly well what it meant: 'S is for skill, C for coping, H for happiness, I for important, Z for being zealously on guard', etc. Christine did not appear to be being playful, or to be engaged in political subversion of oppressive psychiatric labels. Her affect was superficially breezy, yet her casual and unchallengeable dismantling of 'schizophrenia' was thought-stopping for the group. Intolerable meaning – that of a (to her) unbearably shameful diagnosis – was replaced, by autistic fiat, with a distracting and grandiose acrostic. Her utterance was at one and the same time thought-disordered and delusional. It took leave from consensually understood meaning, replacing it – at just that juncture when the terrible fate of her mind was, in effect, under discussion – with something utterly idiosyncratic. Christine would now brook no reasoned engagement, insisting with manic ferocity on the legitimacy of her lexical dismantling. As a result those present felt themselves to be on the edge of a precipice below which was the unthinkable.

One of the signs that Jung came to see as revelatory of the triggering of one of Babette's complexes was her speaking in a stilted manner. Another was her use of neologisms which she herself termed 'power words'. What they were able to do for her, it seems, was to help foster a delusional sense of control. Thus Babette frequently pronounces, in an affected manner, 'I am the double polytechnic irretrievable', or tells us that she lives in the 'double polytechnic' (of both dressmaking and baking) which, as it's a government building, belongs to her. Yet she cannot be brought to see any incongruity between her both being something and living in it. She also proclaims that she both is and has 'the master key' – i.e. the key to the Burghölzli asylum where she lives, the asylum which she also owns since she is 'the threefold world proprietress'. Furthermore, she's 'the finest professorship', 'the Lorelei', 'Schiller's Bell', 'the finest Turkey', etc. On the one hand it's easy to see these as grandiose delusions, compensations for the shattering feelings of worthlessness she feels as an asylum patient. On the other hand we can also see formal thought disorder at play in her both being and owning the master key, the asylum, etc. Her *ownership* gives her a sense of importance amongst people, a sense which is otherwise tragically lacking in her life; her *being* the same phenomena enables her to ward off the fear that they could be taken from her.

Notable too is Babette's nonsensical use of 'affirm' (and 'establish') in a manner that collapses together its two meanings. Babette 'affirms the master-key as my property', she 'establishes a payment', 'affirms the mightiest silver island in the world', etc. Here she demonstrates what Freud called the 'omnipotence of thought' – i.e. the belief, if we may even call it that, that 'thinking makes it so'. To the end of evading her suffering she blurs the distinction between the use of such verbs for the making of empirical judgements and for the unassailable avowal of declarations. She stresses the former when she's positioning herself in consensual reality, and the latter when she fears a threat to her judgement and so retreats to an omnipotent position. Thought is thereby bent out of rational shape, but an illusion of status is nevertheless fostered, one that keeps at bay her sense of worthlessness. Babette is also able to deal magically with her *distress* (the German for which is *Not*) by exercising her right, as thrice world proprietress, to manufacture *notes* in a bank*note* factory: 'banknotes to alleviate the greatest distress' ('Noten für Linderung der größten Not'). As Jung suggests, here a dreamlike condensation of thought appears to obtain through the sound association of *Not*.

Jung's attempts to ask Babette to explain her neologisms and stock words (Groundpostament, I am the Lorelei and Schiller's Bell, crown, universal, conclusion, oleum, Hufeland, amphi, etc.) result in 'a total failure, for she immediately produced a series of fresh neologisms which resembled a word salad'.[51] But by inviting her to associate to them he is at least able to grasp something of what her use of them is doing for her. He can begin to grasp their psychological function, that is, even if her phrases yet want for speaker's meaning. Words now become used not as means of interpersonal communication but as means for operating on the mind, sealing over such associative pathways as would otherwise lead a subject toward topics too painful for her, their use warding off pain in talismanic fashion.[52] Thus another patient endlessly repeated 'Eseamarrieder', the repetition simultaneously registering and deflecting her awareness from the devastating recognition of that which the term contracts: 'He's a married man'.[53] Such words serve to contain the intolerable affect associated with the recognition, and to thereby make life liveable, but at the same time they bury the real meaning with their incoherence. And so too with the knight's moves, blockages, and general disarray of psychotic discourse: all of this serves to steer the mind away from a recognition of that which can't be tolerated.

As will be recalled from Chapter 1, mental illness can essentially involve not only mental suffering but also an impairment to reason driven by the motivated avoidance of that suffering. We're now in a position to see how not only delusion but also thought disorder constitute paradigmatic symptoms of mental illness. For whilst some of the mentally ill subject's disordered thoughts may arise merely from a schizotaxic disposition which in itself is no illness, some may arise from a breakdown caused by suffering, some may be products of a mind which is in retreat from a painful world, and some may even constitute attacks on the recognition of reality. And to return briefly to a topic raised earlier, it's in terms of these relations to suffering and its motivated avoidance that formal thought disorder may be distinguished from aphasia. For whatever the linguistic similarities of certain instances of schizophrenic and aphasic discourse, it's essential to the latter *qua* symptom of an organic disorder that its occurrence not be motivationally intelligible. The pure aphasic possesses an un-tortured innocence that we don't find in the schizophrenic.

Before concluding this survey of thought disorder's causes and ends, the suggestion should also at least be registered that the obscurity of someone's motivated thought-disordered discourse may sometimes arise not simply from his wish for distance but also from his desire for intimacy, or rather be a result of a compromise:

> between his intense desire for, and equally intense fear of, an extraordinarily intimate relationship. It represents an ambivalent desire for the intimacy of a private language, like the language of lovers, whose shared private meanings of words remain obscure to outsiders. But, at the same time, the patient, by his very obscurity, defends against the risk of the intolerable rebuff of someone's understanding him and then refusing his desires.[54]

As with the other motivational readings, what would warrant considering such a suggestion in a particular instance cannot be the disordered discourse considered simply by itself, but rather its behavioural context. Does the ambivalent longing for intimacy manifest itself in how the subject interacts with his interlocutor? Another psychiatrist describes a psychotic inpatient coming into the consulting room, shaking him warmly by the hand, looked piercingly into his eyes, and saying to his doctor: 'I think the sessions are not for a long while but stop me ever going out.' Which is to say: he finds difficult the wait between sessions, whilst also feeling they get in the way of his independence. In case we had any doubt about the ambivalence here in play, the patient's very next association may settle it for us: 'How does the lift know what to do when I press two buttons at once?'[55]

Conclusions

We have considered separately the significance, for disordered thought, of disturbed discourse, sociality, and emotion. The forms of understanding involved were seen to differ. With the first two we saw how the linguistic and social disturbances we encounter in the schizophrenic subject present no mere appearance of disordered thought but rather themselves make for the true rational unrecoverability of her thought. We saw too how falling out of the zone of interpersonal connection can itself be understood as a falling apart of thought. With the third we proceeded not through appreciating the impossibility of rationally retrieving her speaker's meaning, but instead through appreciating how that impossibility itself opens the door to psychology proper. (Where rationality fails, there motivational psychology obtains its permit.) In particular, we saw not only what it is for thought disorder to be a causal product of disturbed feeling, but also how tuning into the psychotic wavelength allows us to see such emotional distress in the disordered discourse. But we also saw that tuning into that wavelength enables us to come to see lapses into thought disorder as motivationally intelligible – i.e. as motivated by a desire to avoid mental pain.

There is much about the form of this motivation that has not been discussed. How should we understand an interaction such as when 'someone with schizophrenia . . . begins to lapse into a formal thought disorder or delusional thinking and, after the clinician says, "I'm sorry, but I don't think we have time for that right now, I really need to know what's been happening to you," . . . snaps back and returns to an accurate narrative description'?[56] Are we to understand this as demonstrating that the man had been *intentionally engaging in* nonsensical thought, or that he was instead *lapsing into* a dreamlike state from which he could nevertheless be recalled? Perhaps the safest thing to say is that all that may be ruled out *a priori* is a reading of his motive which took it as one of his *considerations* (i.e. a reason he 'acted from', an 'agential reason').[57] Whilst we can decide for our own reasons to *talk* nonsense, it's simply not clear what could be meant by our deciding for our own reasons to *think* nonsense. (At best we should be imagining someone who inwardly recites a nonsense poem, or who intentionally takes such drugs as render one irrational.) And if all that we meet with is intentionally nonsensical talk we shall have no reason to talk of thought disorder in the first place. That much the critics of the very idea of thought disorder got right, even whilst failing to understand that disordered talk is properly taken to express disordered thought unless we've positive reasons to suspect thought to here be intact.

Earlier chapters of the book stressed the rational irretrievability of psychotic thought, and suggested that it's only through (apophatically) acknowledging such thought's ununderstandability that we can begin to offer apt acknowledgement to the psychotic subject in her brokenness. The present chapter has begun to consider the character of different – psychological rather than rational – forms of understanding, forms which are only made available by the psychotic subject's failure of reason. Tuning into the psychotic wavelength has been shown to involve both our seeing signs of apparent insouciance as signs of emotional disturbance, and seeing how a defensive, i.e. motivated, avoidance of mental pain can drive disordered thought's proliferation. Such understanding doesn't allow us to after all retrieve speaker's meaning in thought-disordered discourse, but instead enables us to see how it too is an instance of that madness in which, as Schopenhauer put it, the mind seeks refuge from such mental suffering as exceeds its strength. There is, however, a third form of intelligibility beyond the affective and the motivational, one which the literature has often presented as enabling the retrieval of speaker's meaning from psychotic discourse. This has to do with the form of intelligibility enjoyed by 'symbolic' acts, and it's to the 'symbolic' character of psychotic thought that we now turn.

9

Psychotic Symbolization

Introduction

It was at the end of the twentieth century that an elderly schizophrenic woman I shall call Angela told me, on the street in Oxford, that she'd 'just been released from Belsen'. Knowing Bergen-Belsen to have been liberated in 1945, naïvely attempting to retrieve meaning from what otherwise appeared unintelligible, and not yet having had experience with psychotic illness, I took Angela's words for metaphor. I asked her, that is, if she was telling me that she'd experienced her sojourn in the Warneford psychiatric hospital, where she had indeed been staying, as akin to imprisonment in a concentration camp. Her response, which we'll get to below, surprised me. For now I wish to register only that delusional discourse often does appear somehow or other *symbolic* in form, and that the concept of 'metaphor' is indeed often used by psychologists when trying to articulate the sense in which, say, 'incarceration in Belsen' functions as a 'symbol' for involuntary psychiatric detainment. Thus Jung, for example, says of that patient of his we met in the previous chapter – Babette Straub – that when she's in her delusion she 'expresses herself in monstrous, grotesque, distorted metaphors'.[1]

Chapter 8 characterized attunement to the psychotic wavelength as involving a living appreciation not only of how psychotic discourse expresses both emotional experience and its motivated avoidance (that chapter's own topics), but also of how such discourse can *symbolically depict* emotionally charged inner and outer predicaments (the topic of this chapter). What now follows considers the cataphatic temptation to attempt reflective understanding of delusional discourse's symbolic form by treating it, as Jung did with Babette, as discourse from which metaphorical meaning may be retrieved. The argument will be that we achieve the deeper appreciation of what it is to be deluded when we apophatically grasp just how and why delusional discourse resists assimilation to the category of metaphorical speech or writing.

The concept of *symbolism* has been used to characterize psychotic thought at least since Pelletier's 1903 treatise on the association of ideas in mania and dementia praecox.[2] So to begin our investigation, let's attune ourselves to further instances of such psychotic behaviour and talk as inspire mention of symbolization:

[Elena] hallucinated that her mother had complained about her to [Elena's] father; then her father 'looked at her in a very strange way.' He thrust a spear into her lower abdomen, at the same time dancing about in a very peculiar fashion. He was all black and completely nude. He often came to her bed like that, all black; and occasionally he also appeared to her in the form of a bull. [Elena] related that her father had often beaten her – and wanted to abuse her sexually. He often played with her genitalia and must have gone even further. Thus the fear of the father was quite understandable. That the attack with the spear was a sexual one is proved by the completely erotic expression of the patient as she related the hallucination which, in its contents, gave no such direct evidence apart from the frequent occurrence of such things in sexual contexts. While [Elena] related her tale, she hid her face with a guilty embarrassed laugh. When she spoke of the real attacks on her by her father she showed the same attitude that a healthy person would have; her tone of voice was objective, somewhat embarrassed, but not with active eroticism.[3]

Ms R, 32 years old and with a diagnosis of schizophrenia ... presented in a child-like way and had a habit of taking all of her clothes off. The ... other patients found this sort of behaviour upsetting, and the nursing staff were becoming exasperated.... The primary nurse said that the patient lived at home with her parents and spent long periods of time on her own, alone in her bedroom. She had shown very little capacity to stick to any education since her late teens or to hold down a job. However, her father still believed she was capable of getting a job and getting married. The ward manager said that the father was a dominant character who believed that his daughter should 'pull herself together and find a husband and a job'. The primary nurse added that the patient expressed a delusional belief that 'a large man is sitting on top of my head', and that this was reported by Ms R in a flat, lifeless way, devoid of any emotion.... My interpretation was that the man sitting on Ms R's head was her father, who was crushing her with his expectations of normal development, which she did not feel able to meet. She experienced her father as trying to force her into a marriage or a job because of his own preoccupations and anxieties. The situation was re-enacted on the ward as the staff team were trying to push the patient to progress with her treatment before really understanding her underlying difficulties. Ms R. was protesting against these expectations by stripping off and demanding that people look at her.... I suggested to the ... nursing team that they convey to Ms R that they understood her need for someone to see her and take her seriously ... [and] to explore her anxieties about being forced into a job or marriage, and to explain that they understood that Ms R felt under pressure to fit in with the ward's demands for progress, as with her parents' expectations.... The following week, the team presented Ms R again, saying that there had been a marked improvement both in her behaviour and in her mental state.[4]

[Jonas, a] masturbating hebephrenic, who desired normal sexual intercourse, finds a high peak in a mountain range so shocking that he gets into a fight with his companion and has to return home. This is an analogy which can hardly be called pathological. But what is certainly pathological is his interpretation of the analogy in the sense of the real sexual organ and the correspondingly violent reaction.[5]

In all these cases, and many others, we find ourselves wanting to say that one thought (a man thrusting a spear at one's groin; a mountain peak; another man sitting on one's head) somehow 'stands for' or is a 'symbol' for another (a sexual act; a sexual organ or secondary sexual characteristic such as a breast; being emotionally oppressed). Rather than presume a meaning for the word 'symbol' and then ask whether the above-described cases are properly thought of as involving symbolization, what follows will take the term 'symbol' to be, in one of its uses, in the business of registering *whatever* it is that such cases involve. The question then arises: how shall we reflectively understand this 'symbolization'?

Delusional expression as metaphoric

A popular suggestion in the psychological literature has it that the delusional symbol may be understood as a metaphor.[6] Now, the literal sense of 'metaphor' is that of a figurative deployment of language by which a speaker refers directly to one matter by referencing another to which the metaphorical expression is literally applied. 'She gave him a frosty smile': here we transfer connotations from what rhetoricians call the vehicle (or figure, or source; i.e. the frosty weather) to the tenor (or ground, or target; i.e. the emotional expression). Metaphor use belongs to the *ars rhetorica* – i.e. it essentially describes a technique used by a speaker or author to encourage and finesse a listener's grasp of speaker's meaning. Thus we may tell of someone uncritically accepting what someone else says, but by using gustatory metaphors – 'He had her eating out of the palm of his hand', 'She was lapping up/swallowing everything he said' – we provide a more potent sense of the power relations at play, showing how the eager listener's loss of self-possession and willing neediness figures into the readiness with which what he says takes root in her mind.

An important precondition for the intelligible description of a speaker's talk as metaphoric is that he in some way grasp the distinction between (what we, if not he, call) the vehicle and the tenor. There must be a fact of the matter regarding what he's *actually* talking about, and it's his prerogative to say what this is. (He's not actually talking about eating out of another's hands, but instead about someone uncritically and cravenly believing what she's told.) Further, if he somehow thought that to swallow or lap something up simply meant to accept it uncritically, and had no understanding of its literal gustatory sense, then it would be at least debatable whether we should consider him to be speaking metaphorically. For not only does the concept of the *metaphorical* presuppose the concept of the *literal* to which it is (through contrastive application) conceptually related, but a proper application of the concept of metaphorical speech would seem to require that the speaker can himself acknowledge that, when he's deploying a phrase we take to express a metaphor, he's not here to be taken literally. Yet it's with respect to just this issue that we encounter the faltering of the idea that delusional discourse may be understood as expressive of metaphor.

When I asked Angela if she was, with her mention of Belsen, meaning to say that being sectioned to the psychiatric hospital was for her like incarceration in a concentration camp, she looked baffled, became somewhat disturbed, and hesitantly said 'It *was* Belsen?' before quickly changing the subject. This surprised me since at that time I'd had very little experience of such matters. Yet her response is in fact just what the psychopathological literature would have us expect; for while it's often suggested there that delusion can be understood as metaphor, we at least as often find the suggestion that, when a delusional subject is in her delusion, we can no longer distinguish literal from metaphorical uses of her terms as they occur in the delusion's articulation. Or, as the psychoanalytic literature has it, delusion involves a failure of symbolism proper and the ascendancy instead of 'symbolic equation' – so that 'concrete' delusional thought now in some sense conflates the symbol with what it symbolizes.[7] (My question to Angela, we might say, itself contained within it all that's wrong with a theory of delusion as metaphor: I took her to be using metaphor, but her psychotic state itself obviated any description of her discourse here as either literal or metaphoric.) The question that arises now, however, is: what makes it apt to still talk of symbols and what they symbolize when the person whose discourse contains such symbols has, when she's in her delusion, a compromised capacity for symbolic thought?

At this point two rescue strategies for the 'delusion as metaphor' conception present themselves.[8] The first locates the making of the metaphor at a time *before* the psychotic collapse of the would-be vehicle and would-be tenor sets in. To borrow a clinical example: a patient seemed at first to be using a concept of 'devil possession' in a non-literal way – perhaps to describe her experience of being out of mental control – but then became psychotic, at which point the metaphor collapsed into the literal locution – i.e. now she suffered the delusion that she was possessed by a devil.[9] In this approach the retrieval of speaker's meaning which we're hoping to effect involves back-extrapolation to a time before delusion sets in. Whilst she may not now be saying something which can intelligibly be taken as metaphor, what she says yet carries the trace of a metaphor she once used – and so could once acknowledge herself to be using – in her own thinking.

One difficulty with this proposal is that, regardless of its adequacy in meeting its own aetiological ends, it doesn't help us with our ambition of retrieving the delusional speaker's meaning; in fact, it asserts that what is being said isn't now intelligible as metaphor. A second is that many delusions involve figurations that don't precede the psychotic state; we often meet not with erstwhile yet now-collapsed metaphor, but rather with some kind of occurrent disturbance in symbolization which yet requires theorization. This is particularly the case when what we have to do with are the delusional perceptions of schizophrenia – i.e. when someone looking at the cross suddenly sees that he himself is Jesus, or looking at the dog raise its leg 'just knows' that the Kaiser has a special message for her, etc. The principal objection to this rescued metaphor theory is then not to its content but to its scope: in saving intelligibility by invoking pre-delusional metaphor use, the theory doesn't yet help us grasp a sense in which delusional figurations can themselves, whether or not historically preceded by topically relevant metaphoric thinking, be understood symbolically.

A second rescue strategy for the 'delusion as metaphor' conception would have us carry over the concept of *metaphor* from its home ground of intentional human utterance and the *ars rhetorica* to deploy it instead for a subconscious mental process studied by the science of psychology.[10] 'Metaphor' is in effect now deployed in a metaphorical sense, and becomes the name of something that happens to one, rather than a rhetorical device one deploys – not something one chooses, but something that (metaphorically speaking) chooses us.[11] Since on this conception we're no longer to unpack the notion of metaphorical meaning by reference to what a speaker intends, it becomes difficult to know what now shall determine what counts as vehicle and what as tenor. Yet let that pass, and suppose that the distinction between vehicle and tenor may somehow be effected post hoc by the theorist independently of the speaker's meaning. The difficulty now will of course be that we can no longer retrieve such meaning as we do when, puzzled by that which, when taken literally, appears nonsensical, we grasp that our speaker was instead speaking both metaphorically and cogently. Furthermore, the psychologist's metaphor – of a 'subconscious metaphorical process' which alters the form of the psychotic subject's thought – now hangs in the air alongside that still un-theorized notion of 'psychological symbolism' which we'd been hoping it would unpack for us.

Delusion and the pre/trans fallacy

Let's recap. The narrator who uses metaphor ('She gave him a frosty smile') knowingly makes play across the domains of vehicle (frosty weather) and tenor (emotional expression). This knowledge manifests itself not so much in any prior intention, formulated *in foro interno*, to use a particular rhetorical device, but in a range of dispositional facts and capacities: our speaker acknowledges when asked that she's here speaking metaphorically, shows appreciation of the difference between talk about the weather and about emotional displays, recognizes that she's here speaking of expressions rather than of weather, etc.[12] Yet the thought of he who is psychotic loses this quality of being clearly either literal or metaphoric. The sane subject who is feeling wretched may express his experience in metaphoric talk of 'having a dark cloud hanging over' him; the psychotic subject, however, hallucinates or delusionally believes that a dark grey cloud follows him around. (Something rather similar appears to characterize our dream life.) In psychopathology we readily recognize this, and dignify it with terms like 'concrete symbolism' or 'symbolic equation'. Our question, however, is how we shall reflectively understand what such phrases intend.

   To begin to answer this in an apophatic mode, consider what's wrong with saying, as we surely may well be tempted to say, that the just-described psychotic subject who deploys 'concrete symbolism' is taking literally what the non-psychotic subject takes metaphorically. Such a description of the situation with the psychotic subject suffers what we've seen in other chapters – namely the trivialization of an ontological disturbance (i.e. a disruption to the very selfhood of the psychotic subject) by redescribing it as a merely epistemic failing (i.e. as some kind of error made by this subject about a matter of fact). Whilst it's clear what's meant by talk of not realizing that someone else is talking metaphorically, it's not clear what's meant by talk of not realizing that one is oneself deploying metaphor.[13] Or at least: we might be able to think of specific instances in which that would be an apt thing to say – as when someone has become so inured to a metaphor that its status as such never strikes her. (Thus are dead metaphors born.) But the subjects in such instances enjoy what the delusional subject fails to manifest, namely a continued capacity to mean one's words in either a metaphorical or a literal sense. Whereas it's in the nature of psychotic discourse that it can no longer be categorized using the either/or of metaphorical or literal.

This apophatic analysis also provides us with an error theory explaining why theorists are prone to misread concrete symbolism as a form of metaphor. For if we look merely at the sentences spoken by a delusional subject ('a dark cloud hangs over me') we notice nothing about their form which demarcates them from sanely spoken metaphorical locutions. It's only when we situate these sentences in the mouths of sane or psychotic speakers that we come to appreciate the difference of delusional from literal discourse. When a subject's reality-testing is insecure, fragile, or collapsed, an important range of conceptual distinctions no longer finds ready application to his thought and experience. These include the metaphorical vs. the literal, the imagined vs. the perceived, the sacred vs. the profane, the playful vs. the serious, wishing vs. enjoying, inner vs. outer, etc.[14] At first glance, however, the difference between she who knowingly makes play across such categories and she for whom they have collapsed may not be apparent. The fallacy of conflating these similar forms – i.e. the 'pre/trans fallacy'[15] – is all too natural, especially since both are clearly marked by the impossibility of being understood as literal assertions. And – given our desire to make sense of the psychotic subject, and the difficulty attendant on truly tolerating the unmooring of his mind – it's no surprise that the conflation typically takes a 'romantic' or 'idealizing' form, in which the regressive (pre-literal) involution of psychotic thought is conflated with the progressive (trans-literal) evolution of the metaphor-making mind, and that notions like 'unconscious metaphor' which instantiate such a conflation abound in the literature.[16]

Consider now how this distinction between post-literal (metaphoric) and pre-literal (mad) thought help us make sense of the following two encounters with madness:

(a) James Joyce wrote in a famously unnerving, seemingly chaotic, highly allusive, literary style replete with neologisms or 'allmaziful plurabilities' ('In the name of Annah the Allmaziful, the Everliving, the Bringer of Plurabilities, haloed be her eve, her singtime sung, her rill be run, unhemmed as it is uneven!'[17]). This greatly exasperated Jung – whose review of *Ulysses* in turn didn't endear him to Joyce.[18] Now, Joyce deeply doted upon his troubled daughter Lucia who also invented her own words. Despite her father's wishful belief in her misunderstood genius, Lucia was in fact suffering from schizophrenic thought disorder, as Jung diagnosed when he met with her in 1934. Father's and daughter's verbal constructions may have been similar in all sorts of ways – Jung considered James Joyce's 'psychological style' to itself be schizophrenic – but as Jung told Joyce's biographer Richard Ellman when Ellman visited him in 1953, Lucia 'and her father … were like two people going to the bottom of a river, one falling and the other diving'.[19] Or, as he expressed it elsewhere: whilst 'the ordinary patient cannot help talking and thinking in such a way, … Joyce willed it and moreover developed it with all his creative forces. Which incidentally explains why he himself did not go over the border'.[20]

(b) In her autobiographical novel *I Never Promised You a Rose Garden*, the writer Joanne Greenberg shares of her inpatient treatment for schizophrenia, aged 16–20, with Frieda Fromm-Reichmann. The Kingdom of Yr was Greenberg's delusional world;

Yr's Fourth Level provided a refuge where 'there was no emotion to endure, no past or future to grind against'. At first to travel in Yr was to be engaged in a relieving distraction from painful reality, but Yr soon became a nightmare – the Pit, for example, was a place where 'gods and Collect moaned and shouted, but even they were unintelligible.... Meaning itself became irrelevant.' Most agonizing was to make the journey between the worlds of sanity and madness: 'The horror of the Pit lay in the emergence from it, with the return of her will, her caring, and her feeling of the need for meaning before the return of meaning itself.'[21] Greenberg was an exceptionally creative and intelligent young woman, and these resources made for a good prognosis and recovery from schizophrenia; she went on to write twenty novels, and taught anthropology and creative writing at the Colorado School of Mines. Yet lest we be tempted to conflate her (pre-factual) psychotic inventions in Yr and her (trans-factual) creative thought, we do well to heed her oft-repeated advice that she described as 'the strongest thing I'd like to say ever to anybody[:] that creativity and mental illness are *opposites,* not complements.... Imagination is, includes, goes *out*, opens out, learns from experience. Craziness is the opposite: it is a fort that's a prison.'[22]

We may say of James Joyce, but not of his daughter, that because he enjoys sufficient reality contact, he also enjoys sufficient reality testing. Such reality testing is the condition of possibility of his enjoying true imagination – of his swimming rather than falling to the bottom of the river – since to enjoy reality testing simply is for thoughts to be structured so as to sustain our happy allocation of them to the categories either of imaginings or of judgements. We may draw a similar contrast between the delusional experiences Greenberg reports in *I Never Promised You a Rose Garden* and the imaginative work she puts into their presentation in this autobiographical novel – and, for that matter, puts into her many other novels. By contrast with genuine imagination, 'craziness' collapses one's aliveness to the difference between what's real and what's feared or wished. What starts out as balm for unmanageable predicament leads to a state in which 'meaning itself became irrelevant'; the fort that keeps one secure from the world becomes a prison which prevents one from being nourished by it.

Psychological symbolization

We may acknowledge that the concept of metaphor, and the project of retrieving speakers' extant metaphorical meanings, are – so long as we take them in the non-metaphoric senses outlined above – out of place when considering psychotic symbolization. Yet the task remains of reflectively understanding such symbolization, even if we must do our best to accommodate ourselves to its *sui generis* form rather than attempt its assimilation to a more tractable extant category.

In order to grasp symbolization's meaning it will help to first lay out certain basic empirical claims about human mental function and then provide examples of non-psychotic symbolization.[23] These claims are that:

i) We are instinctively drawn to fathom, acquire cognitive mastery over, or at least become somehow able to cope with, the situations and predicaments which confront us. Contrary impulses (such as the policy of the ostrich and the impulse to destruction) do of course also exist. But we've only to think on the developmental function of play (to get used to otherwise stressful confrontations and thereby become more adaptive), on the value of storytelling, myth, and ritual (to corral emotion, develop social understanding and cohesion, overcome anxieties, make the world thinkable), or on the nature of curiosity (our 'epistemophilic instinct'), to grasp the widespread character of our instinctual drive for cognitive, behavioural, and emotional mastery.

ii) To be 'sunk into', or unconsciously 'identified with', a predicament means that we can't readily pull it into view so as to bring our cognitive resources to bear upon it. We find ourselves *in* predicaments rather as we find ourselves *in* moods: our cognitive functions are readily subordinated to their grip rather than vice versa, and this lack of mastery entails objectless anxiety and moodiness. Or, whilst I just wrote that we 'find ourselves' in predicaments, this 'finding', if we interpret it to mean a moment of awareness, can be very belated, if it happens at all. For when it comes to the kinds of relational structures we inhabit (our family dynamics, our intimate relationships, the therapeutic transference) we're often unaware of there being any such predicament in play. It is for us as if we had a coloured filter perpetually fixed over our eyes which, from sheer familiarity, from its structuring every experience we have, is itself invisible to us, rendering us unable to now clearly discriminate in our surroundings that colour which it itself bears.

iii) Unless we disentangle our minds from them, our predicaments 'run through' and impact dismally upon us. The freight of unmetabolized predicamental experience can be subterranean in the sense that it need result in no determinate awareness of it or in thoughts about it and its causes. Instead, it often shows itself in diffuse stress responses (tension, psychophysiological disturbance, nervousness, aggressive behaviour, mindlessness, etc.) and at times in acute psychiatric disturbance (as in the reactive psychoses).

iv) To begin to climb out of our paralysing unregistered predicaments our experience of them must be given some determinate expression. Psychoanalytic theorists have invented various terms, or redeployed various terms taken from sundry other contexts, to denote this process: 'mental digestion', 'metabolism', 'dreaming', 'thinking', 'transduction', 'alpha function', 'symbolic transformation', or 'psychological symbolization'. Such 'psychological' symbolization is quite different from the kind of symbolizing we call 'conventional' – i.e. when it's a matter of convention that means that, say, an ichthys symbol represents the Christian faith or a red rose symbolizes love. For in the psychological case what makes it the case that a particular act, utterance, or creative product symbolizes what it does is not a convention but rather the nature of the experience which inspires it. Furthermore, the bodying forth of psychological symbolization from experience need involve no self-consciousness – for example, it can happen in states of dreaming, trance, or absorption.[24]

v) The result of psychologically symbolizing the as-yet-unmetabolized impact of the world on us can be the formation of particular emotions (e.g. sadness and fear), of truthful avowals of these emotions (the previously stuck, aggressive, and stressed child comes to be able to say 'I'm scared ...'), and of associated truth-apt thoughts ('... that my father will leave'). This process has been called 'mentalization', and becoming able to mentalize in this way is the goal of such psychotherapy as aims primarily to inculcate or restore a capacity to own one's feelings and think about and act rationally on one's predicaments.[25]

vi) However, the general process called 'psychological symbolization' can also result in a far wider array of dispositions, expressions, and acts, ones that need show no expression in such truthful avowals of reality-oriented thoughts and feelings as we find in mentalization. For what can matter far more than propositional truth is emotional motility and the capacity to recover an ability for flexible response, rather than submit to paralysis, in the face of unthinkable predicamental experience. Symbolization here involves the corralling of previously diffuse and unmanageable tensions into discrete thinkable structures, and imagination rather than reasoning is its truest aid.

vii) At the collective level a society develops myths which symbolically articulate the major predicaments of its members' lives (coming of age, sexual union, the unknown, enemies, harvest failure, illness, birth, death, etc.). Individuals then collectively participate in enactments of these myths – i.e. they participate in rituals. Diffuse terrors may now be parlayed into discrete imaginary forms and related ritual acts, and life can go on.

viii) At the individual level unconscious and hence indeterminate anxiety takes a more determinate shape as it finds representation in play, painting, song, fiction, etc. Unthinkable relational predicaments, for example, take thinkable shape as they're expressed in the engagements between characters in an author's novel. This author 'externalizes' his conscious and unconscious relational anxieties in the relations between the characters, and can now make free play with them on the page. The reader who identifies with these characters may thereby find relief from his own inner stuckness as and when the identification supports a progressive structuration of his feelingful relation to his world. This progressive structuration of unconscious anxiety also obtains in the night-time dream, yet fails in the nightmare which wakes us.

In what follows 'psychological symbolization' shall be taken to mean non-mentalizing symbolization – i.e. taken to mean only such narrative, gestural, or pictorial expressive articulation of emotional experience as doesn't involve a subject in the ordinary self-ascription of psychological states.[26]

Examples of psychological symbolization

Let's recap. We began by noting the quasi-metaphoric character of some psychotic thought. We then looked at the difference between psychotic and metaphoric thought, and offered as a negative criterion of delusional discourse that it cannot be understood as either literal or metaphorical. The notion of 'psychological symbolization' has been put forward as a designation for our outworkings of predicamental experience. Next, we shall get a clearer fix on this notion by considering in detail some examples from play, ritual, dreaming, and art, before turning to the question of what's specific about psychotic symbolization.

Play

Rosy, a malnourished and tyrannical seven-year-old, is the daughter of a prostitute who works from home.[27] Both her parents had deprived childhoods and were psychologically ill-equipped for parenthood. When she was five and still living with her parents, her mother killed a violent client with a knife and her father took an overdose. She and her half-siblings now live in different children's homes.

Rosy meets with Janet, a play therapist, in Janet's consulting room for eighteen months of once-weekly non-directive play therapy. There are clear rules about the timing of the session, non-violence, staying in the room, not taking toys home, etc. Here Janet narrates a little from their early interactions; Rosy is telling her what to do:

> [R:] 'Pretend you say "I don't want to go to fight". To fight your own battle. I say you have to. You have to or else you won't get nothing. Be a big boy. You're only 11, 13, 23. Come on, don't be scared.' [J:] 'What battle?' [R:] 'Every battle – ghost battle, Dracula battle. I'll get a knife for you.' [J:] 'All right.' She gives me a knife from the dolls' plastic cutlery. [R:] 'You say "I'm going to fight the ghost." Pretend I'm the ghost and you kill me. You say "Oh, I've killed my mother".' By this time I'm walking round the playroom with the small knife. She creeps up and touches my back. I turn round and stick the knife in her and she lies on a cushion. [J:] 'Oh dear, I've killed my mother. I thought she was the ghost. I'll magic her back to life. I'll fetch a special blanket and cover her over and when she wakes up she'll think she's been asleep.' I fetch a blanket and place it over her. Rosy wakes up. [R:] 'Where am I? I thought I was making the dinner. Pretend you're the old man. Oh, not yet, you ain't had your breakfast. Give me egg and bacon. I'm having the last bit. Pretend you say "I want some"' and she gives me plenty more. 'All the sauce gone—we'll buy some tomorrow. You can go back and fight after dinner. What did I say a minute ago? Oh yes, you're the old man and you change back into my little girl.'[28]

Here Rosy, in the rule-governed safety of the consulting room, instinctively and unreflectively acts out the un-integrated traumas of her life. But rather than directly taking up her own role, it's Janet who's invited to play this part. A couple of months later, however, and Rosy spontaneously performs in her own character, allowing herself now to be a baby who can trust in the availability of Janet's care. After this she's able to 'play out and work through' the unmanageable sexual scenes she has witnessed at home; Janet is relieved when she manages to deflect much of this onto the play room dolls. By the end of therapy Rosy's school and children's home report that the behavioural and emotional problems she evinced at the start have significantly dwindled.

The objects and events in the playroom symbolize the traumatic encounters Rosy has experienced. Even so, it's not so much that she intends them to stand for such experienced people and relations. Their symbolic function is established by no convention, not even a minimal convention that belongs to an intention known to Rosy alone. Instead, the symbolizing function is one that bubbles up spontaneously in such a way that unmanageable and unthinkable experience now receives an outworking with a definite shape.

Myth and ritual

Myths and rituals seem to arise, to become adopted, to be elaborated, and to be maintained, in an organic fashion. Mythic narratives enjoy a certain coherence, yet sometimes portray their scenes with a curious dislocation of the normal associations: the mood may change dramatically, characters and places may suddenly switch, etc.[29] In short they share aspects of what Freud called the 'primary process' characteristics of dream thoughts and, to now make use of a picturesque analogy, may be considered these cultures' collective dreams.[30] The enactment of these 'dreams' are what we call 'rituals'.[31]

Consider Claude Lévi-Strauss's reading of the shamanistic ritual conducted by native Cuna Americans to facilitate difficult childbirth.[32] A *nele* (shaman) sings to the distraught mother-to-be a long incantation which describes how her *purba* (soul) has been captured by *Muu* (the power responsible for embryogenesis). The song begins with the shaman focusing minutely on the recent arrival of the midwife and the experience of labour, with the effect – Lévi-Strauss suggests – that the mother-to-be relives her pains in what is now a precise and tolerable manner. It moves on to tell of the winning back of her *purba*, something that requires the defeat of many spirits, monsters, and magical animals. These creatures are the denizens of the abode of *Muu* and of the *Mu-Igala* (the passageway to *Muu's* abode), and the incantation oscillates dizzyingly between articulations of this mythic domain and passageway and literal talk of the womb and birth canal. Once defeated, relations with *Muu* once again become friendly, her parting words to the shaman being 'Friend *nele*, when do you think to visit again?' Lévi-Strauss theorizes the efficacy of this symbolic treatment as follows:

> The cure would consist, therefore, in making explicit a situation originally existing on the emotional level and in rendering acceptable to the mind pains which the body refuses to tolerate.... The tutelary spirits and malevolent spirits, the supernatural monsters and magical animals, are all part of a coherent system on which the native conception of the universe is founded. The sick woman accepts these mythical beings or, more accurately, she has never questioned their existence. What she does not accept are the incoherent and arbitrary pains, which are an alien element in her system but which the shaman, calling upon the myth, will re-integrate within a whole where everything is meaningful.... The shaman provides the sick woman with a *language*, by means of which unexpressed, and otherwise inexpressible, psychic states can be immediately expressed. And it is the transition to this verbal expression – at the same time making it possible to undergo in an

ordered and intelligible form a real experience that would otherwise be chaotic and inexpressible – which induces the release of the physiological process, that is, the reorganization, in a favorable direction, of the process to which the sick woman is subjected.[33]

Let's accept, for the sake of our discussion, that the ritual incantation is sometimes causally efficacious. How then might we understand it? Lévi-Strauss tells us that the 'cure' – i.e. the progression to a successful labour – consists in 'making explicit a situation originally existing on the emotional level', by providing a 'language' by means of which 'unexpressed, and otherwise inexpressible, psychic states can be immediately expressed'. Yet this so far is but a gesture towards understanding, since what we now need to grasp is what here is meant by 'language', 'making explicit', 'psychic state', and 'expression'.

Here's one way to understand that of which Lévi-Strauss writes. A certain woman at term is, let's imagine, too psychologically unprepared, too sunk into her predicament, too overwhelmed, to be able to cope with labour. Too overwhelmed, in fact, even for separate feelings of pain, fear, and hope to stand a chance of developing; and too overwhelmed to spontaneously situate her experiences within an intelligible temporal progression which stretches from pregnancy via parturition to future motherhood. Her labour pains therefore remain 'incoherent and arbitrary', and she cannot remain a self-same, reality-oriented subject whilst bearing them. Without the capacity to bear her feelings of pain, fear, and hope, she is equally unable to acquiesce in the birth process and bear her baby.[34]

One way to develop such an understanding is through a mentalization-deploying form of cognition which makes explicit one's fears and feelings. Yet as with Rosy and her playing, such a form of cognition may be unnecessary, unavailable, and undesirable. Not necessary, since non-mentalizing versions of symbolization which engage neither the will nor self-reflection may rekindle and steer emotional resources by themselves, making them newly available for life's encounters. Unavailable if the subject is either too young to master, or too distraught to engage in, verbal avowals of thoughts and feelings. And undesirable if the direct light from the headlights of the birth experience is just too bright to see in, or if mentalizing efforts all too easily become hijacked by intellectualizing defences, so that verbal self-ascriptions of thoughts and feelings fail to truly express that which they nevertheless declare. This would-be mentalizer now merely talks about putative feelings (rather as if they belonged to someone else), and a pseudo-mature verbal carapace covers over the failure of emotional experience to take coherent shape.

The woman who's utterly overwhelmed by labour may however be helped by a ritual to develop coherent analogue thoughts and feelings concerning the less overwhelming, analogue adventures in Muu's abode, and these may in turn enable her participation in the birth experience. An analogy which, whilst rather more trivial, nevertheless shares something by way of formal structure, would be the effect turning on a tap has on the disposition to urinate (as also aids those with shy bladder syndrome). The water running from the tap provides an analogue of that urination which, for whatever emotionally incoherent reason, has here become impossible, and thereby causally inspires the urinator to progress with his task.

Dreaming

The psychiatrist Irving Yalom tells of a 45-year-old patient who had remained in deep grief for the four years since his wife's death. He shares two of his patient's dreams:

> I was at my summer house and my wife was there, vague – a mere presence in the background. The house had a different kind of roof, a sod roof, and growing from it was a tall cypress – it was a beautiful tree but it was endangering the house and I had to cut it.[35]

> I was at home and fixing the roof of the house by placing some kind of ornament on it when I felt a big earthquake and could see the silhouette of the city shaking in the distance and saw two twin skyscrapers fall.

Yalom writes of how these dreams related to his patient's grief:

> . . . his associations to 'sod' as well as the roof 'ornament' were his wife's grave and tombstone. It's not unusual for one's life to be depicted as a house in dreams. His wife's death and his unending grief were embodied in the cypress, which endangered his house and which therefore he had to cut. In the second dream his wife's death was represented by the earthquake, which collapsed the twin skyscrapers – the married couple. (This dream, incidentally, occurred years before the Word Trade Centre terrorist attack.) We had been working in therapy on the issues of coming to terms with the fact that the coupled state in which he had lived his life was no more, that his wife was truly dead, and that he had to let go, gradually detach from his wife, and reengage life. The reinforcement supplied by his dreams was instrumental in therapy – they represented to him a message from the fount of wisdom within him that it was time to fell the tree and to turn his attention to the living.[36]

It's one thing for this man to entertain the thought that he needs to re-engage with life, another thing for him to inhabit this as a live possibility. The symbolization of the dreaming mind helps with this: by being cognitively oblique yet affectively direct, by presenting the tasks of living at symbolic remove from the vortex of his grief, it enables new and clear feeling and meaning to emerge.

Art

A classic approach to artistic endeavour considers it 'the creation of forms symbolic of human feeling'.[37] Such feeling may be in the artist's extant emotional repertoire or may arise only when he attempts imaginative involvement with his subject matter. It may be conscious or unconscious, and creating the artwork may be the means by which an artist learns what he feels. Regardless of the form it takes, artistic expression constitutes what we might call the 'symbolic outworking' or (with T. S. Eliot) the 'objective correlative' of that which it expresses.[38] Essential to this outworking is that, far from being the expression of already determinate feeling, it itself makes for such feelings' increasing determinacy.

The different ways in which artistic production may involve symbolization of feeling are articulated by Marion Milner who, in *On Not Being Able to Paint*, describes her difficulties with just that. The first step in unlocking these difficulties proves to be her discovery that 'it was possible at times to produce drawings or sketches in an entirely different way from any that I had been taught, a way of letting hand or eye do exactly what pleased them without any conscious working to a preconceived intention'.[39] With this in mind she resolves to express in her art the feelings enlivened in her by the scenes before her. Thus:

> when sitting in a buttercup field one Sunday morning in June, watching the Downs emerging from the mist ... I concentrated on the mood of the scene, the peace and softness of the colouring, the gentle curve of the Downs, and began to scribble in charcoal, letting hand and eye do what they liked. Gradually a definite form had emerged and there, instead of the peaceful summer landscape, was a blazing heath fire, its roaring flames leaping from the earth in a funnel of fire, its black smoke blotting out the sky.[40]

This surprises Milner, and at first she imagines it to be due to a failed mastery of her medium. But the same thing keeps happening in other experiments. She notices too that although she made her drawings in an absent-minded mood, by the time they were finished she usually had a definite story in mind about what they depicted. Something is taking shape, but she's not yet clear about what it is.

Later Milner looks back at a new series of drawings which, she comes to realize, always contain a nasty, greedy attacking figure (a frightful blood-sucking half-mosquito/half-bat; a serpent; a shark) and an innocent and harmless one (an innocent donkey; a frugal mouse; a baby mermaid). The thought then occurs to her that these pictures make manifest 'angry attacking impulses' that are an essential, yet hitherto denied, part of herself.

When reading a book on art theory, Milner comes across a passage describing how an artwork's vitality depends upon 'the emphasis in each symbol of the living forces, the vital character, of the thing represented ... This vitality must also be accompanied with the tenderness and subtlety born of long and earnest insight into nature, or the symbol, though spirited, will be shallow ...'.[41] She then understands how her previous failure to symbolize her own inner angry and greedy feelings – which is not something other than the failure of such feelings to take adequate shape – was what prevented her from being able to give symbolic form in her painting to the vital scenes about her:

> ... now I understand something of the kind of denials in oneself that could prevent that subtle tenderness. In order to experience such a tenderness for nature outside, in all her forms, one has surely to have found some way of coming to terms with nature inside; or rather, with those parts of nature inside that one had repudiated as too unpleasant to be recognised as part of oneself. Otherwise the unadmitted opposites of the frugal mouse and the innocent donkey would be liable to make

nature hated instead of loved, the peaceful summer morning could turn into a raging fire or a blasting blizzard.⁴²

The psychology of psychological symbolization

The above examples give us a sense of how symbolization dares venture in terrains where mentalization fears to tread. A patient recounting his dreams, a child in her play, and a Sunday painter in the field give symbolic articulation to feelings which they may as yet be unable to mentalize. The examples also make clear how far the notion of psychological symbolization is from the traditional notion of symbolic production: the ordinary symbol stands for or represents that which it symbolizes, whereas a subject's symbolization of his experience involves his use of a medium wherein his experience may itself begin to take determinate shape.⁴³

It's easy enough to see why someone looking at the above examples may be drawn to say that the child, artist, dreamer, or woman in labour is using symbols to represent experience that already enjoys determinate form. If, that is, we take the notion of a symbol in its ordinary sense – namely 'something that stands for, represents, or denotes something else' – and if we take as our paradigm of emotional experience those mature feelings which are already clearly structured and apt for avowal, then the relation of a moment of child's play or of a painted figure's facial expression to particular emotions will naturally appear as one of representation. Yet this appears a clear instance of a pre/trans fallacy: a state which is prior to mentalization is here conflated with one which presupposes it to have already obtained.

We may even here hazard an error theory as to why Freudian psychoanalysis has typically considered psychological symbolization in terms of substitution.⁴⁴ On that conception the mind in conflict represses out of awareness emotions or urges which nevertheless lie determinately within it, and in a moment of bad faith offers up for itself substitutes which provide at least some of the gratification which the repressed emotions or urges would, in happier circumstances, themselves have provided. This conception, if it's not to straightway fall foul of the contradictions inherent in the very idea of a mind which must somehow know what it yet disavows, must also make use: of an inner 'censor', of inner mental 'partitions' to keep the repressed feeling apart from the self-knowing subject, and of some kind of 'introspective' faculty for enabling access to the symbolic substitute – all of which quickly leads us into a complexified, reified and alienated characterization of mental life.⁴⁵ If, however, we consider unconscious emotion not as extant yet hidden, but instead as an inchoate dispositional force which has not yet taken shape (either partly in symbolization or fully in mentalization) – then we may avoid a conception of the symbol as a substitute for that which is 'known yet repressed'. Any notion of substitution, or of a determinate unconscious content for which the symbol is substituted, may now be seen to pertain not to the symbolizing subject but instead merely to the form of our representation of her predicament. An 'unconscious' feeling now becomes that which, along with a high load of anxiety, would unfold in a determinate manner were certain defensive strategies not deployed – rather than something extant but somehow squirreled away within the recesses of a self-concealing mind. And a symbol now becomes not a stand-in for an emotional thought extant yet gone into hiding, but instead a somewhat inarticulate expression of unconscious feeling. Affect is now mobilized, even though its expression doesn't take a mentalizing shape and so doesn't voice that thought which a subject better able to metabolize her predicament would voice ('I'm frightened of father'), but instead voices something analogous ('This toy monster terrorizes this doll').

Consider too the different senses of 'articulate'. One sense considers articulation to be the voicing of that which is already structured. Another considers it to be the development of such discrete structuration. A third considers it in terms of such jointedness as now permits movement. It's these second and third senses which are relevant when we're considering what's meant by psychological symbolization. A subject too sunk into her predicament to be able to give it voice, too identified with it to be able to develop feelings about it, develops instead some feelings in relation to what we naturally consider its analogue. Through imaginative involvement in play, through ritual, dreaming, or artistic production, she imaginatively bodies forth feelings in articulate form and becomes more given to flexible response in the face of her predicament. Now the ghost will be killed with a knife, the denizens of Muu's abode will be defeated, the cypress will be cleared from the roof of the house, and angry attacking impulses will be allowed their breathing space alongside loving and tender feelings. As a consequence, agitation decreases, labour or mourning proceed, artistic vision is rendered incarnate – and life once again unfolds without inhibition.

Psychotic symbolization

Having elucidated the collapse of the literal and the metaphoric in psychotic thought, and outlined the nature of psychological symbolization, we're now in a position to bring these together in a fresh understanding of psychotic symbolization. This understanding, if it's to be of value, should allow us to make reflective sense of what's readily intuitively grasped in the following:

> One of our hebephrenics had to be returned to the hospital twice because, in addition to other things, she cut branches off a *Quittenbaum* (quince tree) in order to signify that she was 'quits' with the pastor. She threw these branches into the creek; they were her sins which would be carried down to the sea.[46]

Here Bleuler's patient engages in an act which, superficially at least, resembles a rite. Yet by contrast with our appreciation of religious acts, we readily recognize it as psychotic. Regularly encountered explanations for this difference include: (i) religious acts are in fact themselves essentially psychotic, but because we're attached or habituated to them we give them a special pleading they've not earned; (ii) religious acts are necessarily participated in by many people, and are not just individual inventions, and it's this which makes it incorrect to consider them psychotic; (iii) what in a religious rite is treated metaphorically is here treated literally, and this is what makes it right to designate it psychotic. Yet if the understanding of psychosis and of psychological symbolism advanced in this chapter is right, we can begin to see our way to an alternative understanding of such acts.

To make clear the character of this understanding, let's invent a plausible empirical setting for the Quittenbaum delusion. Thus let's imagine that here we meet with an unhappily married woman who has become erotically attached to her caring pastor. She now finds herself in intolerable conflict – both because her desire is unrequited and because her conscience can't condone it. Rather than being able to develop this predicament in clear thought, allowing both for a lucid articulation of the desire and for the acknowledgement of the impossibility of its fulfilment, Bleuler's patient is instead – let's imagine – overwhelmed and becomes psychotic. That's to say, her thought is no longer rooted in and calibrated by reality, so she enters a 'waking dream' in which her thoughts no more belong properly either to imagination or to judgement but instead manifest a collapse of the two into each other. Her concrete equation of the quince branches and her sins is not a matter of her treating literally what a non-psychotic rite participant would treat as metaphor. What has instead happened is that she has psychologically symbolized her predicament – i.e. given it a non-mentalistic verbal elaboration – whilst in a psychotic state. Her acts cannot be seen by her as play, art, or ritual, nor can either she or we clearly approach her thought and experience using the categories of the literal or the metaphorical, for her state of mind is such as to make such distinctions void.

Or consider this:

> Another schizophrenic in an advanced stage of her illness, passed the time making hats for herself. She had made 16 of them. One day, she lost two of them. As a form of retaliation against this she decided to break two of her mother's 16 cups.[47]

Let's again invent a backstory to psychologically fill out this brief clinical report. Imagine then that, when young, the patient's mother suffered an insufficient degree of reliable nurture and emotional containment. She's unable to mentalize this deprivation, but finds refuge in collecting symbolic substitutes for (what psychoanalysis calls) the 'absent breast'. With these cups she can feed herself; they enable her to become quasi-self-satisfying; unlike the absent breast, they're reassuringly within her control, hanging as they do on the dresser hooks. Nevertheless, her impoverishing early experience, and her self-involvement, in turn impair her capacity to provide adequate emotional containment to her daughter. To tolerate her own exclusion from the domain of care symbolized by the mother's relationship with her precious cups, the daughter in turn creates her own substitute 'breast' – i.e. she knits herself a hat for each of her mother's 16 cups. With these hats for comfort, she can avoid becoming angry at her mother's emotional neglect. Losing two of them, however, threatens the fragile emotional balance they provide. She can mentalize none of the emotional meaning, but her painful loss is nevertheless mitigated by breaking two of her mother's cups: this breakage perfectly demonstrates what we might call the 'logic' of delusional symbolization.

There's no such thing as our developing here a rational (or what Jaspers called 'empathic') understanding of the patient's breaking of her mother's cups, since this poor patient is not engaged in a rational act. She might say 'I broke them because I lost two of my hats' – yet this, *qua* reason, makes no sense. Minkowski – the author of this report – articulates her vandalism as something done 'in retaliation for' the loss, and it's this which reveals for us the delusional quality of the act. For if something's properly said to be 'done in retaliation', that which is suffered must be understood by the revenging party to be something done to her by the one on whom revenge is taken. It's by bringing the breakage under the description of 'revenge' whilst not providing any such understanding for us that Minkowski helps us appreciate the short-circuiting, delusional, character of that which here confronts us. Yet whilst we can't enter empathically into this act *qua* rational act – i.e. whilst we've no idea how to make 'because I lost two of my hats' into a genuine reason for breaking two of one's mother's cups – we can nevertheless psychologically grasp the act's motivated character: the act functions to restore mental equilibrium.

Near the beginning of this chapter we met three patients, the first of whom was Elena who hallucinates and delusionally believes that her father, 'all black and completely nude', frequently comes to her bed thrusting 'a spear into her lower abdomen and dancing about in a very peculiar fashion'. This, Bleuler tells us, is the same father who does in fact frequently abuse her sexually. At the start of her psychosis she hallucinates her mother complaining about her to her father. When she speaks of his abuse her tone is embarrassed and objective, but when she articulates her hallucination and delusion she wears a 'completely erotic expression'. This all provides a clue to the nature of what would have been more comprehensively repressed had her mind not been so damaged by her abusive upbringing and illness. Her natural heterosexual desires, that is, are awakened by her father, but since she is, like many a healthy teenager, still too sunk into the predicament of the inevitability yet impermissibility of oedipal desires, they can't take a straightforward mentalized form. They instead take a symbolic shape, but do so when she's in a state of waking dream, with the result that she neither straightforwardly believes, nor wishfully imagines, but instead delusionally believes, that her naked black father thrusts his spear into her abdomen.

Following Elena we met Ms R whose father was oppressive in his expectations, obtuse about his daughter's difficulties, and utterly unrealistic about her ability to find or cope with a job or marriage. Like Elena, Ms R is too sunk into her predicament and so can't develop fully mentalized feelings – at first about her father's impossible expectations, and later about the ward staff's equally unhelpful expectations of her progress. The feelings therefore remain merely potential or 'unconscious' – 'trapped', as it were, within the very structure of her relationships rather than condensing out into discrete sufferable experiences. And like Elena, Ms R – due to whatever predisposition she carries, along with the unbearableness of the home situation – becomes psychotic. Nevertheless, the general drive towards psychological symbolization still remains in her, and because she's lost touch with reality it now naturally manifests in delusion: 'a large man is sitting on top of my head'. In someone who had not lost reality contact this thought would naturally be seen as a metaphor, one more naturally expressed in the form of a simile: 'It is for me as if a large man were sitting on my head.' Yet, at least in the ambit of her waking dream, the metaphorical/literal distinction no longer finds instantiation in Ms R's mind – and so to treat her expression as metaphorical would be to commit the pre/trans fallacy. Luckily for Ms R, a psychotherapist sensitive to the meanings of psychological symbolization is able to help the ward staff understand that this large man 'is' her father. Which 'is' is to say: her delusional expression is a psychological symbolization of the stifling predicament she is in, a predicament which, were she able to extricate herself from it for a moment so as to bring it into view, would naturally be expressed in such terms as 'my father is oppressing me'. The ward staff can now take a mentalizing attitude towards Ms R, one which conveys an accepting understanding of her experience, which refrains from repeating the oppression, and which, in making clear that such experiences can be discussed, allows Ms R to begin to mentalize her own suffering.

After Ms R we encountered Jonas, the 'masturbating hebephrenic, who ... finds a high peak in a mountain range so shocking that he gets into a fight with his companion and has to return home'. The analogy, writes Bleuler, 'can hardly be called pathological. But what is ... pathological is [Jonas'] interpretation of the analogy in the sense of the real sexual organ and the correspondingly violent reaction.' Such examples abound in the literature, and testify to the impact of an unintegrated sexuality and unsatisfactory sexual life on psychopathology.

Jonas, let's imagine, struggles both to integrate his sexual desires and to tolerate the shame and frustration of their unfulfilment. He is shy, unconfident, awkward, and doesn't know how to go about finding and attracting a sexual partner. Such a predicament is, after all, not humanly unknown, perhaps especially amongst those at risk of developing mental illness. For Jonas, we hypothesize, the predicament is simply too much to bear. He is lost in it; it courses through him, determining his actions – rather than being something he can pull into view or get a handle on. He can only move dynamically in the world – go walking in the Alps with a companion, say – by rigidly defending against his sexual fears and frustrations. At times mere repression and distraction serve the purpose, but at other times the affective load of his predicament is too great: now he simultaneously dissociates and loses his footing in reality. Yet now that he's slipped into a delusional mode, the frustrating situation can at least take some kind of expressive form: a mountain peak offers an opportunity for Jonas to develop outrage. Unbearable inner turmoil now takes an outward shape; relief is thereby obtained; ersatz sense is made. Such outrage is however impossible to empathically grasp in the terms in which it expresses itself. We could make something of it were it not a mountain peak but an exposed sexual characteristic that was under discussion. We could make something of it too if Jonas were using a metaphor to articulate himself. In the absence of these, however, empathic intelligibility in Jaspers' sense is unavailable. We don't come to understand Jonas in his predicament and in his delusion by grasping his speaker's meaning, since his outraged expression conveys none. Instead, we come to understand him by grasping psychologically how the breakdown of such meaning bespeaks the diremptive power of such complexes as are betrayed by his delusional symbolization.

Before concluding the discussion it's important that we consider the dangers for the patient of openly translating their psychological symbolization to them. This chapter began with mention of Angela who, you will recall, told me, at the end of the twentieth century, that she had just been released from Belsen (which was liberated in 1945).

Interpreting her as using a metaphor (for being discharged from the psychiatric hospital, as indeed she had been) provoked in her a reaction of bafflement and disturbance. This already shows how caution is required when interpreting symbolically freighted psychopathology in the absence of a containing therapeutic relationship. The patient needs to be treated with (moral) understanding even when her discourse is (rationally) unintelligible – yet it can be deeply undoing to receive the kind of (psychological) understanding which renders him defence-less. Showing psychological understanding is often lauded, and indeed is essential for any psychotherapy that not only helps a patient through his psychosis but also helps him work through his underlying complexes and ameliorate his underlying vulnerability. Even so, and especially for the patient whose psychosis is itself a flight from intolerable shame, knowing oneself to be psychologically understood can be a fearful business. To return once again to Schopenhauer: if 'such painful knowledge or reflection is so harrowing that it becomes positively unbearable, and the individual would succumb to it, then nature, alarmed in this way, seizes upon madness as the last means of saving life'. Carelessly undoing this can then constitute an assault on existential life itself.

In this chapter we also met both the notable psychiatrist Frieda Fromm-Reichmann and her patient Joanne Greenberg whom she treated for four years at Chestnut Lodge. In Greenberg's words now: 'People would tell you what perceptive things a patient had said. The thing is I want to choose my perceptions. I don't want them to come out of some kind of unconscious soup. I want it to be something I choose to say, not something that says me.' She adds here too how being understood in that state can feel horrifically dangerous. Whilst Fromm-Reichmann's instruction that 'you must take me with you' was welcome to her, it felt 'horrifically dangerous' to be understood thus. 'I don't know how Frieda got around that. I remember the danger.... It's bigger than you are. It's more powerful. It can kill.'[48]

10

The Politics of Insanity Ascription

Introduction

To judge another mad is in part to judge her rationally unreachable. Yet we often find others unintelligible without designating them insane.[1] And isn't our own lack of understanding simply far too subjective a criterion to use in arriving at such putatively objective determinations as insanity ascriptions? Might it not be, then, that those deemed mad simply live in (what could be called) another logical, metaphysical, or conventional country – a country which we may conceive of if yet not inhabit, one perfectly meaning-sustaining for its inhabitants if not for those who proclaim themselves sane? For that matter, why should it be that, just because I can't find my feet with you, it's you rather than I who's to be classified insane? Is all this not just a power play by me, a political ruse by one unimaginative self-appointed guardian of sanity to exclude from rational discourse those who through necessity or inclination go their own way? And if it's not to be deemed such a power play, mustn't there be some independent, objective, criterion by reference to which our intuitive findings of insanity may themselves be ratified or debunked?

In this final chapter the focus will be not on answering, but instead on dissolving, the above questions. Along the way we shall come to see how the temptation to ask them itself stems from the psychiatric theorist's alienation from, and failure to take responsibility for, his own words. But let's begin where psychiatric training proper often begins, on a ward round. The consultant is asking one of the trainee psychiatrists for a mental state examination and diagnostic workup of Mrs Thomas. The trainee decides that Mrs Thomas is likely suffering from schizophrenia, and notes – amongst other things – both her delusion that her husband is trying to kill her, and that her thought is formally disordered. To further his trainee's learning the consultant asks him to justify his decisions: 'What are your grounds for thinking Mrs Thomas schizophrenic, and what grounds do you have for thinking her claims about her husband to be delusional rather than reasonable?' In giving his reasons the trainee refers to specific facts about Mrs Thomas' general presentation, mood, actions, reasoning, and responses.

Two hours later the ward round is over, and the medical team retreat to the consultant's office. The conversation turns from the practical to the philosophical. Our consultant muses: 'I appreciate that the questions I asked earlier were well-answered by your reference to the specific facts of the case. Now, however, I should like to set before you some more fundamental questions: To what general facts should we appeal to justify our profession's claims that *any* of our patients truly suffer delusion, thought disorder, psychosis, and mental illness? And with what right do we presume ourselves sane whilst proclaiming our patients delusional? It has been said that "Leaving the determination of whether mental illness exists strictly to the psychiatrists is like leaving the determination of the validity of astrology in the hands of professional astrologers."[2] In the face of such critique how should we justify our belief in the validity of our discipline's fundamental categories?' The trainees struggle to know what to do with these questions but, as is the polite presumption in teaching situations, take them for good ones, and so set about trying to answer them. Quite soon they find themselves dividing into two camps, each camp taking a fundamentally different tack whilst trying to justify the validity of such concepts as 'mental illness', 'psychosis', and 'delusion'. A trainee who's studied some philosophy labels them the 'Realists' and the 'Idealists'.

Realism

The Realists find themselves attracted to claims such as the following: 'If our use of psychiatric terms like "psychosis" or "delusion" is to be properly counted as defensible or valid, there must be some bona fide natural facts which they each pick out.' 'All cases of schizophrenia must surely involve the same neurological lesion or the same genetic basis if our concept is picking out anything real.' 'The diverse utterances which in each case warrant a diagnosis of thought disorder must all stem from a breakdown in the same cognitive or neurological mechanism if our concept of "thought disorder" is to command respect.' When pressed over what they mean by 'natural facts', or why they're tempted to reach for genes or cognitive and neurological disruptions, they tell us that we surely can't truly validate the category of 'delusion', say, by appealing to other notions that are pretty much of a piece with it – like 'madness' or 'loss of reality contact'. Someone who's sceptical about the validity of psychiatry's basic conceptual apparatus will need to be convinced by appeals to concepts which don't presuppose a psychiatric sensibility – i.e. a sensibility already shaped by, and constituted by seeing people through, concepts like 'delusion'. And the same too for diagnostic categories like 'schizophrenia', 'schizoaffective disorder', or 'delusional disorder': if they're to be considered valid, some non-psychiatrically-inflected description should be available for what they essentially involve. And reference to genetics, neurobiology, or cognitive psychology may seem to do just that. Our consultant, however, quotes from twenty-first-century psychiatric scholarship: 'not one laboratory marker has been found to be specific in identifying any of the DSM-defined syndromes. Epidemiologic and clinical studies have shown extremely high rates of co-morbidity among the disorders, undermining the hypothesis that the syndromes represent distinct etiologies'; 'our genes seem neither to have read DSM-IV nor to particularly respect the diagnostic boundaries it established'; and 'there is just a weak correlation between general cognitive performance and the presence of ... delusions ... [and] the vast majority of patients with even severe difficulties do not develop delusions.'[3] Some of the trainees start to wonder whether they've made a mistake in their choice of speciality.

At this point it may help to note that our self-styled Realists need have brought with them no prior assumption that psychiatric illnesses are characterizable in cognitive, neurological, or genetic terms. That they find themselves reaching for such notions may of course have something to do with today's culturally prevalent temptations of scientific naturalism (the wish to partake of the prestige or funding of the natural sciences, or the belief that it's somehow only 'natural science that tells us what's real'), or something to do with the prime place of science in much of the rest of medicine. Yet our Realists were led to reach for their lesions and mechanisms here in answer to a quite particular – and, in truth, quite a peculiar – question. This question asked for grounds for thinking that any of the patients they've been meeting with – many of whom surely provide *paradigms* of the delusional, the thought-disordered, the psychotic – *really do* suffer in such ways. In short, the question invited them to consider that use of their specialism's vocabulary is to be counted problematically unwarranted unless warrant for it is providable and provided. Taking on board the question's tacit sceptical presumption – that accusations of unwarrantedness may only reasonably be staved off by provision of warrant – the Realists start to do what anyone attempting to provide such warrant would do. That is, they look around for natural facts to which appeal can be made when justifying the psychiatric use of language.

We shall return below to the question of the reasonableness of the guiding sceptical presumption. But let's first consider how the Idealists answer the consultant's question.

Idealism

Like many psychiatrists before her, one of our Idealist trainees was inspired in her choice of profession by reading R. D. Laing's *The Divided Self*. She recalls from that book a passage suggesting that:

> when two sane persons meet, there is a mutual and reciprocal recognition of each other's identity. . . . However, if there are discrepancies of a sufficiently radical kind remaining after attempts to align them have failed, there is no alternative but that one of us must be insane. I have no difficulty in regarding another person as psychotic, if for instance:
>
> > he says he is Napoleon, whereas I say he is not;
> > or *if* he says I am Napoleon, whereas I say I am not;
> > or *if* he thinks that I wish to seduce him, whereas I think that I have given him no grounds in actuality for supposing that such is my intention . . .
>
> I suggest, therefore, that *sanity or psychosis is tested by the degree of conjunction or disjunction between two persons where the one is sane by common consent.* . . .
> The 'psychotic' is the name we have for the other person in a disjunctive relationship of a particular kind.[4]

Laing's text too can be read as an attempt to take seriously the consultant's question. But unlike the Realists, Laing here justifies psychiatric judgement not by reference to some independent fact about patients' minds or brains, but rather by reference to the degree of disjunction between the doctor's and the patient's understandings. Here they are of a mind with seventeenth-century playwright Nathaniel Lee who remarked, as he was being taken to the Bethlem Hospital, 'They called me mad, and I called them mad, and damn them, they outvoted me.'[5] This, then, is the Idealists' understanding of the warrant for ascriptions of psychosis, delusion, thought disorder, and mental illness: an ascription's ground is not an independent fact about the patient's mind or brain, but the disjunction of the patient's thought with that of those from their families, communities, and doctors who deem one another sane. With their 'Copernican revolution' these Idealists no longer try to show how their judgements about the patient are warranted because they genuinely conform to the actual nature of the mentally ill mind. Instead, in a reversal of the Realist's guiding presupposition, they judge a person to be mentally ill just in so far as her acts and utterances don't conform to the judgement characteristic of those who enjoy a 'common' sense.[6]

At first the Idealist trainees are reassured by their profession's apparent insulation from the Realist's predicaments. But once again their consultant brings them up short by quoting from twenty-first-century scholarship:

> The problem with this distinction is that, far from making the borderline between normality and madness more objective, it introduces an alarming degree of subjectivity. For Jaspers, the empathic attitude of the psychiatrist towards the patient functions as a kind of diagnostic test.... However, behaviours and experiences may vary in degree according to how amenable they are to empathy. By not empathizing hard enough, we may fail to recognize the intelligible aspects of the other person's experiences.[7]

In short, if we can't understand the delusional person, might this not be our problem rather than theirs? Surely our own inability to make sense of someone shouldn't be made a criterion of their unintelligibility? And doesn't such a non-objective way with psychiatric diagnosis leave it open to the kind of abuses that have been documented in psychiatric history – from the suggestion that fugitive slaves be diagnosed as suffering from the mental disorder of 'drapetomania', to the inclusion until 1973 (when dropped from the DSM) or 1990 (when removed from the ICD) of homosexuality as a mental disorder, to the diagnosis in the 1950s and 1960s of USSR political dissenters with a 'sluggish schizophrenia' in which 'seemingly normal' individuals suffer subtle behavioural changes along with 'reformist delusional ideas', 'over-estimation of their own personalities', and 'poor adaptation to the social environment'?[8] If we could instead follow the Realists and make reference to an objective criterion, we could use it to ratify our challenge of such diagnostic abuses. Furthermore, who gets to say who the 'we' is that ratifies itself as sane? Are we really going to let our sense of what is sane hang on the 'common consent' of those who deem one another to enjoy a 'common sense' – i.e. who make meaning in a socially prevalent manner? It can be hard to see as anything but oppressive conformism that psychiatric philosophy which insists individuals must conform to the pattern of a majority's thought in order to not be counted psychotic.[9]

Relativism

Given the failures of Realism and Idealism to articulate a plausible grounding for descriptive psychopathology – but continuing for now with the assumption that psychopathology requires some such grounding if it's to be counted a rational science – some of the trainees now find themselves tempted instead by a radical anti-psychiatric stance which they call Relativism. 'For sure', they say, '*we* can only understand those who share *our* ways of thinking. But perhaps those we judge "psychotic" have their *own* ways of thinking which are, within their own terms, just as valid as ours. So perhaps all we can do is point out the disjunction between our way of thinking and theirs, and accept that whilst we live in one logical country, as it were, they live in another with its own customs and laws.' In fact if we read the above-quoted passage from Laing as enjoying an ironic tone, we might find in his suggestion that the 'psychotic' is the name we have for the other person in a disjunctive relationship of a particular kind, to be nothing more than a critique of the very idea of 'the psychotic'.

Historical precedents for such a conception are not hard to find:

a) The anti-psychologistic logician Gottlob Frege describes the 'psychological logician' as someone who construes logical laws as descriptions of how we happen to think – so that we should have had different laws if, as a contingent matter of fact, we had thought differently. In presenting an implication of the thought of the 'psychological logician' Benno Erdman, Frege asks: 'What ... if beings were even found whose laws of thought directly contradicted ours, so that their application often led to opposite results? The psychological logician could only accept this and say: for them, those laws hold, for us these.'[10]

b) The psychiatrist Eilhard von Domarus – who like Erdman is a psychological logician – develops a theory of the schizophrenic subject as following alternative ('paralogical') laws of thought: whereas the sane 'logician accepts identity only upon the basis of identical subjects, the [schizophrenic] paralogician accepts identity based upon identical predicates.' Thus a 'schizophrenic patient of the Insane Asylum of the University in Bonn ... identified a saint with a cigar box and the male sex'. He did so 'because of what he could predicate [of] each one of these different subjects; and, because this predicate was the same for the three subjects, they were held to be identical.'[11]

c) The philosopher John Campbell, drawing on Wittgenstein's notion of the 'hinge' or 'framework' proposition, proposes that delusional subjects may enjoy alternative logical foundations to their thought. To set the scene: In his last writings Wittgenstein suggested that we do well to distinguish between such propositions as can readily be imagined to be falsified by empirical enquiry and those which articulate our basic certainties and set the scene for any such enquiry. 'The world has existed for quite a long time', 'There are some tables and chairs in this room', and 'This is one hand and this is another': these belong to thought's framework, forming the background required by our attempts to test or disprove more readily falsifiable empirical propositions. These framework propositions are unfalsifiable by us not because that of which they talk is too removed from us to inspect, but rather because it's too close, instead forming the vantage from which we look at the world. As Campbell sees it, since accepting these framework propositions helps constitute our very grasp of their terms' meaning, to relinquish one for another would also involve a change in the meaning of their terms. His suggestion, then, is that we may reconcile ourselves to the peculiarities of delusional discourse by supposing the psychotic subject to have the edifice of her thought grounded in alternative framework propositions.[12]

All such strategies aim to 'solve simultaneously for understanding and utter strangeness' as Naomi Eilan nicely puts it[13] – i.e. aim to do justice to our sense of delusion's unfathomable strangeness whilst simultaneously showing how those in it could both mean what they say and cleave to it with unabashed certainty. (We may not ourselves be able to understand these alternative frameworks, but we do at least now seem to be able to help ourselves to the idea that this is but a function of our thought being inexorably constrained by our own laws of thought or framework propositions.) The question, however, is whether understanding can, in principle if not in practice, really be solved for by the strategies on offer.

Consider: von Domarus has his patient 'holding the opinion' that Jesus, cigar boxes, and sex are identical since for him they're all bound together by a 'feeling of identity'. And this 'feeling' is inspired by a recognition that all three are encircled: 'the head of Jesus, as of a saint, is encircled by a halo, the package of cigars by the tax band, and the woman by the sex glance [*sic*] of the man.' The difference between normal and schizophrenic thinking is, as von Domarus sees it, that whereas 'for a normal person the particular of being encircled is only one of many accidentals, for the schizophrenic patient it is the quality expressing essence'. The question remains, however, as to what it means to suggest that their all being encircled could provide for someone a sufficient condition for three things in fact being identical.

To discern this suggestion's meaning we might attempt an explication such as: 'When the patient says that Jesus or the saints, cigar boxes, and the male or female sex are all identical, what he means is what we mean when we instead say they share a particular property (that of being encircled).' But the problem with such an interpretation is that it solves rather too well for understanding yet dispels rather than honours the strangeness, since now both psychiatrist and patient once again reside in the same logical universe. That is, they now both simply use different words to make the same points, so that all that's required of us to understand the patient is to remember to substitute 'X shares a property with Y' whenever the patient says 'X is Y'. This is akin to what's required of two scientists who find differences in their calculations of the average of a particular data set. Discussion reveals one of them to have meant 'mean', and the other 'median', by 'average'. Having sorted this out, clear communication once again proceeds.

In fact matters aren't quite so straightforward – since we ought to ask just why the patient can't bring his words into conformity with ours. Can we really ascribe clear, albeit alternative, thoughts to him despite his inability to adjust himself to us and to his own mother tongue?[14] But perhaps we can let this pass, and try instead to keep a clear fix on the Relativist's idea that patient and psychiatrist don't merely use their terms differently but somehow live in different logical universes. One of the first things we notice now is that, in order to aim at this possibility of radical difference we shall, paradoxically enough, need reason to believe that both patient and psychiatrist do nevertheless in some sense *share* an understanding of what's meant by 'identity', 'is', 'the same', 'accidental property', 'essence', etc.[15] After all it's said that the patient 'holds the opinion' that Jesus and cigar boxes are as one, and makes use of a different logic of identity – a different logic, that is, of the *same* thing (i.e. identity) that others also reference with their use of 'is' and 'same'. And in order for this 'opinion' of his to represent more than an idiosyncratic use of 'is' or of 'identical' – in order for us so much as to get off the ground even the mere appearance of a different logic of *identity* – we must suppose our patient to in some sense mean what we do by 'is' or 'identical'. Just as our two scientists, despite their having unwittingly talked past each other with their 'means' and their 'medians', both intend to be talking of averages, so too must 'the logician [who] accepts identity only upon the basis of identical subjects, [and] the paralogician [who] accepts identity based upon identical predicates' both mean to be aiming at identity.

Now, however, the question arises of what we could possibly appeal to so as to secure our sense of the intelligibility of this idea of the logician and the paralogician both aiming at a shared 'identity'? To the extent that we have any genuine sense that our patient's – or anyone's – words are to be treated as meaningful, we're surely forced to find them some kind of a place within what the Relativist has been calling our own 'logical country' or 'logical scheme'. But once we do that then we're once again back to assimilating his delusional world to our own, failing to respect its distinctive strangeness, and undermining the very idea that he even has an alternative logical scheme.[16]

In this way we start to see that the sense of our talk of someone living in an alternative logical world to our own is none too clear. To the extent that we're to think of them as actually enjoying thoughts, it seems we must have already assimilated them to our own scheme. However, we can also ask, if we're really supposed to be offering acknowledgement to an alternative logical scheme, whether we can really even make sense of the idea of *our own* thought being constrained by such a scheme. The idea of a logical scheme is after all supposed to be the idea of a particular form that reason is to take, one set of rules for what is to count as valid thought, an understanding as to what shall count as valid inference, what identity and difference are to amount to, etc. And to have such a scheme just is for one's thought to be constrained by it; there is no such thing as thinking which does not employ a logic. And yet here we're to supposedly find intelligible the notion of a genuine alternative to that which is supposed to constrain and inform the very intelligibility of any thought that's thinkable to us. But with what logical scheme are we now to frame this very thought about even the bare idea of different schemes? We seem here to be invited to take up a position both inside and outside our scheme at the same time. The problem is not so much that we can't ourselves occupy this other country, but that, since all of our thoughts – theoretical and practical – are supposedly shaped by our own abode, we can't even conceive of it. And yet there we supposedly are – thinking up the idea of alternative logical countries or schemes, which idea our very own theory should make unintelligible. That notions of 'other logical schemes' seem to remain utterly empty ought to bother us. But here it's as if we're to imagine that, whist we can't provide them with any content at all, we can nevertheless mean something by invoking the barest outline of their bare form. Against that we may (with Kant) remind ourselves that 'thoughts without content are empty'.[17] Or perhaps we might (with Frege) urge that whereas 'other persons presume to acknowledge and doubt a law in the same breath, it seems to me an attempt to jump out of one's own skin against which I can do no more than urgently warn them'.[18]

In short, although it looks as if von Domarus is expressing a thought with his suggestion that 'for a normal person the particular of being encircled is only one of many accidentals, [whereas] for the schizophrenic patient it is the quality expressing essence', it is, when we consider it, utterly opaque as to what the thought is that's thereby expressed. Taken one way it looks like an invitation to redefine either 'essence' or 'accidental'; taken another it looks like straightforward self-contradiction, the self-contradictory suggestion being that someone could meaningfully (not mis-take but) take accidental for essential properties. The relativizing ambition of the psychological logician was to humbly make room in the world for different forms of thought than his own, rather than (as he sees it) to arrogantly judge as awry such cognition as merely doesn't conform to the pattern of his own. When we think it through, however, what we find instead is, ironically and hubristically enough, that it's the psychological logician who, with his over-reaching thesis of 'paralogical thought', has offered us empty words whilst presumptuously proclaiming their meaningfulness.

Rethinking the question

We're now back in the post-ward round discussion, and the dispirited trainees are taking stock of what they've learned. They began by accepting their consultant's question – 'What justifies our saying of ourselves that we are sane, and our allocating our patients to the status of delusional (or thought-disordered, psychotic, or mentally ill)?' – as a good one, and so set about trying to answer it. The Realists hoped to find what we might call an 'objective criterion' for the obtaining of that which descriptive psychopathology references, something which could be used to separate the psychopathological goats from the non-psychopathological sheep – some natural fact about, say, the mind or brain of the delusional subject. Disappointed by what they found, they started to worry that their specialism's categories were wanting for validity. The Idealists then offered their own inability to make sense of the patient as a criterion for the patient's genuine delusionality. This suggestion was shot down as alarmingly subjective and open to abuse: why should one person's failure to understand another be criterial for the latter's delusionality? In despair at finding such a criterion, a relativistic, anti-psychiatric suggestion was explored: the patient is not lacking in, but instead resourced with a different form of, reason. Even here, however, it proved difficult to spell out a coherent thesis: in attempting to give shape to the bare idea of a deeply alternative meaning for their patients' words, the Relativists failed to control the meaning of their own.

Our consultant, however, has further lessons for his trainees. The first thing he does is re-draw their attention to von Domarus' patient's delusional suggestion that Jesus, cigar boxes, and sex are identical because they're all encircled. Whilst we don't do well to understand this in terms of some alternative logic of identity, we can, he notes, understand it perfectly well in terms of the illogic of the dream. For our night-time dreams are typically marked by what Freud called 'condensation': the authoritarian man who was just now our uncle is now of course instead our father, except he is somehow also at the same time that rather authoritarian teacher we had in first grade. Or: you were swimming in the pool at your aunt's house, except that you were also somehow swimming in the British Museum, both of them having, you now notice, just the same kind of marble flooring. That psychotic thought should share dream's confusional aspect isn't surprising, given the lack of reality contact which marks them both.

The next lesson our consultant offers concerns the importance of the trainees thinking for themselves: 'I asked you a question about the validity of our descriptive psychopathological categories, and you dutifully – perhaps rather too dutifully – set about answering it. Your struggles to answer it then led you to become sceptical about your profession's very validity. But why did nobody stop to interrogate my question's validity?' Recall: his question took its lead from an appreciation of the legitimate request for warrant for any particular psychiatric judgement regarding psychopathology: if a trainee couldn't provide context-relative grounds for his judgement that Mrs Thomas was delusional in her belief about her husband's murderousness, then – the thought goes – we shouldn't respect his judgement. But it then attempted to extrapolate this request for warrant to the fundamental categories of descriptive psychopathological thought, asking what general reason there is to think they themselves enjoy any validity. And the force of the question's sceptical bent was such as to drive those in its grip to a complacent idealism or to bite the bullet of anti-psychiatric relativism.

To loosen this grip, let's consider what requests for rational grounds typically bring along with them. An implication of my asking you to provide me with reasons for thinking and acting as you do is that your actions and utterances aren't to be counted rational unless grounds for them can be provided. What this presumption ignores, however, is the possibility that your actions and utterances are themselves paradigm-providing instantiations of rational thought or activity. Consider: you're engaged in deductive inference, and move from 'Socrates is a man' and 'All men are mortal' to 'Socrates is mortal'. If I ask you to justify your drawing of that conclusion from those premises, you'll be hard pressed to come up with grounds. The reason for this is that to move from those premises to 'Socrates is mortal' just is to do what here we call 'engage in deductive reasoning'. We do not, that is, here take it as rational because it conforms to some further paradigm of reason. So too when we're thinking not of deduction but of, say, declarations of will ('I'm going to the shops'). It makes no sense to ask you for your grounds for thinking that that truly is your will. (At best we could point to the absence of signs of self-deception.) And, to turn now to descriptive psychopathology, we find a similar lack of room for meaningful requests for grounds when what we're considering are general categories such as 'delusion'. 'A dog lay in wait for me as he sat on the steps of a Catholic convent. He got up on his hind legs and looked at me seriously.

He then saluted with his front paw as I approached him.'[19] Once we've established that such an utterance in such a context is as paradigmatic an expression of delusional perception as anything is, it makes no sense to now ask 'but is there really such a thing as delusion?' Rather: to believe, in this context, as this man believes just is to be deluded.

This point about the reality of delusion may be generalized. Descriptive psychopathological discourse prescribes the meaning of terms like 'delusion', 'thought disorder', 'psychosis', 'hallucination', etc. Because psychiatric initiates have grasped what it is to be counted delusional, they can cogently ask whether, say, Mrs Thomas really is delusional. Now, such words as 'really is', 'real', and 'reality' occur and obtain their sense within diverse discursive contexts (real delusion vs. delusion-like idea; real money vs. counterfeit; a real smile vs. a phony smile; a real oasis vs. a mirage). What is not evident, however, is that such words enjoy a meaning in abstraction from their contexts – so that we could intelligibly ask whether these various discourses themselves correspond to anything real or not. For it's not as if we give a meaning to 'delusion' or 'money' or 'smile' by means of mysterious acts of pure intellectual intuition, and only then go on to ask what grounds we have for thinking that anything 'in reality' actually corresponds to such terms. Or, it's not as if we learn them as we do terms like 'Loch Ness Monster' or 'fairy' – i.e. independently of referential usage. Instead, we learn their meaning in and through our engagements with the diverse psychiatric, economic, and emotional contexts of our lives. If anyone wants to know what 'delusion' means, then we refer them to such specific contexts, rather than offer up a definition that could be understood by the uninitiated. And given all this, it's simply not clear what it could even mean to ask whether delusion or psychosis ever 'really obtain'.

A further questionable implication of the consultant's original question is that we do well to construe our patients' perceivable acts and utterances as surface appearances pointing beyond themselves to a separable underlying psychopathological reality. To ask whether or not anyone's ever actually delusional is to rather presuppose that our encounter with clinical reality is first of all available to us under descriptions like 'aberrant behaviour', 'disordered discourse', etc., and only secondarily under notions like 'delusional notion' and 'formally disordered thought'. The idea here would be that these latter properly psychiatric symptoms are to stand behind the former merely behavioural ('natural') phenomena – perhaps as 'inner causes' hypothesized by psychiatric theory and inferred to, from their putative 'outer effects', by psychiatric practitioners. But nothing in either (i) our descriptive psychopathological discourse or our ordinary discourse about thoughtful speech, or (ii) the phenomenology of our experience of interpersonal communication, supports this conception of thought and meaning as transcending their expressive manifestations. Instead, ordinary thought and meaning ordinarily appear to us as immanent within acts and utterances considered in context – and so too do disturbances of thought and meaning. I listen to you and in so doing hear what we call 'that which you have to say', and it's in doing just this, rather than in making any secondary acts of inference from what's said to what's meant, that I grasp what, if any, are your thoughts on that matter about which you speak.[20]

For these reasons we're no more of the reasonable or unreasonable *opinion* that delusion or thought disorder obtain than we're of the *opinion* that human minds and bodies, trees and rivers, clouds and economies exist. Such terms ('trees', 'economies', 'delusions') don't signify posits of our minds to explain our experiences, but instead 'dignify' or 'voice' the diverse beings, and characters of the beings, we meet with.[21] To be sure we don't encounter delusions in the way that we encounter arm movements or isolated vocalizations: the acts which warrant description as 'delusional expressions' are embedded in a weave of life which includes a whole historical and situational context. We encounter patterns – or in the case of delusion, characteristic disruptions to the rational patterns – in such lives just as much as we encounter these lives' temporally isolable moments. (We don't first encounter moments and later string them together using posits that go beyond what is encountered; instead, our encounters are with patterns, and are themselves patterned.) We use our terms ('tree', 'person', 'delusion') to mark or voice these encounters and embodiments; we're not, that is, of the *opinion* that we have bodies, that certain utterances express delusion or formal thought disorder, that the coloured patches we see belong to trees growing at the end of the garden.[22] It's true that some terms ('person') are readily grasped by every normally developing child, whilst others ('formal thought disorder', 'legato') require a more specialist education. It's also true that sometimes, in our judgements of individual cases, and when we've already learned to operate with a concept like 'delusion' or 'thought disorder', we make misleading assumptions, and take ourselves to encounter delusion or thought disorder when we do not; in such cases we may surely talk of opinions. But none of this is to say that when we don't make such assumptions, or when we're learning the ropes of psychiatric discourse and judgement through exposure to what effectively are paradigms of particular psychopathology, we're in the opinion-holding business. Nor that a psychiatrist's education in descriptive psychopathology consists primarily in the learning of theories, the taking up of others' posits, or the making of inferences to the best explanation. Instead, it's readily understood as getting our psychopathological eyes and ears in in the midst of the encounters we have with those whose minds are falling apart.

Psychiatric responsibility

At the end of their discussion the trainees take leave of their consultant's question, thereby relinquishing their spurious ambition of justifying or legitimizing such fundamental psychopathological concepts as dignify or mark the disclosure of psychopathological reality. Yet to their dismay, as soon as they're relieved of this impossible justificatory task, they start to experience a new, deeper anxiety. For now what they're more starkly thrown up against are the profound responsibilities of their profession. But why should this be so? In what ways may we understand the Idealist, the Relativist, and the Realist be on the run from the responsibilities of genuine, accountable, psychiatric judgement?

At least when we're considering Idealism, the avoidance of responsible accountability may be easy to see. For as the Idealist psychiatrist might take it, the question of the difference between, say, genuine delusion and delusion-like idea may be collapsed simply into the question of whether he's moved to make the one determination or the other. So long as he's been designated sane and competent by the common consent of his community, whatever he feels like saying now passes psychiatric muster, and the idea of accountability in judgement is thereby nullified.

The Relativist clinician avoids the authoritarianism of the Idealist by proposing an all-shall-have-prizes solution: now the subject hitherto called 'insane' is to be thought of as meaning-making in her own way, as the self-ratifying ruler of her own subjective dominion. Talk of 'insanity' becomes at best merely an uncharitable way to mark the disjunction between the logical form of the patient's thought and one's own. 'I can't now understand you because your expressive life no longer instantiates meaning' collapses into 'I can't now understand you'. But in this way the psychiatrist deprives herself of any rational basis for determinations of insanity, both in the clinic and in the law court. The insanity defence is left without rational basis, and the rationale for involuntary detention collapses into the mere registration of dangerousness. In short, the Relativist avoids the dangers of paternalism whilst also jettisoning what's of value in it – namely, the valuable task of making treatment decisions on behalf of that subject who's currently not in his right mind. Decisions such as these may well be ones for which he, were we to ask him before or after he lost his mind, would express considerable gratitude. It's in stepping up to, rather than avoiding, the task of making such decisions, and shouldering such psychiatric responsibility, that the psychiatrist best performs her duties. Under the guise of a liberal ethic the Relativist in effect refuses to declare the fact of any of the patient's brokenness that escapes the patient's ken. In this way he deprives himself, and us, and his patient, of the possibility of seeing such brokenness as revelatory of what the patient suffers by way of both mental pain and damaged dignity.

To turn now to the Realist: how does he too shirk the responsibilities of psychiatric judgement? The clue to an answer comes from noticing the way he hopes to devolve the normative authority regarding the proper use of descriptive psychopathology's terms from himself and his peers, as exemplary members of the psychiatric profession, to rules which anyone, trained or untrained, could deploy. He hopes, that is, to provide criteria for the making of psychiatric determinations that require no specifically psychiatric sensibility but instead reference only what above were called 'natural facts'. Or, to put it otherwise, what the Realist is trying to do is to obviate the need for clinical judgement, and to find a rule for the use of, say, 'delusion' which will make redundant the need for any special expertise in judging delusion. The natural facts which the Realist is hoping to provide as criteria for some or other psychopathology are not simply the facts of someone's being, say, delusional or hallucinated. (If that is all that's meant by Realism, then we should surely all be Realists, although we may wish to dub ourselves 'realists' with a small 'r'.) Nor are they the specific facts that we may appeal to in justifying a particular psychiatric judgement. (That Mrs Thomas is to be judged delusional about her husband may be something for which justification surely can be given: her husband shows no signs of murderousness, she is peculiarly insistent yet blithe in her conviction at different times, etc.) They're rather facts the recognition of which requires no distinctively psychiatric judgement (since it's just such judgement which is here to be justified), and which may be appealed to in justifying the general use of any particular piece of psychiatric vocabulary (and so can't simply be the psychopathological facts themselves, since that would make the justification circular).

It's for this reason, I suggest, that psychiatry has been tempted to try to find simple rules for the use of terms like 'delusion'. Mrs Thomas, it's now suggested, can properly be said to be deluded only if she entertained belief that was (in an ordinary sense) false, atypical, poorly reasoned, and intransigent. Or perhaps it's said that to be properly judged psychotic is really for one to be in a state in which a particular dysregulation obtains in such limbic and cortical regions as subserve ordinary perception, emotional experience, and thought. The terms 'delusion' or 'psychosis' then become justifiable by reference to judgements regarding matters that are not intrinsically psychopathological but instead have to do with the recognition of ordinarily illogical or fallacious reasoning or the reading of brain scans. The psychiatrist can now devolve his normative authority to the semantic rules given in his textbooks or to the scan-reading neurologist; the justificatory buck need no longer stop with him and his clinical judgement.

One of the reasons the Realist demurs at the suggestion that he give up the requirement, on the use of psychiatric categories, that such use be positively justifiable, is that the alternative seems to introduce an unacceptable degree of subjectivity into the heart of psychiatric judgement. Without the objectivity in judgement that Realism promises, the practices of such judgement not unnaturally seem to him to collapse into the subjectivity of a 'because I say so' Idealism. And the costs of courting such subjectivity naturally strike us as high: on the one hand we fear incurring the ethical cost of that authoritarianism in judgement at which the Relativist baulks; on the other we seem to risk an anarchy of incoordination in the judgements of different psychiatrists. With his ambition of a determinate set of general criteria for the deployment of central psychopathological terms, the Realist considers himself to be – far from shirking the task of himself making responsible psychiatric judgement, as claimed above, instead – responsibly staving off the risks of whimsy and unreliability in pursuing his clinical duties.

One way to describe the problem with this Realist's reaction is to note how he mistakes the non-objectivity of psychiatric concept use for a problematic subjectivity. To understand what this means, consider the conceptual distinction we can draw between such judgement as warrants one or other of the descriptors 'subjective' and 'objective', and such judgement as warrants neither; let's call the first set of judgements 'opinions', and the latter set 'originary judgements'. 'Opinion' here stands for that which may usefully be said to be either justified or unjustified, and which, when it's unjustified, is properly said to be wanting. So consider: Our trainee considers Mrs Thomas a risk to others, so suggests she be sectioned under the Mental Health Act. That she exemplifies such a risk is his opinion. It may just be based on a feeling or hunch of his, in which case we can call it a 'subjective opinion'. On the other hand he may go on to justify it by considering the scientific evidence – that those with certain levels of agitation in combination with certain degrees of psychosis are likely to commit violence – or it may have been arrived at only through consideration of such evidence. In such cases we may call his opinion 'objective'. In the use of the term 'subjective opinion' here under consideration, we shall only call an opinion 'subjective' if it would at least make sense to think of that very same judgement as objective. If, however, it didn't even make sense to talk of the judgement in question as being provided with grounds, then we should call it neither objective nor subjective; it's these other forms of judgement which I here refer to as 'originary'.[23] By way of example we might consider the trainee's judgement that Mrs Thomas, with her jumpy reactions, hand wringing, pacing, fist clenching, constant movement, failure to allow others to speak, etc., is showing signs of agitation. Since to speak of her visible agitation simply is to speak of that particular gestalt of such visible signs which is here evident to him, it makes little sense to describe our trainee as 'of the opinion' that Mrs Thomas is agitated. His judgement regarding her agitation is neither justified nor unjustified; we might instead call it non-justified.

Perhaps it be suggested that, precisely because they may also be justified, justifiable judgements are simply preferable to non-justifiable judgements when it comes to psychiatric practice. Justification is after all of the essence of genuine science; why should it not also be an essential part of responsible practice?[24] Yet what this suggestion, which would make rather a cult of justification, overlooks is the fact that all opinion actually presupposes, and so can hardly supplant, originary judgement. I'm of the opinion that you've broken your arm. The basis of my judgement? The way your arm is hanging. But now what of my judgement that your arm is hanging strangely? Well, that's simply my originary judgement. If someone weren't to grasp the fact of it I should simply show it to her, perhaps alongside pictures of other broken limbs, and say 'see, this is what here is meant by "hanging strangely"'. My judgement is perfectly rational, but it isn't to be counted rational because it's grounded in a reason; rather, it itself exemplifies what rational judgement here looks like. And so too for psychiatric judgement. All that would be achieved by a requirement on psychiatric judgement that it be always and everywhere justifiable would be the evisceration of psychiatry of its distinctive meaning. How so? Because it would amount to a refusal to allow psychiatry's own categories to instantiate their own authentic disclosure of psychopathological reality. For if psychiatry is to retain descriptive categories such as 'delusion', 'psychosis', 'hallucination', 'agitation', etc., they must either be allowed to be those distinctive *sui generis* revelations of aspects or forms of mental illness which we ordinarily take them to be, or be explicable in terms that aren't psychiatry's explicit preserve (belief, truth, error, mistake, inference, perception, etc.). And in this latter case, psychiatry collapses as a distinctive discipline, enjoying no self-possession when it comes to its own conceptual categories, the buck of conceptual accountability having been passed to the disciplines (psychology, neuroscience) on which it's to now rely for its validation.

Despite its radical failure, the Realist approach to psychiatry does at least offer a general scheme for rendering psychiatric practice accountable. Should a question ever arise about the validity of a psychiatric judgement, the Realist psychiatrist offers a general rule by reference to which the question may be answered. ('What makes it right to say of anyone that she's deluded?' 'Because her thought has such and such psychological features.') But without such a rule book to fall back on – with only case law rather than casuistry to guide her, as it were – how is the psychiatrist to responsibly discharge her duty to both patient and society?

In one sense what's required of her is no more than we require of any competent speaker of what we might call 'non-technical' language (i.e. of language not regulated through strict definitions). We pick up words in particular contexts and more or less spontaneously project them into other contexts. Others do the same. In so doing we're all learning – yet also renewing, vivifying, and elaborating – our living language, rather than cranking the handle of a mechanism within which the correct answer to these words' use is somehow already stored up.[25] Nothing ensures that we shall make the same projections as one another, but we hopefully share enough by way of sensibility – i.e. share enough of what Stanley Cavell calls that 'whorl of organism' constituted inter alia by our 'routes of interest and feeling, senses of humour and of significance and of fulfilment, of what is outrageous, of what is similar to what else, what a rebuke, what forgiveness, of when an utterance is an assertion, when an appeal, when an explanation'[26] – to be sufficiently commensurate in our originary judgements.[27]

Yet such a shared projective facility isn't all there for us from the get-go. We refine and elaborate it through the progressive trying out, in contexts such as clinical supervisions and case conferences, of fine distinctions regarding different psychological states. We deepen it through discerning how to apply it to lives described in increasingly rich biographical and phenomenological detail. We finesse it through paying an increasingly close attention to our counter-transference, thereby distinguishing more clearly between such perturbations and mishaps in our clinical interviews as are due to ourselves and such as belong to our patients. We work through our own psychological blind spots and complexes, relinquish our repressive defences, and thereby become better able to take the psychological temperature of those we encounter. We carefully listen to and evaluate the complaints of those outside the profession who feel that their capture within our categories is unhelpful. We increase our capacity to distinguish the disturbed (mad) from the culpable (bad) as we ourselves morally grow, withdrawing our defensive projections of guilt and shame, taking more responsibility for our actions, and maturing in our moral discernment. We attend to when our professionalism or scientism, ambition or insecurity, get the better of us – and strive to put that right. We come to better locate and offer acknowledgement to the humanity of the patient as we learn to tolerate the vulnerability we experience when seeing through the lens of love – truly wanting the best for them, and meeting them in their individuality – rather than merely through that of knowledge. We also come to better tolerate our own doubt and confusion, and in this way prescind from hasty judgement, allowing ourselves to not know what we think, to be surprised by what we find ourselves wanting to say, so as to come gradually to more discerning answers. Or we try to notice not only what confirms, but also what disconfirms, our particular intuitions. Finally, we make greater space for human nature's constitutive indeterminacy, thereby accepting there won't always be right answers to our questions.

In all these ways our duties to use our clinical terms wisely are discharged; our terms are now truly inhabited by us, made more fully our own, and we become in our pronouncements more fully the living embodiments of psychiatric meaning. Now there's no more wishful imagining of ourselves as Realist followers of a law residing outside ourselves and containing its own answers coiled up within itself. Nor do we collapse into either the omnipotent fantasies of Idealism or the impotence of Relativism. Instead, we become a true part of psychiatry's body politic: with our constantly refined and enriched linguistic sensibilities we become repositories of psychiatric wisdom. We learn how to judge – rather than to merely follow such judgements of others as have been codified into rules. This – and not some tallying up of an already determinate word use to a singular and independently established medical fact (Realism), nor some mere undisciplined pronouncement by he who has charitably been deemed sane by his peers (Idealism) – is psychiatric responsibility in judgement. And to this project of accountable clinical growth – a project at once linguistic, psychological, and moral – there is no end.[28]

Notes

Introduction

1 Brown (1944: 97) describes himself as amanuensis, but it's more probable that the 'manic-depressive psychosis' of which he writes is his own (Peterson 1982: 214).

2 Schmidt ([1940] 1987: 120).

3 For an introduction to apophatic theology, see Turner (1995).

4 Murdoch (1999: 75).

5 Deflection: Cavell (1969); Diamond (2003). See also Wittgenstein (2013: 86): 'What makes a subject difficult to understand, if it is significant, important, is not that some special instruction about abstruse things is necessary to understand it. Rather it is the contrast between the understanding of the subject and what most people want to see. . . . What has to be overcome is not a difficulty of the intellect, but of the will.'

6 Recovery: Phillips (2000). Retrieval: Wollheim (1980c).

7 Which isn't to say that psychoanalysis hasn't itself also historically proffered a range of implausible aetiological theories!

8 Something similar can happen in psychiatry, where symptom lists as offered by, for example, ICD-10 or DSM-5, for educational, training or scientific purposes, now get treated as providing definitive criteria – rather than mere indices – for what it means to suffer, say, a schizophrenic or depressive illness. (An index is an empirically reliable indicator rather than a logically necessary criterion; it needn't tell us anything about the essential nature of that which it indicates. I owe this distinction to Anthony Fernandez.)

9 Diamond (2003: 2–3).

10 Frith (1992: 95).

11 Lucas (2009: 307).

12 Wittgenstein (1980c: 33e).

13 In this work 'thought' is used not to signal a species of mental activity – i.e. not to contrast with instances of emotion, intention and perception – but instead in its philosophical sense, to specify the 'content' of any such activity. Instances of perception, cogitation, utterance, and feeling have 'content' when they're aptly described by means of a relevant transitive verb followed by 'that' (or followed by 'for', 'with', etc. when such uses may be rephrased in 'that' terms). If, when I hear you bang the drum, I hear that you're banging the drum, then the content of my perception, my thought, is *that you're banging the drum*. If I'm upset when you traduce me, it may well be that I'm upset with you *for* traducing me; the content of my upset, my thought, then is *that you traduce me*. If I hope for rain, then I hope *that it will rain*. It's essential in all such cases that the subject *understands* what is felt, said, wished, seen, etc. – in the sense that they understand that *that* (that you are banging the drum, for instance) was what was encountered or meant.

14 Jaspers ([1959] 1963: 778).

15 To 'normalize' may mean to help someone feel less uniquely damned (a point I owe to Allen Francis), to therapeutically restore an order the subject has herself lost, or to deconstruct the theorist or clinician's distinction between psychotic and non-psychotic orders so that the subject deemed psychotic may once again be understood in an ordinary fashion. Here the term is deployed in the third sense.

16 The importance of not normalizing (in the third sense outlined by the previous footnote) psychotic symptoms is registered in the following exchange, in Dublin, 1947–48, between the philosopher Ludwig Wittgenstein and his friend the newly qualified psychiatrist M. O'C. Drury. Drury: 'Some of the patients I am seeing present symptoms which I find extremely puzzling. I often don't know what to say to them.' Wittgenstein: 'You must always be puzzled by mental illness. The thing I would dread most, if I became mentally ill, would be your adopting a common-sense attitude; that you could take it for granted that I was deluded' (Rhees 1984: 152).

17 Roger Squires, quoted by Hamilton (2006).

18 Laing (1965) and Kusters ([2014] 2020) sometimes write in this vein.

19 Eilan (2000: 97).

20 E.g. Wittgenstein (1969); Midgley (1973).

1 Mental Illness

1 Heavily condensed from Schmidt (1941) by Jaspers ([1959] 1963: 101–102); translation amended.

2 Champlin (1981). 'Disease' has shifted its sense over time, no longer meaning that lack of ease which could hardly afflict a plant.

3 Such sickness behaviour in animals may be mediated by release of the pro-inflammatory cytokine interleukin-1 (Hart 1988).

4 Ward (2020).

5 Fulford (1989: ch. 7). 'Illness' has to do with 'failure of what is here called "ordinary" doing in the apparent absence of obstruction and/or opposition' (ibid: 109). The fuller analysis considers illness as something wrong with, rather than done by or to us, and sees the painful sensations it often involves as being ineradicable by moving away from a source.

6 Another aspect of this radicalization is considered below in the section on suffering.

7 Champlin (1996).

8 See Wittgenstein (1958a: §§67ff).

9 Rushton (1988).

10 A related distinction concerns what have variously been called 'functional' or 'organic', 'exogenous' or 'endogenous', 'psychiatric' or 'neurological', mental disorders. The meaning of 'functional' varies considerably across and within psychiatric and neurological contexts. Sometimes its use can reflect an ill-considered (functionalist, software vs. hardware) philosophy of mind's relation to brain. At other times, 'organic' means 'due to another, non-psychiatric, medical condition', or 'due to manifest tissue damage' (e.g. stroke, brain injury, neurodegenerative disease, etc.). 'Functional', meanwhile, may sometimes refer to the function played by symptoms in maintaining the emotional economy of the patient; in this use it implies the availability of a form of intelligibility not enjoyed by 'organic' disorder. Sometimes the organic/functional distinction may be best understood as a matter of historical contingency, relating only to the profession which happens to treat the condition in question (neurologists for

organic, psychiatrists for functional). And at other times organic mental disorder may be best understood as localizable to discrete regions of the brain, whilst functional disturbance may be more widespread. See Bell et al. (2020) and de Haan (2020: ch. 4, §6).

11 Ventricles may be enlarged, grey and white matter may be reduced, neuronal connectivity may be altered. Whether this is a cause, an effect or a part of the illness, or when or whether it's due to the use of neuroleptics or to lifestyle, is of course another, empirical, matter.

12 Aristotle ([4th century BC] 1998: book V, part 2).

13 Wittgenstein (1958b: 24–25).

14 Pickering (2006); Szasz (1987: ch. 5).

15 Champlin (1996, 2008) provides further critique of the idea that mental illness is metaphorical illness. His own very nice analogy compares the relation between 'mental illness' and 'physical illness' with that between 'rhymes for the eye' (when the ends of poetry lines are spelled the same) and 'rhymes for the ear' (i.e. ordinary rhyme).

16 Wittgenstein (1958a: §282, p. 216). The notion of the sense of 'mental illness' as secondary sense has been developed by Champlin (1996); the present section draws on his account.

17 Wittgenstein (1958b: §137).

18 Some early examples: Emily Brontë's Catherine suffers from 'nerves'; hopes are expressed of 'a favourable crisis in Catherine's mental illness' (Brontë [1847] 1991: 176); the physician Thomas Arnold described how 'during the courſe of the ſame illneſs, it not unfrequently happens that Mania and Melancholy alternate repeatedly with each other' (Arnold 1782: 58).

19 Pickering (2006).

20 See Jeronimus (2019) and de Haan (2020) on alternative stable states.

21 Hence the duration indices in ICD-10 and DSM-5.

22 For elaboration of a (motivational) 'madness as strategy' versus (disturbance-based) 'madness as dysfunction' distinction, see Garson (2019: ch. 11). See also de Haan (2020: ch. 7).

23 What is meant by 'reality contact' is the topic of Chapter 4; non-psychotic forms of damaged reality contact are not discussed here.

24 Minkowski (1953: 212–213) describes how the schizophrenic retreat to a devitalized state may, 'if we attribute it to the activity of the subject', be described in terms of 'suppression . . . without this in any sense referring to a deliberate and conscious act. The difference between this state of affairs and putting your head in the sand is here particularly clear.'

25 This is particularly obvious in neurotic cases. The phobic patient knows full well the irrationality of his fear, and the way in which his fear-driven avoidance behaviour is ruining his life. Even so, we and he will acknowledge the propriety of describing his behaviour as motivated, even if not chosen or intended.

26 Many schizophrenic subjects do of course feel pain; a patient with a Messianic delusion feels head pain due to an imagined 'crown of thorns'; another feels that a lack of sexual contact has led to a 'building of bones in the spine'. Watson, Chandarana and Merskey (1981).

27 The significance of this sense of suffering as tolerating or allowing ('suffer the little children, and forbid them not, to come unto me' – Mt: 19:14) has been explored by Wilfred Bion; see Abel-Hirsch (2006).

28 Freud ([1924] 1961: 151).

29 Hayward and Taylor (1956: 236).

30 Laing (1963: 203) citing Minkowski.

31 Schopenhauer ([1819] 1969: 193). The following clinical extract shows the dynamic in question. A patient of mine changed his social environment and suffered extreme anxiety. Rather than remain in touch with this, he instead developed the delusion that I was a research scientist who could fund either his eternal isolated flight into outer space, from where he could report back to earth by means of a one-way radio, or his complete neurological immersion in the internet, where there would be no differentiation between his own mind and the rest of humanity. When I rashly shared my intuition that his delusion-driving difficulty was rooted in a struggle to tolerate the uncertainties of ordinary human connection, such that he opted now either for total remove (in outer space) or utter fusion (with the internet), he responded by becoming momentarily reality-oriented and anguished, angrily exclaimed 'of course that's why I need to be mad right now', before quickly lapsing back into the more comfortable, delusional, mode.

32 Kirkbride et al. (2012); Nielssen and Large (2010); Appleby et al. (2019); Milton et al. (2001).

33 Smith (2013). By way of analogy, consider that nobody is cured of the fear of flying by examining the data on flight mortality.

34 The nature of inner integration and reality contact are explored in Chapters 3 and 4.

35 Gaita (2000: ch. 1).

36 Corrigan et al. (2001).

37 This is not measured by such studies as examine our attitudes towards those already described as mentally ill; it's better reflected in the socio-historical move from inhumane incarceration to humane hospitalization.

38 I here intend no implication that we do better to talk of 'people *with* mental illness' or 'person *with* bipolar disorder' rather than talk of 'the mentally ill' or 'bipolar person'. To refer to someone by their profession (he's a psychologist, she bakes), affliction (she's a diabetic, he's schizophrenic) or nationality (he's an American, she's Scottish) is not in itself to invite a reduction of the person to their descriptor. And to insist upon the preposition risks underplaying the extent to which professions, significant afflictions and nationalities are often not extrinsic to but partly constitutive of identity (Sass, 2007).

39 Radden (2019).

40 Spitzer, Endicott and Franchi (2018).

41 For critique of approaches to mental disorder which treat of 'underlying mechanisms' and ignore the existential dimension, see de Haan (2020).

42 Included here are many naturalistic accounts, both scientific and relaxed, such as Wakefield (1992); Murphy (2012); Bolton (2008); Thornton (2007).

2 Delusion's Rational Irretrievability

1 Jaspers ([1959] 1963: 93).

2 Examples adapted from Jaspers ([1959] 1963: 99, 98, 103); Kopelman, Guinan and Lewis (1995: 72). See also Jaspers ([1959] 1963: 99): 'In fact there is no kind of experience with a known object which we could not link with the word "delusion" provided that at the level of meaning, awareness of meaning has become this experience of primary delusion.'

3   By describing the delusional subject as not acknowledging the non-objectivity of her delusional belief, I'm not meaning to imply that she's helpfully thought of as mistaking her delusional belief for objective knowledge. See Chapter 4.

4   Coate (1964: 31–35).

5   Harrison et al. (2018: 8); APA (2013: 87); Campbell (2009: 263); Kring et al. (2007: 351); Ray (2015: 209).

6   Jaspers ([1959] 1963: 95–96).

7   Jaspers ([1959] 1963: 93, 95, 96). For corrective, see Walker (1991); Gorski (2012).

8   Jaspers ([1959] 1963: 106).

9   See case 7 in Fulford and Radoilska (2012).

10 E.g. APA (2013: 87).

11 Beck and Rector (2000) describe cognitive therapy techniques used to inspire doubt in psychotic subjects about their fixed delusions. Manfred Bleuler ([1972] 1978: 489–490) describes how delusions may at least readily go underground even if not being truly relinquished: '. . . delusional assertiveness is not something entirely absolute. In one instance, the schizophrenic relies on his delusions, but the next time he will do without them. He can see in me the concocter of poisons, his murderer, Satan himself, and morally spit at me; yet at the same time, he will point out his aching tooth to me, and cooperate fully by positioning his jaw for local anesthesia and the extraction, and then thank me as warmly as any normal person would. . . . Only in old textbooks is the schizophrenic delusion depicted as an unalterable, rigid condition; in reality, it adapts itself to the patient's inner needs and desires.'

12 Jaspers ([1959] 1963: 195).

13 Jaspers ([1959] 1963: 104); also at p. 411: 'the incorrigibility of delusion has something over and above the incorrigibility of healthy people's mistakes. So far, however, we have not succeeded in defining what this is.'

14 'Definition', Jaspers suggests, 'will not dispose of the matter' (Jaspers ([1959] 1963: 93).

15 Jaspers ([1959] 1963: 778).

16 See Gorski (2012). As far back as 1883 Kraepelin told us that, 'Every delusional idea is a pathologically distorted notion' but, as noted in 'Aschaffenburg's critique of 1915, the word "pathological" pre-empts the very search for those criteria which make it pathological' (Schmidt [1940] 1987: 119–120).

17 Jaspers ([1959] 1963: 704, 408, 96, 98).

18 See Jaspers ([1959] 1963: 28).

19 Phenomenological (Sass 1992: 16–19, 26–27, 78, 215); Constructivist (Geekie and Read 2009: 106, 112); Existential (Laing 1964; Kirsner 1990); Psychodynamic (Evans 2016: 2); Cognitivist (Bentall 2003: 28–29, 95, 300, 495); Neuropsychiatric (Kendler and Campbell 2014).

20 Garety and Freeman (1999: 116); Maher (1988).

21 Bentall (2003: 300).

22 Laing (1964: 593).

23 Geekie and Read (2009: 106, 112).

24 Trepper and Shean (2013: 59).

25 Sass (1992: 16–17).

26 Jaspers ([1959] 1963: 106).

27 Jaspers ([1959] 1963: 639, 641). 'Anlage': constitution or temperament; the 'sum-total of all the endogenous preconditions of psychic life' (Jaspers [1959] 1963: 455). On the relationship between personality and schizophrenic process, see also Stanghellini (2004).

28 Jaspers ([1959] 1963: 639, 640).
29 Jaspers ([1959] 1963: 196). With thanks to Sanneke de Haan for re-translating this
    passage. The remark may appear to contradict what Jaspers says at pp. 302–303:
    'Psychic events "emerge" out of each other in a way which we understand.... Thus we
    understand psychic reactions to experience, we understand the development of
    passion, the growth of an error, the content of dream and delusion, the effects of
    suggestion [etc]....' However, in this later passage Jaspers is discussing not our grasp
    of what someone means by their delusional expression but rather our grasp of what in
    the dynamic context motivated this content's emergence.
30 Jaspers ([1959] 1963: 811). On the 'limits to psychotherapy': Jaspers ([1959] 1963:
    804–805).
31 Stanghellini and Fuchs (2013: xviii) suggest that Jaspers' descriptive 'psychopathology
    attempts to use empathy as a clinical instrument to recreate in the psychopathologist
    the subjective experience of a patient to obtain a valid and reliable description of his
    experience.' Walker (1991: 100) offers that 'Understanding (Verstehen) is my empathic
    access to the other person's subjective experience using the analogy of my own
    experience.'
32 Jaspers ([1959] 1963: part 1, ch. 4, §1); Heidegger ([1927] 1962: div. 1, part IV);
    Merleau-Ponty ([1945] 2012: part 2, ch. 4). See also Wittgenstein (1980b: §170): 'In
    general I do not surmise fear in him – I *see* it. I do not feel that I am deducing the
    probable existence of something inside from something outside; rather it is as if the
    human face were in a way translucent and that I were seeing it not in reflected light
    but rather in its own.'
33 For an exception, consider that we do occasionally have cause to say that we
    understand someone *as* saying *what* she says. For example, Morag asks me to buy
    some milk, and when you ask me what I took her to be getting at, I reply that I
    understood her as asking me to buy some milk. Yet the function of this particular
    'understanding as' locution is just to ward off the implication that here we have to do
    with anything other than simply, empathically, getting/grasping/seeing what she's
    doing.
34 In fact, Jaspers always rejects the notion that our ordinary meaning-grasping involves
    the adding of interpretation or other such acts of thought to an intrinsically meaning-
    denuded perceptual experience: 'Perceptions are never mechanical responses to
    sense-stimuli; there is always at the same time a perception of meaning. A house is
    there for people to inhabit; people in the streets are following their own pursuits. If I
    see a knife, I see directly, immediately a tool for cutting.... We may not be explicitly
    conscious of the meanings we make when we perceive but nevertheless they are
    always present' (Jaspers ([1959] 1963: 99).
35 NKJV, Jn. 10: 14–15.
36 The significance of such non-methodical ability and expectation as constitutes the
    basic form of our comprehension, a form that constitutes our reality contact as such, is
    treated of in Chapter 4. It bears mention that Jaspers distinguishes between 'rational'
    and 'empathic' understanding, reserving the former term for designating inferential
    validity (as may be intact even in delusional systems: Jaspers ([1959] 1963: 307). In the
    present work, however, I deploy the terms 'rational' (and 'reason') more inclusively – to
    also designate that which manifests reality contact.
37 Jaspers ([1959] 1963: 302–303).
38 I.e. 'Anlage': Jaspers ([1959] 1963: 363).
39 Jaspers ([1959] 1963: 196).

40 Jaspers ([1959] 1963: 97, 196, 195).
41 Jaspers ([1959] 1963: 99).
42 Jaspers ([1959] 1963: 196).
43 See Jaspers ([1959] 1963: 96–97).
44 NIMH (2021).
45 Whether the cause of such cognitive deficits and negative symptoms is defensive withdrawal, a primary neurological disorder, depression, or the use of major tranquilizers, is another matter.
46 Garety and Freeman (1999).
47 See Moritz and Woodward (2005). Since Huq, Garety and Hemsley (1988) first used the 'beads task' to test for a 'jumping to conclusions' reasoning style in delusional subjects, over *sixty* papers have been published showing various correlations between making a quick judgement on the beads task and diagnosis, level of delusionality, cognitive style, etc. in schizophrenic, delusional, other psychiatric, and non-clinical populations (Dudley et al. 2016). As with all such studies that merely track correlations between experimental and non-experimental variables, what we never learn, since the studies are not resourced to tell us, is why the experimental results obtain. Researchers typically find that delusional subjects are more likely to jump to conclusions, and suggest that this in turn implies that a tendency to jump to conclusions results in delusions. (It appears that delusional subjects are not – on average – irrationally precipitate, but rather that *non-delusional* subjects are – on average – *irrationally conservative*; even so, this literature still categorizes delusional subjects as 'jumping to conclusions'. Furthermore, *delusional* subjects have been found more likely than non-delusional subjects to *revise* their beliefs in the face of potentially disconfirmatory evidence (Garety, Hemsley and Wessely 1991). How 'jumpiness' is supposed to relate to delusionality is, then, not at all clear.) But perhaps the correlations found between promptness of decision on the beads task and degree of delusionality are instead because an effect (rather than a cause) of currently being psychotic or delusional is that one tends to precipitate judgement, or because delusional subjects can't bring themselves to rationally override their intuitions, or because they're more disinhibited and so more in touch with their disdain for the task and with their desire for it to soon be over, or because a preoccupation with enthralling delusions leads you to not bother trying to put your mind to mundane experiments, or because delusional subjects are also more likely to be in a state of existential despair incompatible with putting one's mind to such tasks, or … Finesse the experimental design to measure all these and other possibilities, so as to see what degree of the relation between delusion and beads task performance was 'explained' only by a jumping to conclusions bias and not by the other factors: the result, I suggest, is likely to be that a small effect remains. But what of it? In this way, such experimental designs in psychology as uncover correlations between variables usually lead to a death by a thousand qualifications, along with the inevitable 'more research is needed' refrain. Stepping back from such experimental studies what we can't help but notice is the depersonalizing distance they *all* take from their subjects. Someone *has become psychotic in the face of what to them are life's intolerable predicaments* – and the interest they receive from the psychologist now takes the form of an inquiry into *how many coloured beads they feel should be inspected before deciding which jar they come from*. In this way, the studies may tell us rather more about the banalizing and deflective zeitgeist of experimental psychology than about their subjects.
48 See Maher (1974, 1988), who also posits that the delusional belief is reinforced by the decrease in anxiety that explanation brings.

49 A survey of the ambitions and shortcomings of cognitive psychological theories of delusion is provided by McKenna (2017: ch. 5); see also Cutting and Musalek (2015).

50 Jaspers ([1959] 1963: 97).

51 Jaspers ([1959] 1963: 196).

52 On interventionism in the psychiatric context, see Woodward (2008) and Kendler and Campbell (2009; 2014).

53 Jaspers ([1959] 1963: 97).

54 Thompson (2008).

55 Jaspers ([1959] 1963: 778).

56 Jaspers (1968: 1318).

57 Jaspers ([1959] 1963: 704).

58 Schopenhauer ([1819] 1969: 193).

59 Jaspers ([1959] 1963: 704).

60 Coate (1964: 119–121).

61 Jaspers ([1959] 1963: 308).

62 Jaspers ([1959] 1963: 363). Emmanuel Levinas (1969) describes as the 'face of the other' that locus where we must stop short if we're to resist the colonizing urge to penetrate the other with understanding and thereby assimilate him to ourself rather than respect him in his alterity.

63 Cp. the saying often attributed to Martin Luther: 'Here I stand; I can do no other.' In one sense, of course, Luther could perfectly well do otherwise – but not if he's to remain true to himself. Jaspers ([1959] 1963: 308) considers the matter of our unaccountable Existence in relation to what he calls our 'freedom', a freedom disclosing itself in 'free decisions, in a grasp of absolute meanings, and in that basic experience where . . . we are roused from ordinary existence into an autonomous self-hood'.

64 Jaspers ([1935] 1955: 118); translation amended.

65 Coate (1964: 122).

3 Reality Contact

1 Séchehaye ([1950] 1951); translation amended. Düss ('Renée'), Séchehaye's patient, is in truth this book's principal author. Düss was ultimately adopted by Séchehaye, and later became a psychologist and author in her own right.

2 'Representation' is not here offered as an explanatory concept, but instead intended merely stipulatively – as signalling such thought (i.e. judgement) and reasoning (i.e. inference) as may be assessed correct or incorrect.

3 Bortolotti (2010); Radden (2011); Currie and Ravenscroft (2001); Hamilton (2006); Bermudez (2001); Bayne and Pacherie (2005). The question of whether delusions are or are not beliefs appears largely ill-conceived, since it typically fails to first consider what the actual point is of our psychopathological talk of delusional belief (on which see the introduction to Chapter 2). As to whether delusional beliefs are truly beliefs, we might equally ask whether a bridge that has been hit by a bomb and now lies in pieces on the river bed is or is not a bridge. Or whether a man who turns the ignition, engages the gear, and depresses the accelerator – in a car which has been raised on bricks – is or is not accelerating the car. Just like such metaphysical debates as can only gather steam because they refuse to first say what they even mean by the questions

they attempt to answer, the doxastic/non-doxastic debate (as to whether Louisa's delusional claims – that the school was a vast barracks filled with children compelled to sing, that things were tricking her, that she was the earth's only inhabitant, that she was nine centuries old, that this meant she wasn't yet born, that the police were trying to put her to death, that her hands turn into cats' paws – are or are not expressive of belief) is also insufficiently motivated.

4   Bortolotti (2010: 259).
5   Schmidt ([1940] 1987); Gorski (2012).
6   Jaspers ([1959] 1963: 106). It might be said that, delusions being confusional, there's not really any such thing as drawing rational implications from them. Against this, consider that we know perfectly well how to answer nonsensical questions such as: if the number 2 is red whilst 3 is green, which of these numbers is the colour of the poppy's flower? See Teichmann (2021).
7   Bortolotti (2010).
8   Sass and Pienkos (2013); Sass (2014b); Porcher (2019).
9   Bleuler ([1911] 1950: 129); for more on double bookkeeping, see ibid: 127–130, 147 and 378.
10 Cp. the phenomenon of blindsight; Hyman (1991).
11 Schreber ([1903] 1988: 301).
12 Sass and Pienkos (2013: 646–648).
13 Jaspers ([1959] 1963: 284).
14 Since doubt presupposes certainty for its intelligibility, global scepticism is incoherent. Wittgenstein: 'If you tried to doubt everything you would not get as far as doubting anything. The game of doubting itself presupposes certainty' (Wittgenstein 1969: §115); 'If I want the door to turn, the hinges must stay put' (ibid: §343). See also Merleau-Ponty: 'To wonder if the world is real is to fail to understand what one is saying' (Merleau-Ponty [1945] 2012: 360).
15 Wittgenstein (1958a: §217, §648; 1993 §498; 1969: §204, §253).
16 Wittgenstein (1969: §341; see also §343, §655).
17 As Moyal-Sharrock (2016: 98) has it, actual hinges 'are really animal or unreflective ways of acting which, once formulated (e.g., by philosophers), look like propositional beliefs'.
18 See Campbell (2001); Eilan (2001); Rhodes and Gipps (2008); Bardina (2018). For critique: Thornton (2007, 2008); Bellaar (2016).
19 Campbell (2001: 96). Campbell goes on to write that the delusional subject treats his delusional beliefs 'as the background assumptions needed for there to be any testing of the correctness of propositions at all' (ibid: 96). Yet whilst some hinge propositions articulate what *might* be called assumptions ('the sun shall rise again'), others are too close to demonstrations of a grasp of semantic meaning ('these are my hands') or are awkwardly wordy conveyances of living certainties ('the ground will continue to support my weight') to readily count as expressive of assumptions. We might put it like this: if an *assumption* is something which I could coherently – but in fact don't – doubt, then it's unclear that what a variety of framework propositions articulate are assumptions. See also Wittgenstein (1969: §§342–345): 'it isn't that the situation is like this: We just *can't* investigate everything, and for that reason we are forced to rest content with assumption' (ibid: §343); and Thornton (2008).
20 The argument is well made by Thornton (2008).
21 See again Thornton (2008).
22 Bardina (2018) disputes Thornton's (2008) argument against identifying delusional utterances with hinge propositions by herself arguing that expressions of delusion

meet the six defining features of hinges outlined by Moyal-Sharrock (2004). But on Moyal-Sharrock's conception, hinge expressions are living certainties given voice in grammatical rules – which rules articulate what it so much as makes sense to think, say and do. Bardina effectively offers us a psychologistic conception of hinges statements: they become articulations of what someone refuses to doubt in practice, rather than of what it makes no sense to doubt..

23 The same difficulties attend Szasz's view that 'Sexual self-stimulation (masturbation), unlike copulation, is a sex act intended to involve and be enjoyed by the self only, not someone else (as well). Similarly, semantic self-stimulation (schizophrenese) is a speech act intended to involve and be understood by the self only, not someone else (as well)' (Szasz 1996: 534).

24 See Kant ([1798] 2006: 113–114) and Wittgenstein (1958a: §§243–315). Kant describes 'the loss of *common sense* (*sensus communis*) and its replacement with *logical private sense* (*sensus privatus*)' as the 'only universal characteristic of madness'. Wittgenstein's argument runs deeper, challenging as it does the coherence of the very idea of 'logical private sense'. Kant's argument, in effect, and because of the way it articulates itself, still holds out hope for a cataphatic approach to madness – a hope which Wittgenstein's argument subsequently dashes.

25 Wittgenstein (1958a: §265).

26 Wittgenstein (1958a: §258).

27 On 'radical interpretation': Davidson (1973).

28 Contra Dreyfus and Taylor (2015: ch 4).

29 *Locus classicus*: Hume ([1739] 2000: book 1, part iii).

30 Wittgenstein calls such conditioning 'training'; Ryle styles it 'wont'. See Wittgenstein (1981: §318, §419; 1969: §279; 1958a: §5, §441); Ryle ([1945] 2009; [1962] 2009).

31 Hume ([1739] 2000: §5.ii.21).

32 Here I repurpose Wittgenstein's offering of 'absence of surprise' as criterion for voluntary action (Wittgenstein 1958a: §628), and reference in particular Merleau-Ponty's ([1945] 2012) conception of the 'grip' (*la prise*) that we have on the world in perception, a grip partly constituted by our lived expectations.

33 Wittgenstein (1969: §254): 'Any "reasonable" person behaves like *this*.'

34 See Wittgenstein (1958a: §289): 'To use a word without a justification does not mean to use it without right.'

35 Wittgenstein (1958a: §217): 'If I have exhausted the justifications, I have reached bedrock and my spade is turned. Then I am inclined to say: "This is simply what I do."'

36 See Wittgenstein (1958a: §16): 'It is most natural, and causes least confusion, to reckon the samples among the instruments of the language.'

37 Wittgenstein (1958a: §216).

38 Husserl ([1952] 1989) uses the term 'protention' to describe such anticipations as structure our experiences; Merleau-Ponty ([1945] 2012: 112) offers us 'lived' rather than 'known' protentions that part-constitute our 'motor intentionality' (*intentionalité motrice*). The concept of 'motor intentionality' is that of 'something *between* movement as a third person process and thought as a representation of movement'; 'an anticipation of, or arrival at, the objective' that is 'ensured by the body itself'. See Morris (2012: ch. 3).

39 O'Regan and Noë (2001); Buhrmann, Di Paolo and Barandiaran (2013).

40 Sass (1994: 21).

41 Wittgenstein (1958a: §250, §540, §583, §584); Wittgenstein (1980b: §776); Wittgenstein (1981: §587).

42 Williams ([1976] 1981: 18).

43 Bleuler (1955: 377).

44 Minkowski (1953); Urfer (2001); Rümke ([1941] 1990); Kimura (1992); Kupper et al. (2015); Howes et al. (2017); Fuchs and Röhricht (2017); van Duppen (2017); Sprong et al. (2007); Bora, Yucel and Pantelis (2009). On the character and development of these interactional capacities in infancy and childhood: Reddy (2008); Hobson (2002).

45 '[It] is a subjectively necessary touchstone of the correctness of our judgments generally, and consequently also of the soundness of our understanding, that we also restrain our understanding by the *understanding of others,* instead of *isolating* ourselves with our own understanding and judging *publicly* with our private representations, so to speak.' To take 'something merely subjective (for instance, habit or inclination) [for] something objective . . . is precisely what the illusion consists in that is said to deceive us, or rather by means of which we are misled to deceive ourselves in the application of a rule. – He who pays no attention at all to this touchstone, but gets it into his head to recognise private sense as already valid apart from or even in opposition to common sense, is abandoned to a play of thoughts in which he sees, acts, and judges, not in a common world, but rather in his own world (as in dreaming)' (Kant [1798] 2006: 113–114).

46 We owe the metaphor of the world's flesh (*la chair du monde*) to Merleau-Ponty ([1964] 1968). On 'fusion', see Wittgenstein (1969: §558).

47 Consider what Wittgenstein (1958a: §16) wrote of samples: '. . . are they part of the *language*? Well, it is as you please. They do not belong among the words; yet when I say to someone: "Pronounce the word 'the'", you will count the second "the" as part of the sentence. Yet it has a role just like that of a colour-sample . . . It is most natural, and causes least confusion, to reckon the samples among the instruments of the language.' What we might be tempted to represent as part of the world (e.g. a colour swatch) functions, once it has been baptized by ostensive definition, equally as a part of language. The suggestion regarding hinges provides the reverse complement of this thought: at its hinges thought belongs to the world rather than to a separate order of representation.

48 Our feelings may of course be apt or misguided. And if we're self-alienated we may engage in non-expressive voicings of these feelings which voicings are correct or incorrect. But if instead we're in a position to actually express our feelings in our voicings of them, we can't still be said to get them right or wrong: now we're not expressing (correct or incorrect) judgements about our feelings but instead expressing the feelings themselves. So too when, by dwelling tightly within our situation, we lend our voice to it, and do not impede it as it courses through our embodied life.

49 Boncompagni (2018).

50 Blankenburg ([1968] 2001).

51 Garety and Freeman (2013).

52 Laing (1960: 153).

53 Gibson (1965).

4 A World of One's Own

1 'Apophany' has to do with the revelatory dawning of a new delusional world of meaning (Conrad 1958; Mishara 2010). Delusional perceptions provide the clearest examples of apophantic revelations (Jaspers [1959] 1963; Schneider 1959).

2   O'Brien ([1958] 1976: 20). The 'sordid . . . mess of reality' which overwhelmed Barbara's
    fragile psychological resources, and which led to her psychotic flight, was the
    emotionally toxic environment of her workplace.
3   O'Brien ([1958] 1976: 147).
4   O'Brien ([1958] 1976: 42–46).
5   Asperger (1944) and Kanner (1943) primarily use the term adjectivally ('autistic') to
    describe the character of certain disturbances of affective contact in children. Kanner
    (1973) describes how he originally borrowed 'autism' from Bleuler, but redeployed it to
    describe children who suffered a deficit in emotionally alive reality contact *ab initio*, by
    contrast with Bleuler's adult schizophrenic patients who had emotionally detached
    from a reality with which they had previously been connected. Haswell Todd (2015)
    provides a comprehensive history.
6   Bleuler ([1911] 1950: 63–67).
7   Minkowski ([1927] 1987).
8   Bleuler ([1972] 1978: 491). On schizophrenic autism: Parnas and Bovet (1991); Parnas,
    Bovet and Zahavi (2002); Gipps and de Haan (2019). Autism is one of several
    self-disturbances that unify schizophrenic presentations; see Parnas and Henriksen
    (2014); Parnas, Carter and Nordgaard (2016).
9   Minkowska (1925: 127). Minkowska's understanding of autism is more subtle than her
    formulation here suggests. Instead she follows her husband Eugene Minkowski's
    theorization, providing the following antitheses to describe autistic transformations of
    consciousness: 'planning replaces habitual life; instinct is opposed by ratiocination;
    thought is substituted for feeling; the analysis of minute details replaces synthetic
    imagination; where one relies on impressions, the autist requires proof; movement is
    abandoned for immobility; objects preferred to people; our intuitive grasp of
    phenomena is replaced by our representation of them; space takes the place of time;
    extension replaces succession' (ibid: 135).
10 Bleuler ([1972] 1978: 493).
11 Bleuler ([1911] 1950: 373).
12 Keats ([1820] 1899).
13 Yeats (1889).
14 Sartre ([1940] 2004).
15 In this Sartre followed the trend of French psychiatry; see Borel and Robin (1925) and
    Minkowski ([1927] 1987). If we take the primary use of 'being away with the fairies' to
    indicate someone's being psychotic, then its use to indicate the ordinary daydreamer is
    a 'complex' (i.e. doubled) metaphor.
16 See Kraepelin (1919); Parnas and Bovet (1991); Parnas, Bovet and Zahavi (2002);
    Minkowski (1953: ch. 4).
17 Sartre ([1940] 2004: 146–148).
18 Wittgenstein (1958a: §§243–315); Sass (1995); Gipps (2021).
19 Bleuler ([1972] 1978: 490). The most significant exploration of this theme is that of
    Sass (1994). In the psychoanalytic literature the matter is considered under the
    heading of 'omnipotence', a term owed to Freud's ([1909] 1979) 'Rat Man' patient. This
    psychoanalytic theory was later transformed by Klein; see Seiguer (1990).
20 A point made clear to me by Sanneke de Haan.
21 On 'pacification': Hopkins (2000). On 'short-circuiting': this chapter's final section.
22 Minkowski (1953) here is drawing on the philosopher Henri Bergson's ([1907] 1911)
    concept of *élan vital*.
23 Laing (1960: 221).

24 The ascription conditions for the content of fantasy are primarily the fantasizer's reports, and the meaning of such reports from his mouth is vouchsafed by his capacity to correctly use their terms in conversation with others and to deploy them correctly should he actually encounter the object of his fantasy in reality (i.e. by his reality contact). Furthermore, we naturally understand genuine fantasy, like genuine metaphor use, to be something which can be acknowledged *as such* by the subject, and it's reasonable to take this capacity to 'own' fantasy to underlie the conceptual distinction we draw between fantasy proper (which can be owned) and delirium or delusion (which cannot).

25 Augustine ([397] 1991: 230).

26 Compare the approach of Sass (1992: 270) who accepts the common psychoanalytic and psychiatric definition of poor 'reality testing'. (As the DSM-III-R had it, someone who suffers a failure in reality testing 'incorrectly evaluates the accuracy of his or her perceptions and thoughts and makes incorrect inferences about external reality, even in the face of contrary evidence'.) He therefore rejects the idea that schizophrenic delusion involves a failure in reality testing. By contrast, he rejects the common psychiatric definition of 'delusion' as false belief, and so allows himself to keep the notion, offering us a new reflective understanding of what it means for the schizophrenic subject to be deluded. In the present work, I reject the standard definitions of both terms and provide new reflective understandings of what they mean, thereby keeping both in lexical play. My disagreement with Sass regarding reality testing is therefore merely verbal.

27 Bleuler ([1911] 1950: 373–374).

28 Freud ([1919] 2003: 10); my italics.

29 The concept makes its first appearance in Freud ([1911] 1979). One such description by him of the alleged activity of reality testing is: 'A perception which is made to disappear by an action is recognized as external, as reality; where such an action makes no difference, the perception originates within the subject's own body – it is not real' (Freud [1916–17] 1957: 232). Throughout his oeuvre Freud employs a seventeenth/eighteenth century empiricist conception of reality contact as mediated by 'presentations' or 'perceptions' or 'mnemic images', these being putative mental states which obtain self-same regardless of whether a subject is actually perceiving or is instead merely hallucinating. (In today's philosophical terminology, Freud typically holds to a *non-disjunctivist* understanding of perception (Hinton 1967; McDowell 1982).) On such a conception the 'ego's' task in reality testing is to assess whether or not any given 'perception' has been caused 'internally' (and so is an hallucination) or 'externally' (and so is a 'veridical' perception). Nevertheless at other points (such as that quoted above in the text, where Freud writes of the patient 'effacing the distinction between reality and imagination') he invites interpretation in a different vein.

30 For example: 'true or psychotic hallucinations are perceptions in the absence of appropriate stimuli that are delusionally believed to be real'; Fulford (2004: 57).

31 To dot our conceptual i's and cross our epistemic t's: To know that one's perceiving X is to perceive X whilst being unencumbered by certain defeaters. The presence of these defeaters requires the true perceiver to have justification for his claim to know he's perceiving, but in their absence he requires no such justification. An example: if what I'm truly perceiving is something very unusual (a pink elephant), and if I've made myself vulnerable to hallucination (I've just taken LSD), then it's reasonable for you to require reasons from me before you take seriously my claim to know that I'm actually seeing a pink elephant.

32   We may also use idiomatic forms of perceptual verbs and say that Barbara, when hallucinating, is 'seeing things' or 'hearing voices' when, in the success-related sense of 'seeing' and 'hearing', she's doing no such thing.

33   The idea of psychosis as waking dream has a venerable history: Kant ([1764] 2011: 211): 'The deranged person is thus a dreamer in waking'; Schopenhauer ([1851] 2014: 202): 'the dream can be described as a brief madness, and madness as a long dream'; Wundt (1874: 662): 'we may in dreams experience almost all the phenomena we encounter in the madhouse'; Jung ([1907] 1991: 86): 'Let the dreamer walk about and act like a person awake, and we have the clinical picture of dementia praecox'; (ibid: 85): 'schizophrenics ... continually live in a dream (especially in the acute phases)'; Bergson ([1907] 1911: 204): 'in every way dreams imitate insanity'; Ey (1967: 575): 'It cannot fail to be obvious that dream and madness spurt from the same source.' (Following Bion ([1962] 1978), the post-Kleinians comprehend psychosis as a *failure* of dreaming. However, their concept of 'dreaming' has been revised and given a novel functional significance (to do with the transformation, during both sleep and wakefulness, of inchoate proto-emotional experience into experience with a thinkable form – which process presupposes, and itself helps to create, a delineation between the conscious and unconscious regions of the mind), and for this reason should not be taken to conflict with a pre-Kleinian understanding of psychosis as waking dream.) What is not often noted, but what is yet grist to an apophatic approach's mill, is the essentially paradoxical character of the idea of a 'waking dream'.

34   'Lucid dreaming' is sometimes offered as a condition in which we enjoy reality-oriented thought whilst yet dreaming. However, it has never been made clear how we may conceptually distinguish between realistically regarding the occurrences in the dream from a 'waking point of view' whilst asleep – i.e. as occurrences in a dream – and merely dreaming that you are so regarding them. Without some such distinction we lack grounds for giving up those ordinary criteria for conscious activity that reference our orientation and responsiveness to our environment.

35   Heraclitus ([5th century BC] 1908: §95, p. 153).

36   Minkowski (1953: ch. 3). *La Schizophrénie* has rightly been described as 'probably the best clinical text on schizophrenia ever written' (Parnas, Bovet and Zahavi, 2002: 131–132).

37   Jung ([1907] 1991).

38   In Minkowski's terms, it's 'poor' (i.e. negative symptom dominated clinical pictures) rather than 'rich' (i.e. clinical pictures which like Barbara's are full of florid delusions and hallucinations) autism which most clearly shows us the essence of schizophrenia. Minkowski also follows Bleuler in taking the relevance of fantasy for schizophrenia to be the use made of it by the rich autist – and so, when aptly refusing to consider rich autism the paradigm for schizophrenic psychosis, he also refuses fantasy a central place in his scheme. The present position, by contrast, is that that it's the ontological collapse of fantasy and reality, and neither the substitution of the latter by the former, nor the richness or poverty of the fantasy in question, which makes for schizophrenic autism.

39   Minkowski (1953: ch. 3).

40   Minkowski ([1927] 1987: 208).

41   Minkowski and Targowla (2001).

42   A curiously similar case is provided by Freud ([1917] 1991: Lecture 17), the patient in this case herself acknowledging a psychosexual ground for the preoccupations.

43   Minkowski ([1927] 1987: 210).

44 A follower of Séchehaye (1956) or of Klein (such as Segal (1990)) might interpret the cup as a symbol of maternal container and feeding breast, and understand the patient's delusional hat-making as her deflection from an unbearable experience of mother's unavailability (a mother who keeps the emotional containment, love, nourishment, to herself, who cherishes her cups more than her daughter) through a defensive identification (constructing her own ersatz maternal part-objects), an identification which partially breaks down when two of the hats are lost, leading to a more direct confrontation with the symbol. Whilst the interpretation is not unnatural, we yet do well to acknowledge how little we know of the case. (See Chapter 9 for discussion of symbolism.)

45 Of course we can also become moody if we suffer a bang to the head, are hungry, are pre-menstrual, etc. And endocrinal and neurochemical alterations can induce psychosis in those suffering non-functional psychoses.

46 Thus the inversions of content and object which psychoanalysis traces for us in the paranoid realm, the unthinkable 'I love/hate him' being transformed into the 'He loves/ hates me'.

47 Minkowski (1953: 212–213).

48 Cited by Laing (1963: 203).

49 On schizotaxia, see Meehl (1962). We might alternatively make use of the older, somewhat different, notions of the 'schizophrene' (Kretschmer [1922] 1945) of 'latent' schizophrenia (Bychowski 1953) – or of today's 'schizotypy' (Everett and Linscott 2015).

50 Suggestions similar to these can be found in Minkowski (1953) and Parnas and Bovet (1991).

51 Panksepp (1998).

52 An unquestioned assumption that what's literally inside the head is also inexorably what's most explanatorily basic in the science of behaviour may also underlie the tendency of biologically minded psychiatry to privilege neurological abnormalities as 'the underlying causes' of significant mental illness; see de Haan (2020).

53 Jaspers ([1959] 1963: 196), my italics; see also (ibid: 284, 724, 779).

54 Currie (2000).

55 Spitzer (1990: 391).

56 This is a bullet which Spitzer (1990: 393–394), insisting on the 'external reality' criterion, forces himself to bite.

57 See Sass (2014a).

58 Sass (1994); Sass and Parnas (2003).

59 Schreber ([1903] 1988) as discussed by Sass (1994: 8, 24, 33).

60 Sass and Parnas (2003: 427).

61 Sass and Parnas (2003: 432).

62 Sass (1994: ch. 1).

63 For critique of Sass along these lines, see Read (2001) and Thornton (2004). What such critique misses is the significance of our being able to enter into states in which we too find ourselves tempted to describe our experience in the terms offered by the schizophrenic subject. This gives us a powerful insight into the significance both of sensorimotor world-disengagement, and of the breakup of inner sensorimotor coherence, for the generation of schizophrenic autism. (These are discussed in Chapters 3 and 5, respectively, of this book.) And this is the fat phenomenological baby which ought not to be thrown out with the modest metaphysical bathwater in Sass's articulation of schizophrenic self-disturbance. The analogy between

schizophrenia and philosophical solipsism will be successful if it's pursued in terms of the fact of the temptation, the temptation's natural expression, and the temptation's possible causes; it will be unsuccessful if pursued in terms of the putative content of that which one's tempted to say.

64   'Resolutist' interpretations of Wittgenstein, of the sort favoured by Conant and Diamond (2004), suggest that there's altogether no such thing as understanding that which does not make sense. And therefore – contra Sass – that there is no understanding that may be transferred from such (in truth but illusory) intellectual grip as we have regarding solipsism and phenomenalism to the obscure phenomena of formal disturbances of schizophrenic experience. For discussion, see Sass (2003) and Thornton (2004). Other interpreters of Wittgenstein find a more happy place for the idea of 'understanding nonsense', and suggest the resolutist to be more prescriptive as to what may or may not be allowed to count as understanding than is warranted by our ordinary talk of sense and nonsense; see Teichmann (2021). We also do well to distinguish between empathically understanding a person (her feelings and motivations, for example) and comprehending what she says (Diamond 2000; Gipps 2010): the latter becoming unavailable even when the former remains a live possibility.

65   See Chapter 5 for more elaborated critique. We may of course identify with or disidentify from our feelings – for example, we may emphatically deny that one of our hurtful outbursts really meant anything; encouraging the reintegration of such split-off emotion keeps the psychoanalyst in business. But such moments of human life take us nowhere near the kind of experiential objectivization mooted by the phenomenological psychopathologist.

66   On the 'face' of the other: Levinas (1969).

67   On the 'short-circuit': Minkowski (1953); Rossi Monti (1998); Urfer (2001); Fuchs (2005). Minkowski, for example, talks: of the need to help the schizophrenic subject break out of her 'cercle enchanté et sans issue', of 'actes figés, ne cherchant pas à aboutir', of 'actes à court-circuit' (Minkowski 1953: 190, 123, 124).

68   On schizophrenia as lived solipsism, see Sass (1994).

69   See Wittgenstein (1958a: §279, §268).

70   Laing (1960: 222–223).

5 The Divided Self

1   For 'the divided self', see James (1902: Lecture VIII) and, for its psychiatric usage, Laing (1960). The phrase from Yeats, which refers to civilization rather than individuals, occurs in his poem 'The Second Coming' (Yeats 1920); Saks (2007) exemplifies its popular psychiatric usage.

2   Amongst its many meanings, 'alienation' signals a withdrawal of interest and trust, a feeling of estrangement from others, and a derangement of mind. The early psychiatrists were known as alienists; their craft known as alienism.

3   Bleuler ([1911] 1950: 8).

4   Bleuler ([1911] 1950: 33ff). By the turn of the nineteenth century the idea of intrapsychic splitting or dissociation became widespread in psychiatry. Esquirol and Griesinger had already talked of *splitting* (Spaltung) in 1838 and 1845; Stransky of *intrapsychic ataxia* and a *dissociation process* in 1903; Wernicke of a *dissociation*

(Sejunktion) psychosis in 1880; Gross of *dementia sejunctiva* and *dissociative* incoherence in 1904; etc. (Scharfetter 2001; Berrios, Luque and Villagrán 2003).

5　In his *Principles of Psychology*, William James (1890: ch. 10) acknowledges that 'What the particular perversions of bodily sensibility may be, which give rise to [such] contradictions [as are met with in self-alienation], is for the most part impossible for a sound-minded person to conceive' (p. 377). Unable to resist a challenge, James nevertheless quickly sets to work distinguishing a 'me' from an 'I', moreover identifying the 'I' with a personified 'Thought' which now somehow takes states of its thinker for its objects. If this 'Thought', or 'I', finds a 'resemblance' between, or 'continuity' of, bodily feelings experienced over time, then it/I now 'feels' a sense of 'personal identity'. If not, then it asks 'Where is my old me? What is this new one? Are they the same? Or have I two? Such questions, answered by whatever theory the patient is able to conjure up as plausible, form the beginning of his insane life' (p. 378). James' account, whilst clearly *outré*, is by no means the least eccentric of the many attempts that have now been made to 'make sense of' intrapsychic alienation – attempts which only appear to succeed for so long as that profoundly alienated conception of ordinary human subjectivity embedded within them itself goes unremarked.

6　Such self disorders are pathognomonic of schizophrenia, being markedly more prominent in schizophrenia than in bipolar disorder, and strongly predictive of future onset of schizophrenia in non-psychotic clinical populations and in those at high risk of psychosis. For a summary of the empirical research, see Nelson, Parnas and Sass (2014).

7　Graham and Stephens (1994: 91–92); Ratcliffe and Wilkinson (2015: 251).

8　Campbell (1999: 610): 'these reports by patients show that there is some structure in our ordinary notion of a thought which we might not otherwise have expected'. Stephens and Graham (1994: 1–2): 'Our aim is to provide a precise characterization of the disturbance of self-consciousness involved in thought insertion and to explain what the possibility of such disturbances shows about the nature of human self-consciousness.'

9　Bleuler ([1911] 1950: 201–202). (See ibid: 201–205 and 449–452 for his entire account of automatisms.) Psychiatric interest in mental automatisms goes back in France to Pierre Janet (1889) and in Germany to Arnold Pick ([1904] 1996). The French concept (*automatisme psychologique*) differs from the German (*Phenomen des Automatismus*) in that only the latter implies a delusional experience of an agency other than oneself performing those actions with which one is no longer identified (German Berrios, personal communication, 29 November 2018).

10　Gipps (2009: 17).

11　Rodriguez McRobbie (2013).

12　Gipps (2009: 8).

13　Gipps (2009: 18–19).

14　Gipps (2009: 9). For further examples of pathological automaticity: Stanghellini (2004) and de Haan and Fuchs (2010). For discussion of healthy automaticity: Bargh and Chartrand (1999).

15　'Passivity experiences' and 'made thoughts' are Marian Hamilton's translations for what Jaspers ([1959] 1963: 122) acknowledges as 'words coined by [patients] themselves, which psychopathology has had to take over'.

16　Pick ([1904] 1996: 326).

17　Mellor (1970: 17).

18　Jaspers ([1959] 1963: 91, 123); see also Bleuler ([1911] 1950: 204). The Heidelberg School (i.e. Jaspers, Schneider et al.) offer delusional passivity experiences as particularly pathognomonic, 'first rank', symptoms of schizophrenia.

19 Jaspers ([1959] 1963: 122); Schneider (1959: 124).

20 Jaspers ([1959] 1963: 123).

21 Frith (1992: 81, 86); see also Frith and Blakemore (2003); Frith (2007). Frith (1992: ch. 5) also posits a *mechanism* which allows us to tell which of the acts we perform, feelings we feel, thoughts we think, are our own, and which are others – a malfunction of which gives rise to passivity experiences. Yet unless intrusive telepathy were part of our evolutionary landscape, it's hard to see why such a mechanism should have evolved. Furthermore, a mechanism ought to *do* something when it's working correctly; it ought to *have a function*. But in the present case the mooted mechanism's only job is to proffer the tautology that the thoughts in our mind are ours – unless it 'malfunctions' and tells us that they're another's. We can make sense of the idea of a mechanism that would tell us, when it was working, that $1 + 1 = 2$, and when malfunctioning that $1 + 1 = 3$ – but not, surely, of a mechanism which, when working, tells us that $1 = 1$ and, when broken, that $1 = 2$.

22 Wittgenstein (1958a: §622). See also: 'Motricity is thus not, as it were, a servant of consciousness, transporting the body to the point of space that we imagine beforehand' (Merleau-Ponty [1945] 2012: 140).

23 The example is from Frith, Blakemore and Wolpert (2000: 358).

24 Examples from Frith (1992: 66); Sterzer et al. (2016: 5).

25 A regress argument made by Gallagher (2000).

26 Schneider (1959: 121, 124).

27 Jaspers ([1959] 1963: 121–122); see also Fish (1984: 48). Today's phenomenological psychopathologists typically follow the Heidelberg School in positing a lost 'sense of myness' or 'mineness' in passivity experience; see, e.g.: Parnas (2000); Stanghellini and Cutting (2003); Gallagher (2015); Nelson, Parnas and Sass (2014); Zahavi (2000).

28 A regress argument made effectively by Thornton (2002).

29 Cp. 'The . . . normal state is the absence of . . . discontinuity, dissociation and loss . . . [which] can therefore be called the possession of "self-feeling": I record my suspicion that this is identifiable rather by consideration of the abnormal than the normal case' (Anscombe 1975: 61).

30 James (1890: 272–273, fn. 3).

31 See Anscombe (1975: 64).

32 The story about the thirteenth-century Sufi satirist is widely told; here I offer my own paraphrase. The story bears comparison with Frith's (1992) suggestion, not intended comically, that our thoughts come with a label attached which identifies them as ours, a label which is misplaced or overlooked in cases of thought insertion.

33 Cp. 'there is no question of recognizing a person when I say I have toothache. To ask "are you sure that it's you who have pains?" would be nonsensical. . . . To say, "I have pain" is no more a statement *about* a particular person than moaning is' (Wittgenstein 1958b: 67).

34 Graham and Stephens (1994: 98); see also Stephens and Graham (2000); Campbell (1999); for critique: Roessler (2013).

35 Graham and Stephens (1994: 98–99).

36 Wittgenstein (1958a: §621).

37 See, for example, Frith (2012); Pettersson-Yeo et al. (2010).

38 The originator of this conception is perhaps R. D. Laing: 'The individual's being is cleft in two, producing a disembodied self and a body that is a thing that the self looks at regarding it at times as though it were just another thing in the world. The total body and also many 'mental' processes are severed from the self which may continue to

operate in a very restricted enclave (phantasying and observing) or it may appear to cease to function altogether (i.e. be dead, murdered, stolen)' (Laing 1960: 174.) Sass (1992) has worked out the proposal in the greatest detail, but see also Stanghellini (2004) and Fuchs (2005).

39 Read (2001) and Thornton (2004) criticize Sass along these lines, although other readings of Sass are available (Henriksen 2013).

40 Herein the natural human terror at the occult, which in this respect parallels the natural human fear of psychosis (see Chapter 1). What evokes horror or dread is ultimately not the thought of, say, marauding spirits, but rather our empathic sense that in the experience of spirit possession selfhood itself has fallen apart.

41 See Sass (1994: ch. 1).

42 Wittgenstein (1968).

43 See Wittgenstein (1980b: vol. 1, §125): 'The feeling of the unreality of one's surroundings. This feeling I have had once, and many have it before the onset of mental illness. Everything seems somehow not real; but not as if one saw things unclear or blurred; everything looks quite as usual. And how do I know that another has felt what I have? Because he uses the same words as I find appropriate.'

44 See Chapter 4.

45 Mellor (1970: 17).

46 Pick ([1904] 1996: 326).

47 The strategy of Frith (1992).

48 The phenomenon of 'blindsight' involves another such dissociation between criteria for ascribing perceptual competence to someone. The subject sincerely avows complete blindness, but to their own surprise can guess or make movements indicative of seeing. Rather than simply acknowledge such a dissociation in the criteria for ascribing, psychologists aiming at a positive psychological explanation have been apt to posit 'visual percepts' that may or may not 'enter consciousness' (Weiskrantz 1997). As John Hyman (1991: 175–176) notes: 'it appears that we can only do justice [to blindsight] by tearing apart the language of vision ... D.B. denies that he can see, and who are we to doubt him? And yet the experimental evidence is unequivocal. The paradox of blindsight lies in the fact that we want to deny that D.B. is blind *and* that he can see. In other words, the phenomenon seems to demand a nonsensical description.' A further example of a dissociation of criteria will be offered in the present work, Chapter 8, on formal thought disorder.

49 Schneider (1959); Soares-Weiser et al. (2015).

6 Self and Other

1 Psychoanalytically-minded ego boundary theorists include Freeman, Cameron and McGhie (1958); Federn ([1949] 1952); Frosch (1983). Scharfetter (1995) and Fish (1976) provide good examples of somewhat more phenomenologically-oriented psychiatrists who make use of the 'ego boundary' concept.

2 Freeman, Cameron and McGhie (1958: 49, 52).

3 Tausk ([1919] 1933).

4 Bleuler ([1911] 1950: 143).

5 Bleuler ([1911] 1950: 145–146).

6 Laing (1960: 215).

7   Freeman, Cameron and McGhie (1958: 54) citing Storch (1924).

8   Jacobson (1954: 104–105).

9   See Bleuler ([1911] 1950: 299), where he offers transitivistic experience in clear consciousness as pathognomonic of schizophrenia.

10   On transitivism and appersonation: Bleuler ([1911] 1950: 145); Freeman (1976). See also Scharfetter (1995) and sections 4 of the EASE (Parnas et al. 2005) and 3.7 of the EAWE (Sass et al. 2017).

11   Following Frosch (1983: 211–217, 310–316).

12   The theory is complex, the same terms being used in different ways even by the same theorists (Hinshelwood 1991). (Some authors distinguish between projection as an intrapsychic process and projective identification as a relational (controlling) process; British Kleinians, however, have tended to view 'projective identification' simply as a deeper theorization of 'projection'.) My discussion of the psychoanalytic theory here is limited to its bearing on the psychopathology under discussion.

13   'Accidents': those properties a being can lose without ceasing to be itself; contrast 'essential properties'. On 'massive projective identification': Roth (2017). On psychotic identification: Jacobson (1954).

14   Frosch (1983: 211–217). Psychoanalytic theory does not always distinguish carefully between projective identification and introjective identification or dedifferentiation, sometimes styling them all instances of projective identification.

15   From personal experience.

16   Watters and Ofshe (1999).

17   The psychoanalytic theory also tells us that transitivism is the result of not one but two defence mechanisms: the subject splits into two (or more) parts, and projective identification then lodges one (or more) of these in one's experience of another person. It's certainly true that we can find splitting in the absence of projection – perhaps the split-off elements are simply repressed, for example. Even so we surely don't here have two separate mechanisms (splitting, projection) as we might in, say, a sweet factory – where one mechanism adds chocolate to a biscuit and another wraps the product either in tin foil or plastic. We do not, for example, first observe the products of defensive splitting and then go on to see the fate of the split-off part at the hands of some other mechanism. The differentiation and enumeration of the mechanisms of splitting and projection lies, one might say, not in the psyche itself but instead merely in the form of our representations.

18   Freud ([1930] 1985: 253).

19   Federn ([1932] 1952: 64).

20   Freeman, Cameron and McGhie (1958: 33, 51).

21   Bellak and Blaustein (1958: 11); italics added.

22   Both Freud ([1914] 1957, [1917] 1991) and Federn ([1928] 1952) offer the cell membrane as analogy for the ego boundary.

23   On the 'skin ego', see Bick (1968); Anzieu (1989).

24   Federn ([1949] 1952: 222); see also Federn ([1928] 1952: 285).

25   In fact Federn, despite his protestations, vacillates in unstable manner between entitative and non-entitative conceptions of his 'ego boundary'; see Polster (1983) and Landis (1963).

26   See Thornton (2002).

27   See Chapter 5.

28   See de Mijolla (2005: 461–488).

29   See Anscombe (1957: §8).

30 It's sometimes said that proprioception – our knowledge of our bodily posture and movement – may be thought of as a sixth sense (to complement seeing, hearing, etc.). Unlike typical senses, however, it's only passively engaged in. Furthermore, it's unclear why we should need a *sense* to tell us where our body parts are and how they're moving if we don't need one to tell us what and how we're thinking and feeling.

31 Sheets-Johnstone (2020).

32 Such a way with the 'ego boundary' and 'ego boundary disorder' concepts leaves open the question of whether cases of phantom limb or rubber hand illusion – when one experiences bodily sensations in a non-existent or unattached limb – are properly thought of as ego boundary disturbances. (In one sense, the experimental subject of the rubber hand illusion *feels tickle sensations in* the rubber hand; in another sense, the experimental subject of course cannot feel what is actually being done to the rubber hand – he's instead feeling what's being done to his own hand, but finding himself moved to urge that it obtains in the rubber hand.) Somatoparaphrenia and body integrity disorder – when one delusionally or non-delusionally experiences a body part as in some sense ego alien – also constitute conceptually ambiguous cases. We shall also feel the naturalness, if not the obligatoriness, of thinking of prostheses, the tennis racket in one's hand, the wheels of the car one is driving, etc., as in some ways extending the reach of the ego boundary. In Gipps 2020a and 2020b, I offered a less ambiguous conception of ego boundary disturbance, one which moreover has that ego-individuating boundary truly being relocated in all those illusory and psychopathological scenarios considered here. But the flaw with such a way with the concept is that it leaves us without adequate resource to specify what's delusional about the kinds of boundary disturbance met with in schizophrenic psychosis.

33 Rhodes and Gipps (2008).

34 A point emphasized to me by Roger Teichmann. Many of the phenomenological explanations of schizophrenic experience offered by Sass (1992, 1994) appear to be of this form.

35 Botvinick and Cohen (1998).

36 As argued in Chapter 3, such failures of reality testing are a function of a loss of reality contact. It should now be clear why being clearly *distinguished from* the world and from others, and enjoying reality *contact*, are so far from contradicting one another that they're instead better considered conditions of one another's possibility.

37 Schopenhauer ([1819] 1969: 193).

7 Hallucination

1 Bleuler ([1911] 1950: 95ff).

2 From Romme et al. (2009). The case histories of this book make clear the social, developmental and emotional contexts for the hallucinated voices, and inspire the understanding that voices often 'metaphorically express': different types of abuse, people involved in the abuse as abusers or rescuers, unexpressed and problematic emotions such as aggression, shame and guilt, and personal crises. See also Romme and Escher (2012); McCarthy-Jones (2017).

3 Esquirol (1817) cited by Berrios and Marková (2012).

4 Definitions derived from Esquirol (1817); Jaspers ([1959] 1963: 6); Harrison et al. (2018: 6); Gurney, Myers and Podmore (1886: 459); www.nhs.uk/conditions/hallucinations/.

5 Anscombe (1965). 'Material objects' is here meant to include all of cats, puddles, beams of light, klaxon sounds, odours, etc. The identity of the 'intentional object', by contrast with that of the material object, is given by what the perceiver or hallucinator says he sees or seems to see.

6 Taine ([1870] 1889: vol. 1, p. 226). On perception as 'controlled hallucination', see Clark (2013: 25). Hippolyte Taine (1828–1893): a theorist of the 'inner phantom' whose philosophically naïve two volume *On Intelligence* repeatedly proclaims his belief that hallucinatory phantoms obtain during all of veridical perception, illusion, or (what we'd normally call) hallucination. His 'proof' is the following *petitio principii*: 'In order to establish that external perception, even when accurate, is an hallucination, it is sufficient to observe that its first phase is a sensation. – In fact, a sensation, and notably a tactile or visual sensation, engenders, by its presence alone, an internal phantom which appears as an external object. . . . Hence we see that the objects we touch, see, or perceive by any one of our senses, are nothing more than semblances or phantoms precisely similar to those which arise in the mind of a hypnotised person, a dreamer, a person labouring under hallucinations, or afflicted by subjective sensations' (Taine ([1870] 1889: vol. 2, pp. 1–2). Taine's contemporary Hermann von Helmholtz (1821–1894) developed a similar (mis)conception of the relation of sensory stimulation to perception (von Helmholtz [1860] 1962); recent inheritors of this include Gregory (1980), Marr (1982), Frith (2007), Friston (2007), and Corlett et al. (2019). Such a conception typically ties together two equally confused pictures, the one relating mind to body by placing experience as a final inner stage of neurological processing (rather than as including all relevant components of an organism's sensorimotoric engagement with its world), the other tasking the brain with inwardly reconstructing (hypothesizing, picturing, unconsciously inferring) what must have been the outer causes either of the aforementioned inner experiences or of the environmental impingements on the sense organs (rather than with maintaining a tightly coupled, robust, sensorimotorically realized, grip on the world). For critique, see Hacker (1995).

7 On disjunctivism in the theory of perception, see McDowell (1982) and Snowdon (1990).

8 Bleuler ([1916] 1924: 61–62): 'The patients are often cognizant of the hallucinations, not exactly that they are false sensations, but they feel that there is something strange about them. Thus they know them through their different content, they state that they have feelings that they have never experienced before, for the expression of which they have to coin new words. They feel that they see remarkable images and scenes, abnormal localizations, voices in the walls or in their own arms, a light in their own body or in the uterus of a passing woman. They also recognize the strangeness through indefinite projection to the outer world. The patient believes that he hears through his leg and not in his ears; he does not know whether he touches an animal or sees it.' Merleau-Ponty ([1945] 2012: 350): 'The most important fact is that patients distinguish, for the most part, between their hallucinations and their perceptions. . . . [A] schizophrenic, who claims to see a man in the garden stopped beneath his window, and having indicated the location, clothing, and posture of the man, is astonished when someone is actually placed in the garden, at the spot indicated, in the same outfit, and standing with the same posture. He stares attentively: "it's true, there is someone there, but it is another person." And yet, he refuses to count two men in the garden. . . . In an alcoholic mania, the subject who sees the doctor's hand as a guinea pig immediately notices that a genuine guinea pig has been placed in the other hand.'

(Sadly we're not told how or why these doctors rapidly procured such stooges and guinea pigs.)

9 Ratcliffe (2019).

10 Sass and Byrom (2015).

11 Jung and Jaffé ([1962] 1993: 322).

12 One of the several ways in which a conception of veridical perception as involving inner images founders is in its failure to grasp that we can only perceptually relate to images of (say) people because we've first enjoyed perceptual relations with actual people. (Of course, once we've seen enough of the world's denizens, and have enjoyed sufficient practice at seeing them in our pictures of them, we can graduate to perceptually relating to artists' drawings of fantastical beasts.)

13 Freud ([1938] 1964: 285).

14 Frith (1992: 71). An earlier version of the theory has it that 'The error that is hallucination arises from the fact that here the inner speech is an exceptionally strong state, and it is confirmed by the unexpectedness of the phenomenon and the absence of any relationship with the previous series of weak states. Any strong state that is unrelated to the general bent of thought is alienated without hesitation, except in so far as we acknowledge that we have been victims of an illusion and have taken for real voices the phantoms of our sick imagination' (Egger 1881: 106). Relatedly, Pintner suggests that Socrates' daemon and Joan of Arc's voices were but 'inner speech asserting itself with greater insistence than is usual in ordinary individuals', and that 'the voice or call that often seems to us to come from elsewhere is our inner speech that puts into articulate words the vague, indefinite thought. . . . Only in cases of insanity . . . does this inner speech detach itself from the individual and then it appears as some outside being that is talking to the patient' (Pintner 1913: 130). Unfortunately, Egger and Pintner don't provide adequate accounts of what it is for inner speech to become 'alienated' or to 'detach itself from the individual'. For overview of the inner speech theory of hallucination, see McCarthy-Jones (2012: ch. 9) and (2017: chs 28–30).

15 Gould (1949); Green and Preston (1981).

16 McCarthy-Jones (2017: 190).

17 Griesinger (1867: 86).

18 Sacks (2012: ix).

19 Locke ([1690] 1984: book IV, iv. 3, p. 348): 'It is evident the mind knows not things immediately, but only by the intervention of the ideas it has of them.'

20 For a brief summary, see Hacker (2013: ch. 8, §3). See also Overgaard (2020).

21 Brugger, Regard and Landis (1997). Autoscopic experience, which can be understood as due to a disturbance in the integration of proprioceptive and sensory stimulation (i.e. a disturbance of the body schema), has been reported in subjects receiving transcranial magnetic stimulation (Blanke and Thut 2007).

22 Jalal and Ramachandran (2014). Such 'presences' may also be induced by electromagnetic brain stimulation (Blanke et al. 2014).

23 Lacan understands psychotic hallucination to result from what he called 'foreclosure' (Freud's German: *Verwerfung*, Lacan's French: *foreclusion*) rather than projection, such that 'that which has not emerged into the light of the symbolic appears in the real' (Lacan 1966: 388). Freud had it of Judge Daniel Paul Schreber's hallucinations that: "It was incorrect to say that the perception suppressed internally is projected outwards; the truth is rather, as we now see, that what was abolished internally returns from without"; 'Jung . . . has perceived that the deliria and motor stereotypes occurring in

[schizophrenia] are the residues of former object-cathexes, clung to with great persistence. This attempt at recovery ... does not, as in paranoia, make use of projection, but employs a hallucinatory (hysterical) mechanism' (Freud ([1911] 1979: 71, 77). See Gauthier (2000); Lacan (1966: 541).

24 Martindale and Summers (2013: 126).

25 Jones (2012).

26 Powers, Mathys and Corlett (2017).

27 Husserl ([1966] 1991) calls this readiness 'protention'; Blaiklock (2017) provides useful explication. On sensory readinesses as part of the anticipatory aspect of reality contact, see Chapter 3.

28 Gipps (2017).

29 Alternative anticipation-involving understandings of hallucination are available: Gallagher (2005) construes verbal hallucination as unanticipated thought; Ratcliffe (2017) construes verbal hallucination as due to anxiously anticipating an increasingly determinate thought content.

30 What follows draws on McCarthy-Jones (2017: ch. 38). For an introduction to predictive processing, see Wiese and Metzinger (2017).

31 Metzinger (2004: 51–52).

32 For detailed and diverse predictive processing understandings of hallucination, see Notredame et al. (2014), Jardri et al. (2016), and Sterzer et al. (2018).

33 We could of course stipulate something; perhaps we decide that Bolt's acceleration was constituted by the last moments of its efficient causation brought under a formal description – the increasing force and frequency with which his shoes repel the turf. But this isn't to provide an answer to an already understood question ('what's the constitution/material cause of his acceleration?'), but instead to perform the double duty of first providing a sense for an initially empty question and then answering it. Or perhaps we stipulate that his acceleration's material cause is the increasingly rapid movement of his legs or of his body over the track. This, however, gives a new meaning to the 'is' in 'what is his acceleration?', rather than discerns a sense to the question already latently contained, as it were, in the terms (including 'is') in which it's put.

34 Daniel and Mason (2015).

35 Ramachandram and Hirstein (1998). Suffering amputation, especially in traumatic circumstances, leaves you with a more than 90% chance of experiencing a phantom limb with phantom pains. If such pains were due to aberrant afference from the amputation site, then it would be reasonable to expect further surgeries on the stump to resolve the problem; they are not thereby resolved. Mirror box, motor imagery, and virtual reality therapies can however sometimes recalibrate the body schema for the missing limb (i.e. alter the moment-to-moment generation of sensory readinesses), thereby providing relief from painfully frozen phantom limbs (Ramachandram and Hirstein 1998; Herrador Colmenero et al. 2018). The body schema's adjustment to the loss of a limb can be a difficult process: 'phenomenal limbs' may at first attenuate, leaving only the extremities hanging in space, but then can telescope inwards, becoming like those of thalidomide babies; the pain experienced in them can last for decades (Katz 2001).

36 Marschall et al. (2020).

37 Kelleher et al. (2012).

38 Mavromatis (1987: ch. 2).

39 Hughlings Jackson (1884, 1888). Today the 'release' concept is principally used to explain utilization behaviours and echopraxia.

40 West (1975); Sacks (2012). Today the release theory of hallucination is restricted to the explanation of Charles Bonnet syndrome (Schultz and Meltzack 1991).

41 For example, Joseph Zinkin translates the subsection heading 'Auslösung der Halluzinationen' from Bleuler's schizophrenia treatise with 'The release of hallucinations' (Bleuler 1911: 88; [1911] 1950: 107). The 'release' metaphor is also put to effective use elsewhere in psychiatry – as in Fairbairn's ([1943] 1952) compelling discussion of the importance of the psychoanalyst working to release defensively introjected bad internal objects from the unconscious.

42 The short-circuiting metaphor is Minkowski's; see final section in Chapter 4.

43 Noë (2004).

44 Grimby (1993); Olson et al. (1985).

45 Sacks (2012: 232).

46 See Chapter 9.

47 The defensively motivated 'introjection of the bad object' as the first step of significantly disturbed personality development, and then the later 'release' of the bad object in provocative situations, are comprehensively treated by Fairbairn ([1941] 1952; [1943] 1952).

48 Tale 109 from Grimm Brothers ([1812] 1944). The relationship between the experience of ghosts and the vicissitudes of mourning is also explored in Anthony Minghella's film *Truly, Madly, Deeply* (1990); as Juliet Stevenson progressively mourns his passing, Alan Rickman's ghost gradually takes his leave. With thanks to Edward Harcourt for these examples.

8 Disordered Thought

1 Jung ([1907] 1991: ch. 5); Woods (2011).

2 Jung ([1907] 1991: 99).

3 The thought of manic subjects can, like that of schizophrenic subjects, also be vague and insufficiently responsive to context, and loosely linked together ideas may be extravagantly combined in expansive playful discourse. By contrast, more prototypically schizophrenic discourse is marked by schizophrenic autism, may contain neologisms, is more disorganized, deploys concepts which have collapsed into one another, and involves unstable referents and reference frames, thus proving rather harder to follow (Holzman, Shenton and Solovay 1986; Sass and Parnas 2017; Morgan et al. 2017; Bleuler [1916] 1924: ch. II, §3).

4 Meehl (1990); Morgan et al. (2017). Wahlberg et al. (1997) show a gene–environment interaction – children at a high genetic risk for schizophrenia adopted into families with a high degree of communication deviance are more likely to develop thought disorder than those adopted into families with low degrees of communication deviance.

5 Bleuler ([1911] 1950); Bleuler ([1916] 1924); Moskowitz and Heim (2011). 'Of the thousands of associative threads which guide our thinking, this disease [schizophrenia] seems to interrupt, quite haphazardly, sometimes such single threads, sometimes a whole group, and sometimes even large segments of them [i.e. "thought deprivation"]. In this way, thinking becomes illogical and often bizarre. Furthermore, the associations tend to proceed along new lines, of which so far the following are known to us: Two ideas, fortuitously encountered, are combined into one thought [i.e. "condensation"], the logical form being determined by incidental circumstances.

Clang-associations receive unusual significance, as do indirect associations. Two or more ideas are condensed into a single one. The tendency to stereotype [i.e. a general tendency to repetitive rituals] produces the inclination to cling to one idea to which the patient then returns again and again. Generally, there is a marked dearth of ideas to the point of monoideism [i.e. prolonged absorption in a single thought]. Frequently some idea will dominate the train of thought in the form of blocking [i.e. obstruction of thought's flow], naming [i.e. just saying the names of the objects about one], or echopraxia [which here instead means echolalia – just repeating another's utterances]' (Bleuler [1911] 1950: 14).

6   Bleuler ([1911] 1950: 84, n. 27).

7   Rochester and Martin (1979: 106).

8   Whether such avoidance may be motivated will be discussed later in the chapter. Whilst it's impossible to tell from this transcript alone whether it bespeaks motivated avoidance, it's intriguing to note that the fate of the donkey is here replaced by talk of how something is fought off and pushed away so that things may 'go up around it'.

9   Locke ([1690] 1984: book 2, ch. 33).

10 See Thornton (1998: ch. 2, §3).

11 What follows draws on the exploration of the concept of 'thinking' in Wittgenstein (1958a: §§327–342), Arrington (2001), and Teichmann (2015: ch. 3).

12 Ryle ([1966–67] 2009).

13 Contra what the following theorists of thought disorder suggest: Chaika and Lambe (1985: 8): 'speech [is] an overt behavior, [while] thought [is] a cognitive process inferred on the basis of many different overt behaviors including speech'; Andreasen (1982: 296): 'Thought processes cannot be observed directly and can only be inferred from introspection, self-report, or experimental approaches'; Hart and Lewine (2017: 516): 'The study of "thought disorder" assumes that thought processes can be accurately inferred from speech'. Frith (1992: 97): 'The peculiar speech observed in many schizophrenic patients is traditionally labelled "thought disorder". This label suggests that the peculiar things that schizophrenic patients say are a consequence of peculiar thoughts. The label further suggests that the ability to put these thoughts into language is unimpaired. So far this assumption remains unproven. . . . There is a fundamental difference between language and thought, which has received surprisingly little emphasis in the study of schizophrenia. Thinking is a private matter, whereas language is arguably the most important method we have for communicating with others.'

14 Chaika (1982).

15 Andreasen (1982, 1986).

16 Rochester and Martin (1979); Bentall (2003). The psychiatrist here is lampooned for his circularity in allegedly encouraging us both to infer thought disorder from incoherent talk whilst also allegedly explaining schizophrenic talk in terms of disordered thought ('so . . . thought disorder is when talk is incoherent . . . and talk is incoherent when the thought is disordered . . .').

17 Andreasen (1982).

18 The empirical defence proceeds by discovering the correlation of disordered speech with object sorting choices, intrusion of personal preoccupations, and delusions. Harrow et al. (2003).

19 Andreasen (1986); Chaika (1982).

20 It has been suggested that the multiplicity of psychological processes affected to different degrees in different cases of thought disorder might rightly incline one to

think of formal thought disorder as a 'loose family-resemblance concept' (Sass and Parnas 2017). The approach offered here, by contrast, has it that the concept is better understood logically than psychologically – in terms of a disturbance to thought rather than to thinking (attending, remembering, ordering, etc.) – and that its unity is accordingly to be grasped not in terms of any singular psychological process but in terms of the kind of unintelligibility here met with.

21 Chaika (1982: 588–589) offers: 'Until and unless experimentation confirms that thought and speech are identical – and thus far this has not been proven – one cannot assume that a break in one automatically indicates a break in the other. Indeed one's thoughts must be separate from one's speech, preceding it, for how else could one choose the exact words and syntax one wished to convey one's meaning.' Yet given their categorical differences, it's unclear how empirical experimentation could show the identity of thought and speech any more than it could show either the identity or the lack of identity of the hurrying and the breakfasting of the hurried breakfaster (Ryle [1966–67] 2009). As for the requirement that thought must precede speech, or that we're in the business of choosing the exact words and syntax one wishes to convey one's meaning: nothing in the phenomenology of everyday meaningful speech suggests that anything like this usually goes on. Instead, we simply talk, and when we do our thought is immanent within rather than antecedent to our talk, characterizing rather than causing it.

22 Teichmann (2017).

23 Hertzberg (2010). What was said of thinking parallels what Wittgenstein here says about remembering: '"But you surely can't deny that, for example, in remembering, an inner process takes place." – What gives the impression that we want to deny anything? … What we deny is that the picture of an inner process gives us the correct idea of the use of the word "to remember". Indeed, we're saying that this picture, with its ramifications, stands in the way of our seeing the use of the word as it is' (Wittgenstein 1958a: §305)

24 Schizophrenic subjects sometimes report struggling to put their thoughts into words, and psychologists sometimes take this as evidence of a dissociation between thought and language in schizophrenia – without, however, providing alternative criteria for the having of the thoughts. (It's not as if such patients manifest mere word-finding difficulties.) See, e.g. Frith (1992: 97).

25 Searles (1961: 49). Searles was (alongside Fromm-Reichmann, Harry Stack Sullivan and others) a psychiatrist at Chestnut Lodge (Maryland), which, along with the Burghölzli Clinic (Zurich), was an intellectual home of much important work on schizophrenic disturbances of thought.

26 See Chapter 4.

27 See Frith (1992: 100); Rutter (1982: 613).

28 See Gipps (2016).

29 Heidegger ([1927] 1962: §I.5.34).

30 Gipps (2016); Gipps and de Haan (2019).

31 Such a thought is, however, reminiscent of just such attempts at hyper-reflective compensation as may arise in response to that loss of pre-reflective attunement as is due to the depredations of a schizophrenic illness (Sass and Parnas 2003).

32 Sullivan ([1956] 1973: 315–316).

33 Given that many important functions of language – such as the social grooming (bonding by affiliating) that talk affords – often depend little on it instantiating reason, it's no skin off such discourse's conceptual nose that it's mainly driven by association.

34 To bend von Herder's ([1772] 2002) terminology to new ends.

35 Rochester and Martin (1979: 106).

36 Frith (1992: 99).

37 A version of the 'pre/trans fallacy' described in Chapter 9.

38 See Chapter 2.

39 Here as elsewhere we must distinguish reason from reasoning. When I'm merely rationalizing, my drawing of conclusions from premises (i.e. my reasoning) may be impeccable; nevertheless it may be utterly unreasonable of me to engage in *any* such reasoning in the context in question. Consider Bernard Williams' ([1976] 1981) contention (here slightly adapted) that if someone decides to rescue his beloved wife rather than a stranger from drowning on the basis that, say, his wife is the younger of the two, then, without impugning the rationality of this justification, his wife may yet have just cause for complaint that her husband here had 'one thought too many' – since the very fact that *she's his wife* might have been thought to suffice as an explanation for his choice. It's the unreasonableness of engaging in this reasoning which permits us to seek a psychological understanding of his thinking (perhaps he's not really the uxorious fellow he presents himself as being).

40 Bleuler (1982: 591). Manfred, son of Eugen, was director of the Burghölzli asylum from 1942 until 1969 where, like his father, he lived in close contact with his patients.

41 Lucas (2009: ch. 11); Evans (2016: ch. 5).

42 Hayman (1999: 53).

43 Jung ([1907] 1991: 21). On 'complexes': 'A complex is a collection of associations linked together by the same feeling-tone . . . When complexes are touched upon, the person concerned shows evidence of emotional disturbance . . .' (Storr 1991: 21). On 'flight of ideas': Jung refers here not to a manic rush or pressure of speech but rather to such schizophrenic thought as shows an 'absence of directing principle' (Jung [1907] 1991: 14).

44 Docherty et al. (1994); Burbridge and Barch (2002); Minor et al (2016).

45 This is not to say that the emotional disturbance is itself intact. As we saw in Chapter 5, the unity of the emotion has in such cases been compromised, and it has accordingly fallen apart – such that some of the criteria for being upset (the discombobulation) are now satisfied whilst others (the facial and vocal displays, the avowal) remain unsatisfied.

46 On 'seeing in': Wollheim (1980b). Experimental psychologists have sometimes been baffled by psychoanalysts' explanations of thought disorder because the psychologists' conception of psychological understanding restricts its remit to the causal relations between separately assayable stimuli and responses, thereby excluding both expressive relations and the understanding of them met with in 'seeing in'. Thus Chapman and Chapman (1973: 226) argue, contra Jung, that we may question whether schizophrenic thought disorder ever 'occurs in response to specific affective stimuli'; since 'schizophrenics show a greater preoccupation than normal people with their emotional problems, the fact of this preoccupation is not clear evidence that either their thought disorder or schizophrenia in general results from those problems. The deviant speech of paretics [i.e. sufferers from paralytic dementia] also shows their preoccupation with emotional problems. Surely, the only thing that has saved us from psychoanalytic theories of paresis has been the discovery that it is caused by syphilis.' In fact, such arguments fail not only because inner emotional experiences are but unhappily theorized as 'stimuli', nor merely because expressive relations are invisible through this particular psychological lens, nor simply because more recent studies (see

note 421) have shown the causal impact of emotional disturbance on thought's form, but also because the conception of causality it presupposes is itself inadequate. For why shouldn't a neurobiologically explicable disturbance be grasped as the diathesis for – i.e. as a vulnerability to – thought disorder, and emotional disturbance be grasped as the stressor which, together with the diathesis, results in disordered thought? (In fact, the *diathesis-stress model* of psychopathology was first introduced by Paul Meehl (1962) precisely to explain just such schizophrenic disturbances.) For that matter, why shouldn't aspects of the delusions or mania even of a paretic patient become psychologically intelligible once we approach these too with a psychiatric sensibility attuned to the psychotic wavelength?

47 Laing (1960); Fromm-Reichmann ([1958] 1959); Sullivan (1962); Stanghellini (2004).
48 Pienkos and Sass (2016); Sass and Parnas (2017).
49 Nietzsche ([1887] 1969). See also Stanghellini and Ballerini (2007, 2011). Pienkos and Sass (2016) recount one thought-disordered subject saying that he would deliberately speak 'nonsense' but would deliberately insert meaningful phrases into it to check whether his doctors were listening. If that were the most apt self-description then the idea that he was thought disordered would surely have to be revoked. What seems more likely is that he often willingly falls into an autistic, genuinely thought-disordered, mode, but sometimes makes an effort to regain reality contact – and that his description of himself as deliberately speaking nonsense is hyperbolical.
50 Bion (1955) offers a Kleinian conception of thought disorder as resulting from attacks by the psychotic part of the personality on the capacity to think about and relate to reality. More recent Kleinians have speculated that thought disorder results from a failure of early containment (i.e. of the parent's sensitive detoxifying of an infant's overwhelming feelings) (Grotstein 1989).
51 Jung ([1907] 1991: 111).
52 Laffal (1982: 605) offers this: 'Language, for some schizophrenic individuals, appears to have become a means primarily of operating upon the patient's [experiential] world, but only at considerable cost to communication with others.'
53 The example is owed to Karl Kleist, and cited by Leader (2011: 107).
54 Burnham (1955: 70).
55 Bion (1955: 226).
56 Strauss (1991: 86).
57 Sandis (2012).

9 Psychotic Symbolization

1 Jung ([1907] 1991: 145).
2 'It is to be remarked that the symbol plays a very great part in the discursions of the insane.... The symbol could be defined as a false perception of a relation of identity or a very marked analogy between two objects which in reality present only a very vague analogy' (Pelletier, 1903: 129). Pelletier's conception differs somewhat from than those that have settled in psychoanalysis. For Jung (1964: 20), a 'symbol is a term, a name, or even a picture that ... possesses specific connotations in addition to its conventional and obvious meaning. It implies something vague, unknown, or hidden from us.' Laplanche and Pontalis (1988: 443) propose that, in psychoanalysis, 'the term "symbolic" is used to describe the relation which links the manifest content of

behaviour, thought and speech to their latent meaning; it is applicable *a fortiori* where the manifest meaning is most lacking (as, for example, in the case of symptomatic acts that are obviously inexplicable in terms of any of the conscious motives which the subject might adduce).... [We] should only speak of symbolism in psycho-analysis in cases where what is symbolized is unconscious.... [If] a piece of behaviour, say, has at least two meanings, one of which is standing for the other, both concealing and expressing it, then we may describe the relationship between them as a symbolic one.'

3   Bleuler ([1911] 1950: 412); the name Elena is supplied by myself.

4   Evans (2016: 106–107).

5   Bleuler ([1911] 1950: 432). Jonas: name supplied by myself. Hebephrenia: a form of schizophrenia marked by formally disordered thought and flat or inappropriate affect.

6   As well as Jung's remark on Babette's thought reported in this chapter's first paragraph, consider the following examples of psychotic discourse being understood as expressive of metaphor: 'people who think they are God or the devil ... communicate in metaphors that often hint at the heart of their problem' (Breggin, 1993: 55); Frieda Fromm-Reichmann could 'understand a patient's metaphoric language ... It was her special gift not only to understand the nature of the unconscious conflicts hidden behind the patient's delusion and metaphors, but also to use language that indicated to the patient that he was being understood' (Arlow 1989: 181–182); 'Joanne Greenberg, author of *I Never Promised You a Rose Garden* and perhaps Fromm-Reichmann's best-known patient, indicates that from her perspective ". . . if the symptoms are metaphors, the therapist has to be someone who understands those metaphors or at least is amenable to learning them"' (McAfee 1989: 523); 'it is our job to help the patient understand his or her own metaphor and symbolism that have taken on the concretized form of psychotic delusions and hallucinations' (Steinman 2019: 247).

7   See Segal ([1957] 1981), Rosenfeld (1965), Jung ([1907] 1991), and Searles (1962: 23): 'just as the schizophrenic is unable to think in effective, consensually validated metaphor, so too is he unable to think in terms which are *genuinely* concrete'. Other authors have discussed general disturbances in the appreciation of metaphorical meaning in patients suffering psychotic illnesses – e.g. Cutting and Murphy (1990); de Bonis et al (1997).

8   Derived from Rhodes and Jakes (2004).

9   The example also derives from Rhodes and Jakes (2004); see their case 'P1'.

10 Such strategies deploy the influential, psychologized conception of metaphor of Lakoff and Johnson (1980) (for critique see Champlin (1982) and McGlone (2011)) and, in relation to delusion, are exemplified by Rhodes and Jakes' (2004) talk of 'metaphorical processes', of experiences which are themselves 'transformed' or 'permeated' 'by metaphorical meaning', of 'basic cognitive mechanisms' that are themselves 'metaphorical', etc.

11 Stein (2021).

12 There appears to be no sharp demarcation line between cases where true metaphor is being used and cases which should be recognized as instead manifesting merely the polysemous nature of various of our terms. 'Frosty', for example, has achieved recognition in the dictionary as a term for the expression of emotion – but only in a figurative, extended, or allusive sense.

13 A similar difficulty attends Currie's (2000) suggestion that the psychotic subject mistakes his own imaginings for beliefs.

14 It is, I propose, the phenomenological similarity between (i) that infantile mentality which as yet does not instantiate such distinctions and (ii) that psychotic mentality

which has suffered their post-formation collapse, that constitutes the actual, if rarely aptly articulated, positive content of psychoanalytic theories of psychosis as a function of regression. According to Sass (1992: 19–21, 410–411), psychoanalytic regression/ primitivity conceptions of psychotic thought and experience fail to acknowledge the often intact reasoning of the psychotic subject, and encourage a misconception of psychosis which has Dionysian passion here overturning Apollonian reason. We can agree with Sass both that active psychosis may often instead involve an inner dislocation of emotion and instinct along with what may even be a hypertrophy of reasoning, and that we don't do well to posit a quite general mental regression in the psychotic subject. Even so, active psychosis does essentially involve a disturbance of reason (if not of reasoning), and one of the key ways in which the delusional subject 'loses her mind' is that for her, when she is in her delusion, the distinctions between metaphoric and literal, imagined and perceived, etc., inwardly collapse.

15 Wilber (1982).

16 On 'unconscious metaphor', see Langer (1942); Langer is in fact talking of the dreaming (she also talks of 'dream-metaphors') rather than the psychotic mind, but the point stands.

17 Joyce (1939: 104).

18 Jung ([1932] 1966).

19 Ellman (1982: 679).

20 Letter to Patricia Graecen, 29 June 1955, cited in Ellman (1982: 641).

21 Greenberg published *I Never Promised You . . .* under the pen name Hannah Green ([1964] 2004). The true story of her treatment with Fromm-Reichmann is told by Hornstein (2000: 9).

22 McAfee (1989: 527). Greenberg underlines this point elsewhere: 'Creativity makes bridges, bonds, links. Mental illness cuts, surrounds, makes a fort which turns out to be a prison' (Cragg 2006).

23 I describe these claims (i)–(viii) as 'empirical' since it's surely imaginable that matters could have been otherwise (i.e. they are not 'necessary' truths). Even so their status as 'basic' shows itself in the fact that any examples we give of them do not so much constitute evidence that would justify them as instead exemplify their meaning. They are, one might say, 'phenomenological articulations' or 'revelations' of the nature of a central aspect of human experience. (For elaboration of this distinction, see Gipps (2019).)

24 A concept of symbolization along these lines appears to originate in Susanne Langer's (1942) *Philosophy in a New Key: A Study in the Symbolism of Reason, Rite, and Art*. It was developed by post-Kleinian psychoanalysts such as Wilfred Bion (1978), Hanna Segal ([1957] 1981), and Donald Meltzer (Meltzer and Harris Williams 2008), and also by the psychoanalytically-oriented art theorists Adrian Stokes (2014) and Richard Wollheim (1980a). For discussion of this distinctly aesthetic, imagination-focused, British, post-Kleinian approach to psychoanalysis, see Glover (2009). Newcomers to contemporary Kleinian analysis do well to attend to how it has more-or-less self-consciously redefined terms such as 'thinking', 'dreaming', and 'symbol formation' by relating them to the function allocated to them within a modified version of Freud's 'dream work' theory. The additional sense which 'thinking', 'dreaming', etc. now enjoy has to do with the largely unconscious psychological processes by which emotional conflicts and problems seek resolution (Meltzer, 2009). In this sense, even an improvising musician whose playing constitutes an affective outworking of previously blocked emotion could be said to be 'engaged in dreaming' – a thinking or dreaming

involving her temporally separating out, from a previously futile mass, and within the containing function of the temporally extended performance, different emotional experiences. A conception of a dream as a 'container' for anxiety has also influenced the psychoanalytic theory of dreaming; hence Bion's (1978) conception of myth as cultural dream entails within it an understanding of the myth as an anxiety container for the social group.

25 Mentalization: Fonagy and Allison (2012).
26 My precedent here is Jung's (1978: 70) description of the symbol as 'an expression of an intuitive idea that cannot yet be formulated in any other or better way'.
27 West (1983).
28 West (1983: 653).
29 Kirk (1970: 270).
30 Campbell (1968); see also row C of Bion's (1978) grid.
31 Campbell (1988).
32 Lévi-Strauss ([1949] 1963).
33 Lévi-Strauss ([1949] 1963: 197).
34 A possible mechanism: high adrenaline levels in labour's early stages, and low oxytocin levels in its later stages, cause contractions to slow or stop (Buckley 2015).
35 Yalom (2002) doesn't mention it, but the cypress, commonly planted in cemeteries, has since antiquity been a conventional symbol of mourning, death, and everlasting life.
36 Yalom (2002: 232).
37 Langer (1953: 40). See also: "'Living form" is the most indubitable product of all good art, be it painting, architecture, or pottery. Such form is "living" in . . . that . . . it *expresses* life – feeling, growth, movement, emotion, and everything that characterizes vital existence. This expression, moreover, is not symbolization in the usual sense of conventional or assigned meaning, but a presentation of a highly articulated form wherein the beholder recognizes, without conscious comparison and judgment but rather by direct recognition, the forms of human feeling: emotions, moods, even sensations in their characteristic passage. . . . It is this . . . that Mondrian extolled in his reflections: "'Art' is . . . the expression of true reality and true life . . . indefinable but realisable in plastics'" (Langer 1953: 82).
38 Eliot (1920).
39 Milner (1957: xvii).
40 Milner (1957: 6).
41 Milner (1957: 44), citing Holmes (1911: 304–305).
42 Milner (1957: 44).
43 Nagel's (1943) review of Langer (1942) exemplifies what I here urge is a misunderstanding of psychological symbolization.
44 Petocz (1999, 2019) provides a clear articulation of a 'Freudian broad theory of symbolism' in which the symbolizing mind operates in accord with a 'conflict-repression-substitution' formula.
45 For existential-phenomenological critique of traditional psychoanalytic metapsychology, see Boss (1963) and Sartre ([1943] 2018: ch. 2). In this context, it's worth noting that the psychoanalytic theory of dreaming and symbolizing has changed considerably from Freud's, especially under the influence of Wilfred Bion. Bion shifted the emphasis of psychoanalytic dream theory from symbolic substitutions guarding sleep to the creative process of dreaming, a process he equated with the unconscious processing of emotional meaning (Schneider 2010; Ogden 2007). For the idea that dreaming involves what I'm styling as a partial disidentification from

unthinkable predicament, see Bollas (1987: ch. 4). ('I regard the dream as a fiction constructed by a unique aesthetic: the transformation of the subject into his thought, specifically, the placing of the self into an allegory of desire and dread that is fashioned by the ego' (Bollas 1987: 64).) For critique of the idea that self-consciousness (i.e. our ability to self-ascribe thoughts and feelings) requires some kind of introspection or consciousness of oneself, see Narboux (2018); for an account of the making conscious of what is unconscious which doesn't invoke introspection, see Finkelstein (2019).

46 Bleuler ([1911] 1950: 439).
47 Minkowski ([1927] 1987: 210).
48 McAfee (1989: 528).

10 The Politics of Insanity Ascription

1 Think of your reaction to reading Stephen Hawkins' *Brief History of Time*: you might have judged yourself too ignorant to understand it, or thought him a poor explainer – but you probably didn't judge him insane.

2 Caplan (1995: xxiii). The consultant's question here is in effect of a piece with that of Chapter 2 which asked for a *criterion* for delusion or mental illness.

3 Kupfer et al. (2002: xvii); Kendler (2010: 1291); Bell, Raihani and Wilkinson (2021). See also: 'Psychiatry has uncovered very few mechanisms responsible for currently employed diagnoses and modern psychiatric evidence suggests there might not be many essentialist or homeostatic mechanisms out there waiting to be found' (Fellowes 2019: 475).

4 Laing (1960: 36–37). We may also consider the philosopher Stanley Cavell's response to the question 'Who is crazy?': 'I do not say no one is, but must somebody be, when people's reactions are at variance with ours? It seems safe to suppose that if you can describe any behaviour which I can recognize as that of human beings, I can give you an explanation which will make that behaviour coherent, i.e. show it to be imaginable in terms of natural responses and practicalities. Though *those* natural responses may not be mine, and those practices not practical for me, in my environment, as I interpret it. And if I say "They are crazy" or "incomprehensible" then that is not a fact but my fate for them. I have gone as far as my imagination, magnanimity, or anxiety will allow; or as my honour, or my standing cares and commitments, can accommodate' (Cavell 1979: 117–118).

5 Hornstein (2002).

6 For the original Kantian idealist's 'Copernican revolution', see Kant ([1787] 1999: 110 (B xvi–xvii)). The DSM-IV also invokes what I here style an 'Idealist' element when it suggests that delusion is false belief which, amongst other things, is 'firmly sustained despite what almost everyone else believes … The belief is not one ordinarily accepted by other members of the person's culture or subculture … When a false belief involves a value judgment, it is regarded as a delusion only when the judgment is so extreme as to defy credibility' (APA 1994: 765, n. 16). Following Ghaemi (2004), DSM-5 shifts this emphasis on intelligibility to peers from all delusion to such delusion as is styled 'bizarre': 'Delusions are deemed bizarre if they are clearly implausible and not understandable to same-culture peers …' (APA 2013: 87); for critique of this approach, see Gorski (2012).

7 Bentall (2003: 28–29).

8   On drapetomania: Bynum (2000); there's no evidence the diagnosis was actually used
    (Dawson 2021). On the political abuses of psychiatry in the USSR: Bloch and
    Reddaway (1977, 1984).
9   In a later edition of *The Divided Self*, Laing considers that previously he was 'already
    partially falling into the trap I was seeking to avoid . . . still writing . . . too much about
    Them, and too little of Us. . . . In the context of our present pervasive madness that we
    call normality, sanity, freedom, all our frames of reference are ambiguous and
    equivocal. . . . A man who prefers to be dead rather than Red is normal. A man who
    says he has lost his soul is mad. A man who says that men are machines may be a great
    scientist. A man who says he *is* a machine is "depersonalized" in psychiatric jargon. . . .
    A little girl of seventeen in a mental hospital told me she was terrified because the
    Atom Bomb was inside her. That is a delusion. The statesmen of the world who boast
    and threaten that they have Doomsday weapons are far more dangerous, and far more
    estranged from "reality" than many of the people on whom the label "psychotic" is
    affixed' (Laing 1965: 11–12).
10 Frege ([1893] 1964: 14). Frege is not here endorsing, but instead is critiquing, the
    thinking of the psychological logician; the passage continues: 'I [Frege] would say: here
    we have a hitherto unknown kind of madness.'
11 von Domarus ([1944] 1964: 111).
12 Campbell (2001). See also Eilan (2000) and Bardina (2018). For critique: Thornton
    (2008); Bellaar (2016). See also Chapter 3.
13 Eilan (2000: 97).
14 See Chapter 8.
15 See Benoist (2020).
16 See Davidson (1973–74). What Davidson shows is, in effect, that if we succeed in
    making sense of someone else, we thereby have no ground for speaking of their having
    a different conceptual scheme – and that if we fail to make sense of them, we thereby
    have no ground for speaking of their having a conceptual scheme at all. And as
    Davidson goes on to argue, thinking through these considerations shows that in the
    end we must relinquish the very idea of a logical (or 'conceptual', as he has it) scheme.
17 Kant ([1787] 1999: A51/B76).
18 Frege ([1893] 1964: 15).
19 Schneider (1959: 105).
20 See Chapter 8.
21 See Chapter 3; also Gipps (2019).
22 See Wittgenstein (1958a: 178): 'My attitude towards him is an attitude towards a soul
    [i.e. towards a being who can suffer fear, pain, etc.]. I am not of the *opinion* that he has
    a soul.'
23 Other uses of a concept of 'subjective opinion' are available. For example, we can use
    one such concept to articulate matters of personal taste. Such matters of taste are not
    intelligibility described as evidenced or as objective. And here the subjective/objective
    distinction functions not to effect a contrast within a singular category of opinion or
    judgement, but instead to articulate different things that can be meant by 'opinion' or
    'judgement'.
24 Something like this is a large part of what drives the 'scientist practitioner' model of
    clinical psychology.
25 Wittgenstein (1958a: §§218–219).
26 Cavell (1969: 52).

27 See Wittgenstein (1958a: §242). We may note here again the difference between 'agreement in opinions' and 'commensuration in originary judgements'. Wittgenstein writes that the agreement of human beings 'in the *language* they use ... is not agreement in opinions but in form of life' (ibid: §241). I take it that being disposed to commensuration in judgement is part of what it means to share a 'form of life'.

28 This vision of the intrinsically ethical and psychological character of taking responsibility for, and showing accountability in, one's language use has in particular been developed by Cavell (1979).

References

Abel-Hirsch, N. (2006), 'The perversion of pain, pleasure, and thought: On the difference between "suffering" an experience and the "construction" of a thing to be used', in D. Nobus and L. Downing (eds), *Perversion: Psychoanalytic Perspectives/Perspectives on Psychoanalysis*, 99–109, London: Routledge.

American Psychiatric Association (APA) (1994), *Diagnostic and Statistical Manual: DSM-IV*, Arlington, VA: American Psychiatric Association.

American Psychiatric Association (APA) (2013), *Diagnostic and Statistical Manual: DSM-5*, Arlington, VA: American Psychiatric Association.

Andreasen, N. (1982), 'Should the term "thought disorder" be revised?', *Comprehensive Psychiatry*, 23 (4): 291–299.

Andreasen, N. (1986), 'Scale for the assessment of thought, language, and communication (TLC)', *Schizophrenia Bulletin*, 12 (3): 473–482.

Anscombe, G. E. M. (1957), *Intention*, Ithaca, NY: Cornell University Press.

Anscombe, G. E. M. (1965), 'The intentionality of sensation: A grammatical feature', in R.J. Butler (ed.), *Analytical Philosophy – Second Series*, 158–180, Oxford: Blackwell.

Anscombe, G. E. M. (1975), 'The first person', in S. Guttenplan (ed.), *Mind and Language*, 45–65, Oxford: Clarendon Press.

Anzieu, D. (1989), *The Skin Ego*, New Haven, CT: Yale University Press.

Appleby, L., N. Kapur, J. Shaw, I. Hunt, S. Ibrahim, P. Turnbull, L. Bojanić, C. Rodway, S.-G. Tham, N. Richards and J. Burns (2019), *The National Confidential Inquiry into Suicide and Safety in Mental Health. Annual Report: England, Northern Ireland, Scotland and Wales, 2019*, Manchester: University of Manchester. Available online: https://documents.manchester.ac.uk/display.aspx?DocID=46558 (accessed 15 January 2021).

Aristotle ([4th century BC] 1998), *Metaphysics*, trans. H. Lawson-Tancred, London: Penguin.

Arlow, J. (1989), 'Delusion and metaphor', in A.-L.S. Silver (ed.), *Psychoanalysis and Psychosis*, 173–182, Madison, CT: International Universities Press.

Arnold, T. (1782), *Observations on the Nature, Kinds, Causes, and Prevention of Insanity, Lunacy or Madness*, Leicester: G. Ireland.

Arrington, R. L. (2001), 'Thought and its expression', in S. Schroeder (ed.), *Wittgenstein and Contemporary Philosophy of Mind*, 129–149, Basingstoke: Palgrave.

Asperger, H. (1944), 'Die "Autistischen Psychopathen" im Kindesalter', *Archiv für Psychiatrie und Nervenkrankheiten*, 117 (1): 132–135.

Augustine, A. ([397] 1991), *Confessions*, trans. H. Chadwick, Oxford: Oxford University Press.

Bardina, S. (2018), 'Abnormal certainty: Examining the epistemological status of delusional beliefs', *International Journal of Philosophical Studies*, 26 (4): 546–560.

Bargh, J. A. and T. A. Chartrand (1999), 'The unbearable automaticity of being', *American Psychologist*, 54 (7): 462–479.

Bayne, T. and E. Pacherie (2005), 'In defence of the doxastic conception of delusions', *Mind & Language*, 20 (2): 163–188.

Beck, A. T. and N. A. Rector (2000), 'Cognitive therapy of schizophrenia: A new therapy for the new millennium', *American Journal of Psychotherapy*, 54 (3): 291–300.

Bell, B., N. Raihani and S. Wilkinson (2021), 'Derationalising delusions', *Clinical Psychological Science*, 9 (1): 24–37.

Bell, V., S. Wilkinson, M. Greco, C. Hendrie, B. Mills and Q. Deeley (2020), 'What is the functional/organic distinction actually doing in psychiatry and neurology?', *Wellcome Open Research*, 5: 138. Available online: https://wellcomeopenresearch.org/articles/5-138/v1 (accessed 15 June 2021).

Bellaar, R. (2016), 'Understanding Schizophrenia: A Wittgensteinian Approach to Double-Bookkeeping', MSc dissertation, University of Amsterdam.

Bellak, L. and A. B. Blaustein (1958), 'Psychoanalytic aspects of schizophrenia', in L. Bellak (ed.), *Schizophrenia: A Review of the Syndrome*, 279–335, New York: Logos Press.

Benoist, J. (2020), 'Alien meaning and alienated meaning', in S. Miguens (ed.), *The Logical Alien: Conant and His Critics*, 281–292, Cambridge, MA: Harvard University Press.

Bentall, R. (2003), *Madness Explained: Psychosis and Human Nature*, London: Penguin.

Bergson, H. ([1907] 1911), *Creative Evolution*, trans. A. Mitchell, New York: Henry Holt.

Bermudez, J. L. (2001), 'Normativity and rationality in delusional psychiatric disorders', *Mind & Language*, 16 (5): 457–493.

Berrios, G. E., R. Luque and J. M. Villagrán (2003), 'Schizophrenia: A conceptual history', *International Journal of Psychology and Psychological Therapy*, 3 (2): 111–140.

Berrios, G. E. and I. S. Marková (2012), 'The construction of hallucinations: History and epistemology', in J. Blom and I. Sommer (eds), *Hallucinations*, 55–71, New York: Springer.

Bick, E. (1968), 'The experience of the skin in early object-relations', *International Journal of Psychoanalysis*, 49 (2): 484–486.

Bion, W. R. (1955), 'Language and the schizophrenic', in M. Klein, P. Heimann and R. Money-Kyrle (eds), *New Directions in Psychoanalysis*, 220–239, London: Tavistock.

Bion, W. R. ([1962] 1978), *Learning from Experience*, in W. R. Bion, *Seven Servants: Four Works by Wilfred R. Bion*, New York: Jason Aronson.

Bion, W. R. (1978), *Seven Servants: Four Works by Wilfred R. Bion*, New York: Jason Aronson.

Blaiklock, J. (2017), 'Husserl, protention, and the phenomenology of the unexpected', *International Journal of Philosophical Studies*, 25 (4): 467–483.

Blanke, O. and G. Thut (2007), 'Inducing out-of-body experiences', in S. Della Sala (ed.), *Tall Tales About the Mind and Brain: Separating Fact from Fiction*, 425–439, Oxford: Oxford University Press.

Blanke, O., P. Pozeg, M. Hara, L. Heydrich, A. Serino, A. Yamamoto, T. Higuchi, R. Salomon, M. Seeck, T. Landis, S. Arzy, B. Herbelin, H. Bleuler and G. Rognini (2014), 'Neurological and robot-controlled induction of an apparition', *Current Biology*, 24 (22): 2681–2686.

Blankenburg, W. ([1968] 2001), 'First steps toward a psychopathology of "common sense"', trans. A. Mishara, *Philosophy, Psychiatry, & Psychology*, 8 (4): 303–315.

Bleuler, E. (1911), *Dementia Praecox oder Gruppe der Schizophrenien*, Leipzig: Deuticke.

Bleuler, E. ([1911] 1950), *Dementia Praecox or the Group of Schizophrenias*, trans. J. Zinkin, New York: International Universities Press.

Bleuler, E. ([1916] 1924), *Textbook of Psychiatry*, trans. A. A. Brill, New York: Macmillan.

Bleuler, E. (1955), *Lehrbuch der Psychiatrie*, 9th edn, Berlin: Springer.

Bleuler, M. ([1972] 1978), *The Schizophrenic Disorders*, trans. S. M. Clemens, New Haven, CT: Yale University Press.

Bleuler, M. (1982), 'Inconstancy of schizophrenic language and symptoms', *Behavioral and Brain Sciences*, 5 (4): 591.

Bloch, S. and P. Reddaway (1977), *Russia's Political Hospitals: The Abuse of Psychiatry in the Soviet Union*, London: Victor Gollancz.

Bloch, S. and P. Reddaway (1984), *Soviet Psychiatric Abuse: The Shadow Over World Psychiatry*, London: Victor Gollancz.

Bollas, C. (1987), *The Shadow of the Object: Psychoanalysis of the Unthought Known*, London: Free Association Books.

Bolton, D. (2008), *What is Mental Disorder?*, Oxford: Oxford University Press.

Boncompagni, A. (2018), 'Common sense, philosophy, and mental disturbance: A Wittgensteinian outlook', in I. Hipólito, J. Gonçalves and J. Pereira (eds), *Schizophrenia and Common Sense*, 227–238, Cham: Springer.

Bora, E., M. Yucel and C. Pantelis (2009), 'Theory of mind impairment in schizophrenia: Meta-analysis', *Schizophrenia Research*, 109 (1–3): 1–9.

Borel, A. and G. Robin (1925), 'Les rêveurs. Considérations sur les mondes imaginaires', *L'Évolution Psychiatrique*, 1: 155–192.

Bortolotti, L. (2010), *Delusions and Other Irrational Beliefs*, Oxford: Oxford University Press.

Boss, M. (1963), *Psychoanalysis and Daseinsanalysis*, New York: Basic Books.

Botvinick, M. and J. Cohen (1998), 'Rubber hands "feel" touch that eyes see', *Nature*, 391 (6669): 756. Available online: https://doi.org/10.1038/35784.

Breggin, P. (1993), *Toxic Psychiatry*, London: Fontana.

Brontë, E. ([1847] 1991), *Wuthering Heights*, London: Knopf.

Brown, C. (1944), *Brainstorm*, New York: Farrar & Rinehart.

Brugger, P., M. Regard and T. Landis (1997), 'Illusory reduplication of one's own body: Phenomenology and classification of autoscopic phenomena', *Cognitive Neuropsychiatry*, 2 (1): 19–38.

Buckley, S. (2015), *Hormonal Physiology of Childbearing*, Washington, DC: Childbirth Connection Programs. Available online: www.ChildbirthConnection.org/HormonalPhysiology (accessed 25 May 2021).

Buhrmann, T., E. Di Paolo and X. Barandiaran (2013), 'A dynamical systems account of sensorimotor contingencies', *Frontiers of Psychology*, 4: 285. Available online: https://www.frontiersin.org/articles/10.3389/fpsyg.2013.00285/full (accessed 7 March 2021).

Burbridge, J. A. and D. M. Barch (2002), 'Emotional valence and reference disturbance in schizophrenia', *Journal of Abnormal Psychology*, 111 (1): 186–191.

Burnham, D. L. (1955), 'Some problems in communication with schizophrenic patients', *Journal of the American Psychoanalytic Association*, 3 (1): 67–81.

Bychowski, G. (1953), 'The problem of latent psychosis', *Journal of the American Psychoanalytic Association*, 1 (3): 484–503.

Bynum, B. (2000), 'Discarded diagnoses: Drapetomania', *The Lancet*, 356 (9241): 1615.

Campbell, J. (1968), *The Hero with a Thousand Faces*, Princeton, NJ: Princeton University Press.

Campbell, J. (1988), *The Power of Myth*, New York: Doubleday.

Campbell, J. (1999), 'Schizophrenia, the space of reasons, and thinking as a motor process', *The Monist*, 82 (4): 609–625.

Campbell, J. (2001), 'Rationality, meaning, and the analysis of delusion', *Philosophy, Psychiatry, & Psychology*, 8 (2–3): 89–100.

Campbell, R. (2009), *Campbell's Psychiatric Dictionary*, 9th edn, Oxford: Oxford University Press.

Caplan, P. J. (1995), *They Say You're Crazy: How the World's Most Powerful Psychiatrists Decide Who's Normal*, Reading, MA: Addison-Wesley.

Cavell, S. (1969), *Must We Mean What We Say?*, New York: Scribner.

Cavell, S. (1979), *The Claim of Reason*, New York: Oxford University Press.

Chaika, E. (1982), 'Thought disorder or speech disorder in schizophrenia', *Schizophrenia Bulletin*, 8 (4): 588–591.

Chaika, E. and R. Lambe (1985), 'The locus of dysfunction in schizophrenic speech', *Schizophrenia Bulletin*, 11 (1): 8–15.

Champlin, T. S. (1981), 'The reality of mental illness', *Philosophy*, 56 (218): 467–487.

Champlin, T. S. (1982), 'Review: Metaphors we live by', *Philosophical Books*, 23 (2): 111–116.

Champlin, T. S. (1996), 'To mental illness via a rhyme for the eye', in A. O'Hear (ed.), *Verstehen and Humane Understanding*, Cambridge: Cambridge University Press.

Champlin, T. S. (2008), 'Review: The metaphor of mental illness', *Journal of Applied Philosophy*, 25 (4): 353–355.

Chapman, L. J. and Chapman, J. P. (1973), *Disordered Thought in Schizophrenia*, New York: Appleton-Century-Crofts.

Clark, A. (2013), 'Expecting the world: Perception, prediction, and the origins of human knowledge', *Journal of Philosophy*, 110 (9): 469–496.

Coate, M. (1964), *Beyond All Reason*, London: Constable.

Conant, J. and C. Diamond (2004), 'On reading the Tractatus resolutely', in M. Kölbel and B. Weiss (eds), *Wittgenstein's Lasting Significance*, 46–99, London: Routledge.

Conrad, K. (1958), *Die Beginnende Schizophrenie*, Stuttgart: Thieme Verlag.

Corlett, P. R., G. Horga, P. C. Fletcher, B. Alderson-Day, K. Schmack and A. R. Powers (2019), 'Hallucinations and strong priors', *Trends in Cognitive Science*, 23 (2): 114–127.

Corrigan, P. W., L. P. River, R. K. Lundin, D. L. Penn, K. Uphoff-Wasowski, J. Campion, J. Mathisen, C. Gagnon, M. Bergman, H. Goldstein and M. A. Kubiak (2001), 'Three strategies for changing attributions about severe mental illness', *Schizophrenia Bulletin*, 27 (2): 187–195.

Cragg, C. (2006), '"Appearances" in a "Rose Garden"? Interview with Joanne Greenberg'. Available online: https://beta.prx.org/stories/10227 (accessed 18 March 2021).

Currie, G. (2000), 'Imagination, delusions and hallucinations', *Mind & Language*, 15 (1): 168–183.

Currie, G. and I. Ravenscroft (2001), *Meeting of Minds: Thought, Imagination and Perception*, Oxford: Oxford University Press.

Cutting, J. and D. Murphy (1990), 'Preference for meanings in schizophrenics', *Brain and Language*, 39 (3): 459–468.

Cutting, J. and M. Musalek (2015), 'The nature of delusion: Psychologically explicable? Psychologically inexplicable? Philosophically explicable? Part 1', *History of Psychiatry*, 26 (4): 404–417.

Daniel, C. and O. J. Mason (2015), 'Predicting psychotic-like experiences during sensory deprivation', *BioMed Research International*, 2015: 439379. Available online: http://dx.doi.org/10.1155/2015/439379 (accessed 28 April 2021).

David & Lisa (1962), [Film] Dir. Frank Perry. USA: Vision Associates Productions.

Davidson, D. (1973), 'Radical interpretation', *Dialectica*, 27 (3–4): 314–328.

Davidson, D. (1973–74), 'On the very idea of a conceptual scheme', *Proceedings and Addresses of the American Philosophical Association*, 47: 5–20.

Dawson, G. (2021), 'Drapetomania: The lack of relevance to psychiatry'. Available online: https://real-psychiatry.blogspot.com/2021/08/drapetomania-lack-of-relevance-to.html (accessed 4 January 2022).

de Bonis, M., C. Epelbaum, V. Deffez and A. Feline (1997), 'The comprehension of metaphors in schizophrenia', *Psychopathology*, 30 (3): 149–154.

de Haan, S. and T. Fuchs (2010), 'The ghost in the machine: Disembodiment in schizophrenia – two case studies', *Psychopathology*, 43 (5): 327–333.

de Haan, S. (2020), *Enactive Psychiatry*, Cambridge: Cambridge University Press.

de Mijolla, A. (ed.) (2005), *International Dictionary of Psychoanalysis*, Detroit, MI: Thomson Gale.

Diamond, C. (2000), 'Ethics, imagination, and the method of Wittgenstein's *Tractatus*', in A. Crary and R. Read (eds), *The New Wittgenstein*, 149–173, London: Routledge.

Diamond, C. (2003), 'The difficulty of reality and the difficulty of philosophy', *Partial Answers*, 1 (2): 1–26.

Docherty, N. M., I. M. Evans, W. H. Sledge, J. P. Seibyl and J. H. Krystal (1994), 'Affective reactivity of language in schizophrenia', *Journal of Nervous and Mental Disease*, 182 (2): 98–102.

Dreyfus, H. and C. Taylor (2015), *Retrieving Realism*, Cambridge, MA: Harvard University Press.

Dudley, R., P. Taylor, S. Wickham and P. Hutton (2016), 'Psychosis, delusions and the "jumping to conclusions" reasoning bias: A systematic review and meta-analysis', *Schizophrenia Bulletin*, 42 (3): 652–665.

Egger, V. (1881), *La Parole Intérieure*, Paris: Librairie Germer Baillière.

Eilan, N. (2000), 'On understanding schizophrenia', in D. Zahavi (ed.), *Exploring the Self*, 97–113, Amsterdam: John Benjamins.

Eilan, N. (2001), 'Meaning, truth, and the self: Commentary on Campbell and Parnas and Sass', *Philosophy, Psychiatry, & Psychology*, 8 (2–3): 121–132.

Eliot, T. S. (1920), 'Hamlet and his problems', in T. S. Eliot, *The Sacred Wood: Essays on Poetry and Criticism*, London: Methuen.

Ellman, R. (1982), *James Joyce*, Oxford: Oxford University Press.

Esquirol, J. E. D. (1817), 'Hallucinations', *Dictionnaire des Sciences Médicales*, vol. XX, 64–71, Paris: C. L. F. Panckoucke.

Evans, M. (2016), *Making Room for Madness in Mental Health: The Psychoanalytic Understanding of Psychotic Communication*, London: Karnac.

Everett, K. V. and R. J. Linscott (2015), 'Dimensionality vs taxonicity of schizotypy: Some new data and challenges ahead', *Schizophrenia Bulletin*, 41 (suppl. 2): S465–S474.

Ey, H. (1967), 'La dissolution du champ de la conscience dans le phénomène sommeil-veille et ses rapports avec la psychopathologie', *La Presse Médicale*, 75: 575–578.

Fairbairn, W. R. D. ([1941] 1952), 'A revised psychopathology of the psychoses and psychoneuroses', in W. R. D. Fairbairn, *Psychoanalytic Studies of the Personality*, 28–58, London: Routledge & Kegan Paul.

Fairbairn, W. R. D. ([1943] 1952), 'The repression and return of bad objects (with special reference to the "war neuroses")', in W. R. D. Fairbairn, *Psychoanalytic Studies of the Personality*, 59–81, London: Routledge & Kegan Paul.

Federn, P. ([1928] 1952), 'Ego as subject and object in narcissism', in P. Federn, *Ego Psychology and the Psychoses*, 283–322, New York: Basic Books.

Federn, P. ([1932] 1952), 'Ego feelings in dreams', in P. Federn, *Ego Psychology and the Psychoses*, 60–89, New York: Basic Books.

Federn, P. ([1949] 1952), 'Ego psychological aspect of schizophrenia', in P. Federn, *Ego Psychology and the Psychoses*, 210–226, New York: Basic Books.

Fellowes, S. (2019), 'Scientific realism, antirealism, and psychiatric diagnosis', in S. Tekin and R. Bluhm (eds), *The Bloomsbury Companion to Philosophy of Psychiatry*, 467–484, London: Bloomsbury Academic.

Finkelstein, D. H. (2019), 'Making the unconscious conscious', in R. G. T. Gipps and M. Lacewing (eds), *The Oxford Handbook of Philosophy and Psychoanalysis*, 331–346, Oxford: Oxford University Press.

Fish, F. (1976), *Fish's Schizophrenia*, 2nd edn, Bristol: John Wright.

Fish, F. (1984), *Fish's Schizophrenia*, revised edn, ed. M. Hamilton, Bristol: John Wright.

Fonagy P. and E. Allison (2012), 'What is mentalization? The concept and its foundations in developmental research', in I. Vrouva and N. Midgley (eds), *Minding the Child: Mentalization-Based Interventions with Children, Young People and Their Families*, 11–34, London: Routledge.

Freeman, T., J. Cameron and A. McGhie (1958), *Chronic Schizophrenia*, London: Tavistock.

Freeman, T. (1976), 'On the psychopathology of transitivism and appersonation', *British Journal of Psychiatry*, 129 (5): 414–417.

Frege, G. ([1893] 1964), *The Basic Laws of Arithmetic*, trans. and ed. M. Furth, Berkeley, CA: University of California Press.

Freud, S. ([1909] 1979), 'Notes upon a case of obsessional neurosis (the "Rat Man")', in S. Freud, *Case Histories II*, 33–128, Harmondsworth: Pelican.

Freud, S. ([1911] 1979), 'Psychoanalytic notes on an autobiographical account of a case of paranoia (dementia paranoides) (Schreber)', in S. Freud, *Case Histories II*, 131–223, Harmondsworth: Pelican.

Freud, S. ([1914] 1957), 'On narcissism', in J. Strachey (ed.), *Standard Edition of the Complete Psychological Works of Sigmund Freud*, vol. 14, 67–103, London: Hogarth Press.

Freud, S. ([1916–17] 1957), 'A metapsychological supplement to the theory of dreams', in J. Strachey (ed.), *Standard Edition of the Complete Psychological Works of Sigmund Freud*, vol. 14, 225–235, London: Hogarth Press.

Freud, S. ([1917] 1991), *Introductory Lectures on Psychoanalysis*, London: Penguin.

Freud, S. ([1919] 2003), *The Uncanny*, trans. D. McLintock, New York: Penguin.

Freud, S. ([1924] 1961). 'Neurosis and psychosis', in J. Strachey (ed.), *Standard Edition of the Complete Psychological Works of Sigmund Freud*, vol. 19, 149–154, London: Hogarth Press.

Freud, S. ([1930] 1985), 'Civilization and its discontents', in A. Dickson (ed.), *Civilization, Society and Religion: The Penguin Freud Library*, vol. 12, 251–340, Harmondsworth: Penguin.

Freud, S. ([1938] 1964), 'Some elementary lessons in psycho-analysis', in J. Strachey (ed.), *Standard Edition of the Complete Psychological Works of Sigmund Freud*, vol. 23, 279–286, London: Hogarth Press.

Friston, K. J. (2007), 'Free energy and the brain', *Synthese*, 159 (3): 417–458.

Frith, C. D. (1992), *The Cognitive Neuropsychology of Schizophrenia*, Hove: Lawrence Erlbaum Associates.

Frith, C. D., S.-J. Blakemore and D. M. Wolpert (2000), 'Explaining the symptoms of schizophrenia: Abnormalities in the awareness of action', *Brain Research Reviews*, 31 (2–3): 357–363.

Frith, C. D. and S.-J. Blakemore (2003), 'Self-awareness in action', *Current Opinion in Neurobiology*, 13 (2): 219–224.

Frith, C. D. (2007), *Making Up the Mind: How the Brain Creates Our Mental World*, Chichester: Wiley-Blackwell.

Frith, C. D. (2012), 'Explaining delusions of control: The comparator model 20 years on', *Consciousness and Cognition*, 21 (1): 52–54.

Fromm-Reichmann, F. ([1958] 1959), 'Basic problems in the psychotherapy of schizophrenia', in D. Bullard (ed.), *Psychoanalysis and Psychotherapy: Selected Papers of Frieda Fromm-Reichmann*, 210–220, Chicago, IL: University of Chicago Press.

Frosch, J. (1983), *The Psychotic Process*, New York: International Universities Press.

Fuchs, T. (2005), 'Corporealized and disembodied minds: A phenomenological view of the body in melancholia and schizophrenia', *Philosophy, Psychiatry, & Psychology*, 12 (2): 95–107.

Fuchs, T. and F. Röhricht (2017), 'Schizophrenia and intersubjectivity: An embodied and enactive approach to psychopathology and psychotherapy', *Philosophy, Psychiatry, & Psychology*, 24 (2): 127–142.

Fulford, K. W. M. (1989), *Moral Theory and Medical Practice*, Cambridge: Cambridge University Press.

Fulford, K. W. M. (2004), 'Insight and delusion: From Jaspers to Kraepelin and back again via Austin', in X. F. Amador and A. S. David (eds), *Insight and Psychosis: Awareness of Illness in Schizophrenia and Related Disorders*, 2nd edn, 51–78, Oxford: Oxford University Press.

Fulford, K. W. M. and L. Radoilska (2012), 'Three challenges from delusion for theories of autonomy', in L. Radoilska (ed.), *Autonomy and Mental Disorder*, 44–74, Oxford: Oxford University Press.

Gaita, R. (2000), *A Common Humanity: Thinking About Love and Truth and Justice*, London: Routledge.

Gallagher, S. (2000), 'Self-reference and schizophrenia', in D. Zahavi (ed.), *Exploring the Self*, 203–239, Amsterdam: John Benjamins.

Gallagher, S. (2005), 'Self-reference and schizophrenia: A cognitive model of immunity to error through misidentification', in D. Zahavi (ed.), *Exploring the Self: Philosophical and Psychopathological Perspectives on Self-Experience*, 203–239, Amsterdam: John Benjamins.

Gallagher, S. (2015), 'Relations between agency and ownership in the case of schizophrenic thought insertion and delusions of control', *Review of Philosophy and Psychology*, 6 (4): 865–879.

Garety, P., D. Hemsley and S. Wessely (1991), 'Reasoning in deluded schizophrenic and paranoid patients', *Journal of Nervous and Mental Disease*, 179 (4): 194–201.

Garety, P. and D. Freeman (1999), 'Cognitive approaches to delusions: A critical review of theories and evidence', *British Journal of Clinical Psychology*, 38 (2): 113–154.

Garety, P. and D. Freeman (2013), 'The past and future of delusions research', *British Journal of Psychiatry*, 203 (5): 327–333.

Garson, J. (2019), *What Biological Functions Are and Why They Matter*, Cambridge: Cambridge University Press.

Gauthier, S. (2000), 'Hallucinations ou projection: les hallucinations psychotiques, entre sentiment de présence et allusion à l'absence', *Revue Française de Psychoanalyse*, 64 (3): 831–849.

Geekie, J. and J. Read (2009), *Making Sense of Madness*, Hove: Routledge.

Ghaemi, N. (2004), 'The perils of belief: Delusions reexamined', *Philosophy, Psychiatry, & Psychology*, 11 (1): 49–54.

Gibson, J. J. (1965), 'Constancy and invariance in perception', in G. Kepes (ed.), *The Nature and Art of Motion*, 60–70, London: Studio Vista.

Gipps, R. G. T. (2009), 'Bodily Experience in Psychosis: A Phenomenological Investigation. Section B of Subjective Experience of the Body in Schizophrenia', DClin Psychol dissertation, Canterbury Christ Church University. Available online: www.academia. edu/528492/Subjective_Experience_of_the_Body_in_Psychosis (accessed 20 March 2021).

Gipps, R. G. T. (2010), 'The intelligibility of delusion', *Current Opinion in Psychiatry*, 23 (6): 556–560.

Gipps, R. G. T. (2016), 'Schizophrenic discourse as disturbed relating', *Journal of Psychopathology*, 22: 71–78. Available online: https://www.jpsychopathol.it/wp-content/uploads/2016/05/10_Art_Expressions_Gipps_ok1.pdf.

Gipps, R. G. T. (2017), 'Hallucination as unrelinquished anticipation', *Philosophical Perspectives in Clinical Psychology*, 14 June. Available online: https://clinicalphilosophy. blogspot.com/2017/06/hallucination-as-unrelinquished.html (accessed 4 May 2021).

Gipps, R. G. T. (2019), 'A new kind of song: Psychoanalysis as revelation', in R. G. T. Gipps and M. Lacewing (eds), *The Oxford Handbook of Philosophy and Psychoanalysis*, 433–455, Oxford: Oxford University Press.

Gipps, R. G. T. and S. de Haan (2019), 'Schizophrenic autism', in G. Stanghellini, M. Broome, A. Raballo, A. V. Fernandez, P. Fusar-Poli and R. Rosfort (eds), *The Oxford Handbook of Phenomenological Psychopathology*, 812–826, Oxford: Oxford University Press.

Gipps, R. G. T. (2020a), 'Disturbance of ego boundary enaction in schizophrenia', *Philosophy, Psychiatry, & Psychology*, 27 (1): 91–106.

Gipps, R. G. T. (2020b), 'When ego boundaries break', *Philosophy, Psychiatry, & Psychology*, 27 (1): 111–113.

Gipps, R. G. T. (2021), 'The narcissism of the private linguist', in M. Balaska (ed.), *Cora Diamond's Ethics*, 223–246, London: Palgrave Macmillan.

Glover, N. (2009), *Psychoanalytic Aesthetics: The British School*, London: Karnac.

Gorski, M. (2012), 'Karl Jaspers on delusion: Definition by genus and specific difference', *Philosophy, Psychiatry, & Psychology*, 19 (1): 79–86.

Gould, L. N. (1949), 'Auditory hallucinations and subvocal speech: Objective study in a case of schizophrenia', *Journal of Nervous and Mental Disease*, 109 (5): 418–427.

Graham, G. and G. L. Stephens (1994), 'Mind and mine', in G. Graham and G. L. Stephens (eds), *Philosophical Psychopathology*, 91–109, Cambridge, MA: MIT Press.

Green, H. aka J. Greenberg ([1964] 2004), *I Never Promised You a Rose Garden*, New York: New American Library.

Green, P. and M. Preston (1981), 'Reinforcement of vocal correlates of auditory hallucinations by auditory feedback: A case study', *British Journal of Psychiatry*, 139 (3): 204–208.

Gregory, R. L. (1980), 'Perceptions as hypotheses', *Philosophical Transactions of the Royal Society of London B: Biological Sciences*, 290 (1038): 181–197.

Griesinger, W. (1867), *Mental Pathology and Therapeutics*, trans. C. L. Robertson and J. Rutherford, London: The New Sydenham Society.

Grimby, A. (1993), 'Bereavement among elderly people: Grief reactions, post-bereavement hallucinations and quality of life', *Acta Psychiatrica Scandinavica*, 87 (1): 72–80.

Grimm & Grimm ([1812] 1944) *The Complete Grimm's Fairy Tales*, New York: Pantheon Books.

Grotstein, J. S. (1989), 'A revised psychoanalytic conception of schizophrenia: An interdisciplinary update', *Psychoanalytic Psychology*, 6 (3): 253–275.

Gurney, E., F. Myers and F. Podmore (1886), *Phantasms of the Living*, London: Trübner.

Hacker, P. M. S. (1995), 'Helmholtz's theory of perception: An investigation into its conceptual framework', *International Studies in the Philosophy of Science*, 9 (3): 199–214.

Hacker, P. M. S. (2013), *The Intellectual Powers: A Study of Human Nature*, Chichester: Wiley-Blackwell.

Hamilton, A. (2006), 'Against the belief model of delusion', in M. C. Chung, K. W. M. Fulford and G. Graham (eds), *Reconceiving Schizophrenia*, 217–234, Oxford: Oxford University Press.

Harrison, P., P. Cowen, T. Burns and M. Fazel (2018), *Shorter Oxford Textbook of Psychiatry*, 7th edn, Oxford: Oxford University Press.

Harrow, M., E. M. O'Connell, E. S. Herbener, A. M. Altman, K. J. Kaplan and T. H. Jobe (2003), 'Disordered verbalizations in schizophrenia: A speech disturbance or thought disorder?', *Comprehensive Psychiatry*, 44 (5): 353–359.

Hart, B. L. (1988), 'Biological basis of the behavior of sick animals', *Neuroscience & Biobehavioral Reviews*, 12 (2): 123–137.

Hart, M. and R. R. J. Lewine (2017), 'Rethinking thought disorder', *Schizophrenia Bulletin*, 43 (3): 514–522.

Haswell Todd, S. D. (2015), 'The Turn to the Self: A History of Autism 1910–1944', PhD dissertation, University of Chicago, Illinois. Available online: https://knowledge. uchicago.edu/record/238?ln=en (accessed 12 January 2021).

Hayman, R. (1999), *A Life of Jung*, London: Bloomsbury.

Hayward, M. L. and J. E. Taylor (1956), 'A schizophrenic patient describes the action of intensive psychotherapy', *Psychiatric Quarterly*, 30: 211–248.

Heidegger, M. ([1927] 1962), *Being and Time*, trans. J. Macquarrie and E. Robinson, Oxford: Blackwell.

Henriksen, M. (2013), 'On incomprehensibility in schizophrenia', *Phenomenology and the Cognitive Sciences*, 12 (10): 105–129.

Heraclitus ([5th century BC] 1908), 'Fragments', in ed. and trans. J. Burnet, *Early Greek Philosophy*, 2nd edn, 143–191, London: A & C Black.

Herrador Colmenero, L., J. M. Perez Marmol, C. Martí-García, M. de los A. Querol Zaldivar, R. M. Tapia Haro, A. M. Castro Sánchez and M. E. Aguilar-Ferrándiz (2018), 'Effectiveness of mirror therapy, motor imagery, and virtual feedback on phantom limb pain following amputation: A systematic review', *Prosthetics and Orthotics International*, 42 (3): 288–298.

Hertzberg, L. (2010), 'Attending to the actual sayings of things', in V. Munz, K. Puhl and J. Wang (eds), *Language and World: Part One: Essays on the Philosophy of Wittgenstein*, 125–134, Lancaster: Gazelle Books.

Hinshelwood, R. D. (1991), *A Dictionary of Kleinian Thought*, London: Free Association Books.

Hinton, J. M. (1967), 'Visual experiences', *Mind*, 76 (April): 217–227.

Hobson, P. (2002), *The Cradle of Thought*, London: Pan Macmillan.

Holmes, C. (1911), *Notes on the Science of Picture-Making*, London: Chatto & Windus.

Holzman, P. S., M. E. Shenton and M. R. Solovay (1986), 'Quality of thought disorder in differential diagnosis', *Schizophrenia Bulletin*, 12 (3): 360–372.

Hopkins, J. (2000), 'Psychoanalysis, metaphor, and the concept of mind', in M. Levin (ed.), *The Analytic Freud*, 11–35, London: Routledge.

Hornstein, G. (2000), *To Redeem One Person is to Redeem the World: The Life of Frieda Fromm-Reichmann*. New York: The Free Press.

Hornstein, G. (2002), 'Narratives of madness, as told from within', *Chronicle of Higher Education*, 25 January. Available online: https://www.chronicle.com/article/narratives-of-madness-as-told-from-within/ (accessed 30 January 2022).

Howes, C., M. Lavelle, P. Healey, J. Hough and R. McCabe (2017), 'Disfluencies in dialogues with patients with schizophrenia', *Proceedings of the 39th Annual Meeting of the Cognitive Science Society*. Available online: https://mindmodeling.org/cogsci2017/papers/0425/index.html (accessed 7 March 2021).

Hughlings Jackson, H. (1884), 'The Croonian lectures on evolution and dissolution of the nervous system. Lecture II', *British Medical Journal*, 1 (1214): 660–663.

Hughlings Jackson, H. (1888), 'Discussion at the neurological society on muscular hypertonicity in paralysis, on July 7, 1888', *Brain*, X: 312.

Hume, D. ([1739] 2000), *A Treatise of Human Nature*, Oxford: Oxford University Press.

Huq, S. F., P. A. Garety and D. R. Hemsley (1988), 'Probabilistic judgments in deluded and non-deluded subjects', *Quarterly Journal of Experimental Psychology A: Human Experimental Psychology*, 40(4): 801–812.

Husserl, E. ([1952] 1989) *Ideas Pertaining to a Pure Phenomenology and to a Phenomenological Philosophy: Second Book*, trans. R. Rojcewicz and A. Schuwer, Dordrecht: Kluwer Academic.

Husserl, E. ([1966] 1991), *On the Phenomenology of the Consciousness of Internal Time (1893–1917)*, trans. J. B. Brough, Dordrecht: Kluwer Academic.

Hyman, J. (1991), 'Visual experience and blindsight', in J. Hyman (ed.), *Investigating Psychology: Sciences of the Mind after Wittgenstein*, 166–200, London: Routledge.

Jacobson, E. (1954), 'On psychotic identifications', *International Journal of Psychoanalysis*, 35: 102–108.

Jalal, B. and V. S. Ramachandran (2014), 'Sleep paralysis and "the bedroom intruder": The role of the right superior parietal, phantom pain and body image projection', *Medical Hypotheses*, 83 (6): 755–757.

James, W. (1890), *Principles of Psychology*, vols 1 and 2, New York: Henry Holt.

James, W. (1902), *The Varieties of Religious Experience*, London: Longmans, Green.

Janet, P. (1889), *L'Automatisme Psychologique*, Paris: Felix Alcan.

Jardri, R., K. Hugdahl, M. Hughes, J. Brunelin, F. Waters, B. Alderson-Day, D. Smailes, P. Sterzer, P. R. Corlett, P. Leptourgos, M. Debbané, A. Cachia and S. Denève (2016), 'Are hallucinations due to an imbalance between excitatory and inhibitory influences on the brain?', *Schizophrenia Bulletin*, 42 (5): 1124–1134.

Jaspers, K. ([1935] 1955), *Reason and Existenz*, trans. W. Earle, New York: Noonday Press.

Jaspers, K. ([1959] 1963), *General Psychopathology*, trans. J. Hoenig and M. Hamilton, Manchester: Manchester University Press.

Jaspers, K. (1968), 'The phenomenological approach in psychiatry', *British Journal of Psychiatry*, 114 (516): 1313–1323.

Jeronimus, B. F. (2019), 'Dynamic system perspectives on anxiety and depression', in E. S. Kunnen, N. M. P. de Ruiter, B. F. Jeronimus and M. A. van der Gaag (eds), *Psychosocial Development in Adolescence: Insights from the Dynamic Systems Approach*, 100–126, London: Routledge.

Jones, B. W. (2012), 'Your brain develops the negative', *Webvision*, 7 June. Available online: https://webvision.med.utah.edu/2012/06/your-brain-develops-the-negative/ (accessed 16 June 2021).

Joyce, J. (1939), *Finnegans Wake*, London: Faber & Faber.

Jung, C. G. ([1907] 1991), *The Psychology of Dementia Praecox*, in C. Jung, *The Psychogenesis of Mental Disease*, trans. R. F. C. Hull, London: Routledge.

Jung, C. G. ([1932] 1966), 'Ulysses: A Monologue', in C. G. Jung, *The Spirit in Man, Art, and Literature*, Collected Works, vol. 15, 163–203, Princeton, NJ: Princeton University Press.

Jung, C. G. and A. Jaffé ([1962] 1993), *Memories, Dreams, Reflections*, London: Fontana.

Jung, C. G. (1964), 'Approaching the unconscious', in C. G. Jung, M.-L. von Franz, J. L. Henderson, A. Jaffé, and J. Jacobi, *Man and His Symbols*, Part 1, New York: Anchor Press.

Jung, C. G. (1978), *The Spirit in Man, Art and Literature*, Princeton, NJ: Princeton University Press.

Kanner, L. (1943), 'Autistic disturbances of affective contact', *Nervous Child*, 35 (4): 100–136.

Kanner, L. (1973), 'The birth of early infantile autism', *Journal of Autism and Childhood Schizophrenia*, 3 (2): 93–95.

Kant, I. ([1764] 2011), 'Essay on the Maladies of the Head', in P. Frierson and P. Guyer (eds), *Observations on the Feeling of the Beautiful and Sublime and Other Writings*, 205–217, Cambridge: Cambridge University Press.

Kant, I. ([1787] 1999), *Critique of Pure Reason*, 2nd edn, trans. P. Guyer and A. Wood, Cambridge: Cambridge University Press.

Kant, I. ([1798] 2006), *Anthropology from a Pragmatic Point of View*, trans. R. B. Louden, Cambridge: Cambridge University Press.

Katz, J. (2001), 'Phantom limbs', in N. J. Smelser and P. B. Baltes (eds), *International Encyclopedia of the Social & Behavioral Sciences*, 11353–11357, Oxford: Elsevier.

Keats, J. ([1820] 1899), *The Complete Poetical Works and Letters of John Keats*, Boston, MA: Houghton, Mifflin.

Kelleher, I., D. Connor, M. C. Clarke and N. Devlin (2012), 'Prevalence of psychotic symptoms in childhood and adolescence: A systematic review and meta-analysis of population-based studies', *Psychological Medicine*, 42 (9): 1857–1863.

Kendler, K. (2010), 'Advances in our understanding of genetic risk factors for autism spectrum disorders', *American Journal of Psychiatry*, 167 (11): 1291–1293.

Kendler, K. and J. Campbell (2009), 'Interventionist causal models in psychiatry: Repositioning the mind–body problem', *Psychological Medicine*, 39 (6): 881–887.

Kendler, K. and J. Campbell (2014), 'Expanding the domain of the understandable in psychiatric illness: An updating of the Jasperian framework of explanation and understanding', *Psychological Medicine*, 44 (1): 1–7.

Kimura, B. (1992), *Ecrits de Psychopathologie Phénoménologique*, trans. J. Bouderlique, Paris: Presses Universitaires de France.

Kirk, G. S. (1970), *Myth: Its Meaning and Functions in Ancient and Other Cultures*, London: Cambridge University Press.

Kirkbride, J. B., A. Errazuriz, T. J. Croudace, C. Morgan, D. Jackson, J. Boydell, R. Murray and P. Jones (2012), 'Incidence of schizophrenia and other psychoses in England, 1950–2009: A systematic review and meta-analyses', *PLoS ONE*, 7 (3): e31660. Available online: https://doi.org/10.1371/journal.pone.0031660.

Kirsner, D. (1990), 'An abyss of difference: Laing, Sartre and Jaspers', *Journal of the British Society for Phenomenology*, 21 (3): 209–215.

Kopelman, M. D., E. M. Guinan and P. D. R. Lewis (1995), 'Delusional memory, confabulation, and frontal lobe dysfunction: A case study in De Clérambault's syndrome', *Neurocase*, 1 (1): 71–77.

Kraepelin, E. (1919), *Dementia Praecox and Paraphrenia*, trans. R. Barclay and G. Robertson, Edinburgh: Livingstone.

Kretschmer, E. ([1922] 1945), *Physique and Character*, trans. W. J. H. Sprott, 2nd edn, London: Kegan Paul, Trench, Trubner.

Kring, A., G. Davison, J. Neale and S. Johnson (2007), *Abnormal Psychology*, 10th edn, New York: Wiley.

Kupfer, D. J., M. B. First and D. A. Regier (eds) (2002), *A Research Agenda for DSM-V*, Washington, DC: American Psychiatric Association Press.

Kupper, Z., F. Ramseyer, H. Hoffmann and W. Tschacher (2015), 'Nonverbal synchrony in social interactions of patients with schizophrenia indicates socio-communicative deficits', *PLoS ONE*, 10 (12): e0145882. Available online: https://journals.plos.org/plosone/article?id=10.1371/journal.pone.0145882.

Kusters, W. ([2014] 2020), *A Philosophy of Madness: The Experience of Psychotic Thinking*, trans. N. Forest-Flier, Cambridge, MA: MIT Press.

Lacan, J. (1966), *Écrits*, Paris: Seuil.

Laffal, J. (1982), 'Language competence and schizophrenic language', *Behavioral and Brain Sciences*, 5 (4): 604–605.

Laing, R. D. (1960), *The Divided Self: An Existential Study in Sanity and Madness*, London: Tavistock.

Laing, R. D. (1963), 'Minkowski and schizophrenia', *Review of Existential Psychology & Psychiatry*, 3 (3): 195–207.

Laing, R. D. (1964), 'Review of Karl Jaspers' "General Psychopathology"', *International Journal of Psychoanalysis*, 45: 590–593.

Laing, R. D. (1965), *The Divided Elf: An Existential Study in Sanity and Madness*, 2nd edn, Harmondsworth: Penguin.

Lakoff, G. and M. Johnson (1980), *Metaphors We Live By*, Chicago, IL: University of Chicago Press.

Landis, B. (1963) 'A Study of Ego Boundaries', PhD dissertation, New School for Social Research, New York.

Langer, S. (1942), *Philosophy in a New Key: A Study in the Symbolism of Reason, Rite, and Art*, Cambridge, MA: Harvard University Press.

Langer, S. (1953), *Feeling and Form,* London: Routledge & Kegan Paul.

Laplanche, J. and J. B. Pontalis (1988), *The Language of Psychoanalysis*, London: Karnac.

Leader, D. (2011), *What is Madness?*, London: Penguin.

Lévi-Strauss, C. ([1949] 1963), 'The effectiveness of symbols', in C. Lévi-Strauss, *Structural Anthropology*, 186–205, New York: Basic Books.

Levinas, E. (1969), *Totality and Infinity*, trans. A. Lingis, Pittsburgh, PA: Duquesne University Press.

Locke, J. ([1690] 1984), *An Essay Concerning Human Understanding*, London: Penguin.

Lucas, R. (2009), *The Psychotic Wavelength: A Psychoanalytic Perspective for Psychiatry*, Hove: Routledge.

Maher, B. A. (1974), 'Delusional thinking and perceptual disorder', *Journal of Individual Psychology*, 30 (1): 98–113.

Maher, B. A. (1988), 'Anomalous experience and delusional thinking: The logic of explanations', in T. F. Oltmanns and B. A. Maher (eds), *Delusional Beliefs*, 15–33, New York: Wiley.

Marr, D. (1982), *Vision*, San Francisco, CA: Freeman.

Marschall, T. M., S. G. Brederoo, B. Ćurčić-Blake and I. E. C. Sommer (2020), 'Deafferentation as a cause of hallucinations', *Current Opinion in Psychiatry*, 33 (3): 206–211.

Martindale, B. and A. Summers (2013), 'The psychodynamics of psychosis', *Advances in Psychiatric Treatment*, 19 (2): 124–131.

Mavromatis, A. (1987), *Hypnagogia: The Unique State of Consciousness Between Wakefulness and Sleep*, London: Routledge.

McAfee, L. (1989), 'Interview with Joanne Greenberg', in A.-L. S. Silver (ed.), *Psychoanalysis and Psychosis*, 513–533, Madison, CT: International Universities Press.

McCarthy-Jones, S. (2012), *Hearing Voices: The Histories, Causes and Meanings of Auditory Verbal Hallucinations*, Cambridge: Cambridge University Press.

McCarthy-Jones, S. (2017), *Can't You Hear Them? The Science and Significance of Hearing Voices*, London: Jessica Kingsley.

McDowell, J. (1982), 'Criteria, defeasibility and knowledge', *Proceedings of the British Academy*, 68: 455–479.

McGlone, M. S. (2011), 'Hyperbole, homunculi, and hindsight bias: An alternative evaluation of conceptual metaphor theory', *Discourse Processes*, 48 (8): 563–574.

McKenna, P. (2017), *Delusions: Understanding the Un-understandable*, Cambridge: Cambridge University Press.

Meehl, P. E. (1962), 'Schizotaxia, schiztypy, schizophrenia', *American Psychologist*, 17 (12): 827–838.

Meehl, P. E. (1990), 'Toward an integrated theory of schizotaxia, schizotypy, and schizophrenia', *Journal of Personality Disorders*, 4 (1): 1–99.

Mellor, C. S. (1970), 'First-rank symptoms of schizophrenia', *British Journal of Psychiatry*, 117 (1): 15–23.

Meltzer, D. and M. Harris Williams (2008), *The Apprehension of Beauty*, London: Karnac.

Meltzer, D. (2009), *Dream Life: A Re-examination of the Psychoanalytic Theory and Technique*, London: Karnac.

Merleau-Ponty, M. ([1945] 2012), *Phenomenology of Perception*, trans. D. A. Landes, Abingdon: Routledge.

Merleau-Ponty, M. ([1964] 1968), *The Visible and the Invisible*, trans. A. Lingis, Evanston, IL: Northwestern University Press.

Metzinger, T. (2004), *Being No One: The Self-Model Theory of Subjectivity*, Cambridge, MA: MIT Press.

Midgley, M. (1973), 'The concept of beastliness', *Philosophy*, 48 (184): 111–135.

Milner, M. (1957), *On Not Being Able to Paint*, Los Angeles, CA: J. P. Tarcher.

Milton, J., S. Amin, S. P. Singh, G. Harrison, P. Jones, T. Croudace, I. Medley and J. Brewin (2001), 'Aggressive incidents in first-episode psychosis', *British Journal of Psychiatry*, 178 (5): 433–440.

Minkowska, F. (1925), 'Troubles essentiels de la schizophrénie dans leurs rapports avec les données de lay psychologie et de la biologie modernes', *L'Évolution Psychiatrique*, 1: 127–141.

Minkowski, E. ([1927] 1987), 'The essential disorder underlying schizophrenia and schizophrenic thought', in J. Cutting and M. Shepherd (eds), *The Clinical Roots of the Schizophrenia Concept*, 188–212, Cambridge: Cambridge University Press.

Minkowski, E. (1953), *La Schizophrénie: Psychopathologie des Schizoïdes et des Schizophrènes*, 2nd edn, Paris: De Brouwer.

Minkowski, E. and R. Targowla (2001), 'A contribution to the study of autism: The interrogative attitude', trans. S. Ziadeh, *Philosophy, Psychiatry, & Psychology*, 8 (4): 271–278.

Minor, K. S., M. P. Marggraf, B. J. Davis, N. F. Mehdiyoun and A. Breier (2016), 'Affective systems induce formal thought disorder in early-stage psychosis', *Journal of Abnormal Psychology*, 125 (4): 537–542.

Mishara, A. (2010), 'Klaus Conrad (1905–1961): Delusional mood, psychosis, and beginning schizophrenia', *Schizophrenia Bulletin*, 36 (1): 9–13.

Morgan, C. J., M. J. Coleman, A. Ulgen, L. Boling, J. O. Cole, F. V. Johnson, J. Lerbinger, J. A. Bodkin, P. S. Holzman and D. L. Levy (2017), 'Thought disorder in schizophrenia and bipolar disorder probands, their relatives, and nonpsychiatric controls', *Schizophrenia Bulletin*, 43 (3): 523–535.

Moritz, S. and T. S. Woodward (2005), 'Jumping to conclusions in delusional and non-delusional schizophrenic patients', *British Journal of Clinical Psychology*, 44 (2): 193–207.

Morris, K. (2012), *Starting with Merleau-Ponty*, London: Continuum.

Moskowitz, A. and G. Heim (2011), 'Eugen Bleuler's "Dementia Praecox or the Group of Schizophrenias" (1911): A centenary appreciation and reconsideration', *Schizophrenia Bulletin*, 37 (3): 471–479.

Moyal-Sharrock, D. (2004), *Understanding Wittgenstein's 'On Certainty'*, London: Palgrave Macmillan.

Moyal-Sharrock, D. (2016), 'The animal in epistemology', *International Journal for the Study of Skepticism*, 6 (2–3): 97–119.

Murdoch, I. (1999), 'Metaphysics and ethics', in P. Conradi (ed.), *Existentialists and Mystics*, 59–75, New York: Penguin.

Murphy, D. (2012), *Psychiatry in the Scientific Image*, Cambridge, MA: MIT Press.

Nagel, E. (1943), 'Review of "Philosophy in a New Key" by Susanne K. Langer', *Journal of Philosophy*, 40 (12): 323–329.

Narboux, J.-P. (2018), 'Is self-consciousness consciousness of one's self?', in O. Kuusela, M. Ometita and T. Uçan (eds), *Wittgenstein and Phenomenology*, 197–247, New York: Routledge.

National Institute of Mental Health (NIMH) (2021), 'Schizophrenia'. Available online: https://www.nimh.nih.gov/health/publications/schizophrenia/index.shtml (accessed 13 June 2021).

Nelson, B., J. Parnas and L. Sass (2014), 'Disturbance of minimal self (ipseity) in schizophrenia: Clarification and current status', *Schizophrenia Bulletin*, 40 (3): 479–482.

Nielssen, O. and M. Large (2010), 'Rates of homicide during the first episode of psychosis and after treatment: A systematic review and meta-analysis', *Schizophrenia Bulletin*, 36 (4): 702–712.

Nietzsche, F. ([1887] 1969), *On the Genealogy of Morals*, New York: Vintage Books.

Noë, A. (2004), *Action in Perception*, Cambridge, MA: MIT Press.

Notredame, C.-E., D. Pins, S. Deneve and R. Jardri (2014), 'What visual illusions teach us about schizophrenia', *Frontiers in Integrative Neuroscience*, 8: 63. Available online: https://doi.org/10.3389/fnint.2014.00063 (accessed 28 April 2021).

O'Brien, B. ([1958] 1976), *Operators and Things: The Inner Life of a Schizophrenic*, London: Sphere.

Ogden, T. H. (2007), 'On talking as dreaming', *International Journal of Psychoanalysis*, 88 (3): 575–589.

Olson, P. R., J. A. Suddeth, P. I. Peterson and C. Egelhoff (1985), 'Hallucinations of widowhood', *Journal of the American Geriatrics Society*, 33 (8): 543–547.

O'Regan, J. K. and A. Noë (2001), 'A sensorimotor account of vision and visual consciousness', *Behavioral and Brain Sciences*, 24 (5): 939–973.

Overgaard, S. (2020), 'How not to think of perception', *Harvard Review of Philosophy*, 27: 121–132.

Panksepp, J. (1998), *Affective Neuroscience: The Foundations of Human and Animal Emotions*, Oxford: Oxford University Press.

Parnas, J. and P. Bovet (1991), 'Autism in schizophrenia revisited', *Comprehensive Psychiatry*, 32 (1): 7–21.

Parnas, J. (2000), 'The self and intentionality in the pre-psychotic stages of schizophrenia: A phenomenological study', in D. Zahavi (ed.), *Exploring the Self: Philosophical and Psychopathological Perspectives on Self-Experience*, 115–147, Philadelphia, PA: John Benjamins.

Parnas, J., P. Bovet and D. Zahavi (2002), 'Schizophrenic autism: Clinical phenomenology and pathogenetic implications', *World Psychiatry*, 1 (3): 131–136.

Parnas, J., P. Møller, T. Kircher, J. Thalbitzer, L. Jansson, P. Handest and D. Zahavi (2005), 'EASE: Examination of anomalous self-experience', *Psychopathology*, 38 (5): 236–258.

Parnas, J. and M. G. Henriksen (2014), 'Disordered self in the schizophrenia spectrum: A clinical and research perspective', *Harvard Review of Psychiatry*, 22 (5): 251–265.

Parnas, J., J. Carter and J. Nordgaard (2016), 'Premorbid self-disorders and lifetime diagnosis in the schizophrenia spectrum: A prospective high risk study', *Early Intervention in Psychiatry*, 10 (1): 45–53.

Pelletier, M. (1903), *L'Association des Idées dans la Manie Aigue et dans la Débilité Mentale*, Paris: J. Rousset.

Peterson, D. (ed.) (1982), *A Mad People's History of Madness*, Pittsburgh, PA: University of Pittsburgh Press.

Petocz, A. (1999), *Freud, Psychoanalysis and Symbolism*, Cambridge: Cambridge University Press.

Petocz, A. (2019), 'Symbolism, the primary process, and dreams: Freud's contributions', in R. G. T. Gipps and M. Lacewing (eds), *The Oxford Handbook of Philosophy and Psychoanalysis*, 255–280, Oxford: Oxford University Press.

Pettersson-Yeo, W., P. Allen, S. Benetti, P. McGuire and A. Mechelli (2010), 'Dysconnectivity in schizophrenia: Where are we now?', *Neuroscience & Biobehavioral Reviews*, 35 (5): 1110–1124.

Phillips, D. Z. (2000), *Recovering Religious Concepts, Closing Epistemic Divides*, Basingstoke: Macmillan.

Pick, A. ([1904] 1996), 'On the pathology of the consciousness of the self', trans. R. Vivani and G.E. Berrios, *History of Psychiatry*, vii: 319–332.

Pickering, N. (2006) *The Metaphor of Mental Illness*, Oxford: Oxford University Press.

Pienkos, E. and L. Sass (2016), 'Expressions of alienation: Language and interpersonal experience in schizophrenia', *Journal of Psychopathology*, 22: 62–71.

Pintner, R. (1913), 'Inner speech during silent reading', *Psychological Review*, 20 (2): 129–153.

Polster, S. (1983), 'Ego boundary as process', *Psychiatry*, 46 (3): 247–258.

Porcher, J. E. (2019), 'Double bookkeeping and doxasticism about delusion', *Philosophy, Psychiatry, & Psychology*, 26 (2): 111–119.

Powers, A. R., C. Mathys and P. R. Corlett (2017), 'Pavlovian conditioning-induced hallucinations result from overweighting of perceptual priors', *Science*, 357 (6351): 596–600.

Radden, J. (2011), *On Delusion*, London: Routledge.

Radden, J. (2019), 'Mental disorder (illness)', *Stanford Encyclopedia of Philosophy*. Available online: https://plato.stanford.edu/entries/mental-disorder/ (accessed 16 February 2021).

Ramachandram, V. S. and W. Hirstein (1998), 'The perception of phantom limbs', *Brain*, 121 (9): 1603–1630.

Ratcliffe, M. (2017), *Real Hallucinations: Psychiatric Illness, Intentionality, and the Interpersonal World*, Cambridge, MA: MIT Press.

Ratcliffe, M. and S. Wilkinson (2015), 'Thought insertion clarified', *Journal of Consciousness Studies*, 22 (11–12): 246–269.

Ratcliffe, M. (2019), 'Auditory verbal hallucinations and their phenomenological context', in G. Stanghellini, M. Broome, A. Raballo, A. V. Fernandez, P. Fusar-Poli and R. Rosfort (eds), *The Oxford Handbook of Phenomenological Psychopathology*, 789–802, Oxford: Oxford University Press.

Ray, W. (2015), *Abnormal Psychology*, London: Sage.

Read, R. (2001), 'On approaching schizophrenia through Wittgenstein', *Philosophical Psychology*, 14 (4): 449–475.

Reddy, V. (2008), *How Infants Know Minds*, London: Harvard University Press.

Rhees, R. (ed.) (1984), *Recollections of Wittgenstein*, Oxford: Oxford University Press.

Rhodes, J. and S. Jakes (2004), 'The contribution of metaphor and metonymy to delusions', *Psychology and Psychotherapy*, 77 (1): 1–17.

Rhodes, J. and R. G. T. Gipps (2008), 'Delusions, certainty, and the background', *Philosophy, Psychiatry, & Psychology*, 15 (4): 295–310.

Rochester, S. and J. R. Martin (1979), *Crazy Talk: A Study of the Discourse of Schizophrenic Speakers*, New York: Plenum Press.

Rodriguez McRobbie, L. (2013), 'The strange and mysterious history of the Ouija board', *The Smithsonian Magazine*, 27 October. Available online: www.smithsonianmag.com/history/the-strange-and-mysterious-history-of-the-ouija-board-5860627/ (accessed 14 April 2021).

Roessler, J. (2013), 'Thought insertion, self-awareness, and rationality', in K. W. M. Fulford, M. Davies, R. G. T. Gipps, G. Graham, G. Stanghellini and T. Thornton (eds), *The Oxford Handbook of Philosophy and Psychiatry*, 658–672, Oxford: Oxford University Press.

Romme, M., S. Escher, J. Dillon, D. Corstens and M. Porris (2009), *Living with Voices: 50 Stories of Recovery*, Ross on Wye: PCCS Books.

Romme, M. and S. Escher (eds) (2012), *Psychosis as a Personal Crisis: An Experience-Based Approach*, Hove: Routledge.

Rosenfeld, H. (1965), *Psychotic States: A Psychoanalytic Approach*, London: Hogarth Press.

Rossi Monti, M. (1998), 'Whatever happened to delusional perception?', *Psychopathology*, 31 (5): 225–233.

Roth, M. (2017), 'Projective identification and relatedness: A Kleinian perspective', *Psychoanalytic Perspectives*, 14 (3): 350–355.

Rümke, H. C. ([1941] 1990), 'The nuclear symptom of schizophrenia and the praecox feeling', *History of Psychiatry*, 1 (3): 331–341.

Rushton, P. (1988), 'Lunatics and idiots: Mental disability, the community, and the poor law in north-east England, 1600–1800', *Medical History*, 32 (1): 34–50.

Rutter, D. R. (1982), 'Language in schizophrenia: A social psychological perspective', *Behavioral and Brain Sciences*, 5 (4): 612–613.

Ryle, G. ([1945] 2009), 'Philosophical arguments', in J. Tanney (ed.), *Collected Essays of Gilbert Ryle 1929–1968*, 203–221, Abingdon: Routledge.

Ryle, G. ([1962] 2009), 'Abstractions', in J. Tanney (ed.), *Collected Essays of Gilbert Ryle 1929–1968*, 448–458, Abingdon: Routledge.

Ryle, G. ([1966–67] 2009), 'Thinking and reflecting', in J. Tanney (ed.), *Collected Essays of Gilbert Ryle 1929–1968*, 479–493, Abingdon: Routledge.

Sacks, O. (2012), *Hallucinations*, London: Picador.

Sandis, C. (2012), *The Things We Do and Why We Do Them*, New York: Palgrave Macmillan.

Saks, E. R. (2007), *The Center Cannot Hold*, New York: Hyperion.

Sartre, J.-P. ([1940] 2004), *The Imaginary: A Phenomenological Psychology of the Imagination*, London: Routledge.

Sartre, J.-P. ([1943] 2018), *Being and Nothingness*, trans. S. Richmond, London: Routledge.

Sass, L. A. (1992), *Madness and Modernism: Insanity in the Light of Modern Art, Literature, and Thought*, New York: Basic Books.

Sass, L. A. (1994), *The Paradoxes of Delusion: Wittgenstein, Schreber, and the Schizophrenic Mind*, Ithaca, NY: Cornell University Press.

Sass, L. A. (1995), 'Antonin Artaud, modernism, and the yearning for a "private language"', in K. S. Johannessen and T. Nordenstam (eds), *Culture and Value* (papers from 18th International Wittgenstein Symposium), Kirchberg, Austria: Austrian Ludwig Wittgenstein Society.

Sass, L. A. (2003), 'Incomprehensibility and understanding: On the interpretation of severe mental illness', *Philosophy, Psychiatry, & Psychology*, 10 (2): 125–132.

Sass, L. A. and J. Parnas (2003), 'Schizophrenia, consciousness, and the self', *Schizophrenia Bulletin*, 29 (3): 427–444.

Sass, L. A. (2007), '"Schizophrenic person" or "person with schizophrenia"? An essay on illness and the self', *Theory & Psychology*, 17 (3): 395–420.

Sass, L. A. and E. Pienkos (2013), 'Delusion', in K. W. M. Fulford, M. Davies, R. G. T. Gipps, G. Graham, J. Z. Sadler, G. Stanghellini and T. Thornton (eds), *The Oxford Handbook of Philosophy and Psychiatry*, 632–657, Oxford: Oxford University Press.

Sass, L. A. (2014a), 'Self-disturbance and schizophrenia: Structure, specificity, pathogenesis', *Schizophrenia Research*, 152 (1): 5–11.

Sass, L. A. (2014b), 'Delusion and double bookkeeping', in T. Fuchs, T. Breyer and C. Mundt (eds), *Karl Jaspers' Philosophy and Psychopathology*, 125–147, New York: Springer.

Sass, L. A. and G. Byrom (2015), 'Phenomenological and neurocognitive perspectives on delusions: A critical overview', *World Psychiatry*, 14 (2): 164–173.

Sass, L. A. and J. Parnas (2017), 'Thought disorder, subjectivity, and the self', *Schizophrenia Bulletin*, 43 (3): 497–502.

Sass, L. A., E. Pienkos, B. Skodlar, G. Stanghellini, T. Fuchs, J. Parnas and N. Jones (2017), 'EAWE: Examination of anomalous world experience', *Psychopathology*, 50 (1): 10–54.

Scharfetter, C. (1995), 'The self-experience of schizophrenics: Empirical studies of the ego/self in schizophrenia, borderline disorders and depression', Zürich: Private Publication.

Scharfetter, C. (2001), 'Eugen Bleuler's schizophrenias – synthesis of various concepts', *Schweiz Archiv für Neurologie und Psychiatrie*, 152: 34–37.

Schmidt, G. ([1940] 1987), 'A review of the German literature on delusion between 1914 and 1939', in J. Cutting and M. Shepherd (eds), *The Clinical Roots of the Schizophrenia Concept: Translations of Seminal European Contributions on Schizophrenia*, 104–134, Cambridge: Cambridge University Press.

Schmidt, G. (1941), 'Zum Wahnproblem', *Zeitschrift für die gesamte Neurologie und Psychiatrie*, 171: 570–590.

Schneider, J. A. (2010), 'From Freud's dream-work to Bion's work of dreaming: The changing conception of dreaming in psychoanalytic theory', *International Journal of Psychoanalysis*, 91 (3): 521–540.

Schneider, K. (1959), *Clinical Psychopathology*, trans. M. W. Hamilton, New York: Grune & Stratton.

Schopenhauer, A. ([1819] 1969), *The World as Will and Representation*, vol. 1, trans. E. F. J. Payne, New York: Dover.

Schopenhauer, A. ([1851] 2014), 'Essay on spirit-seeing and related issues', *Parerga and Paralipomena: Volume 1: Short Philosophical Essays*, 198–272, trans. S. Roehr and C. Janaway, Cambridge: Cambridge University Press.

Schreber, D. P. ([1903] 1988), *Memoirs of My Nervous Illness*, trans. I. Macalpine and R. A. Hunter, Cambridge, MA: Harvard University Press.

Schultz, G. and R. Meltzack (1991), 'The Charles Bonnet syndrome: "Phantom visual images"', *Perception*, 20 (6): 809–825.

Searles, H. F. (1961), 'Schizophrenic communication', *Psychoanalysis and the Psychoanalytic Review*, 48 (1): 3–50.

Searles, H. F. (1962), 'The differentiation between concrete and metaphorical thinking in the recovering schizophrenic patient', *Journal of the American Psychoanalytic Association*, 10 (1): 22–49.

Séchehaye, M. ([1950] 1951), *Autobiography of a Schizophrenic Girl*, trans. G. Rubin-Rabson, New York: Grune & Stratton.

Séchehaye, M. (1956), *A New Psychotherapy in Schizophrenia*, trans. G. Rubin-Rabson, New York: Grune & Stratton.

Segal, H. ([1957] 1981), 'Notes on symbol formation', in H. Segal, *The Work of Hannah Segal*, 49–65, New York: Jason Aronson.

Segal, H. (1990), *The Work of Hanna Segal: A Kleinian Approach to Clinical Practice*, Northvale, NJ: Jason Aronson.

Seiguer, G. H. (1990), 'Omnipotence in the works of Melanie Klein', *Melanie Klein & Object Relations*, 8 (1): 81–98.

Sheets-Johnstone, M. (2020), 'The lived body', *Humanist Psychologist*, 48 (1): 28–53.

Smith, M. (2013), 'Anti-stigma campaigns: Time to change', *British Journal of Psychiatry*, 202 (suppl. 55): s49–s50.

Snowdon, P. (1990) 'The objects of perceptual experience', *Proceedings of the Aristotelian Society, Supplementary Volume*, 64: 121–150.

Soares-Weiser, K., N. Maayan, H. Bergman, C. Davenport, A. J. Kirkham, S. Grabowski and C. E. Adams (2015), 'First rank symptoms for schizophrenia (Cochrane test diagnostic accuracy review)', *Schizophrenia Bulletin*, 41 (4): 792–794.

Spitzer, M. (1990), 'On defining delusions', *Comprehensive Psychiatry*, 31 (5): 377–397.

Spitzer, R. L., J. Endicott and J.-A. Micoulaud Franchi (2018), 'Medical and mental disorder: Proposed definition and criteria', *Annales Médico-Psychologiques, Revue Psychiatrique*, 176: 656–665.

Sprong, M., P. Schothorst, E. Vos, J. Hox and H. van Engeland (2007), 'Theory of mind in schizophrenia: Meta-analysis', *British Journal of Psychiatry*, 191 (1): 5–13.

Stanghellini, G. and J. Cutting (2003), 'Auditory verbal hallucinations – breaking the silence of inner dialogue', *Psychopathology*, 36 (3): 120–128.

Stanghellini, G. (2004), *Disembodied Spirits and Deanimated Bodies: The Psychopathology of Common Sense*, Oxford: Oxford University Press.

Stanghellini, G. and A. Ballerini (2007), 'Values in persons with schizophrenia', *Schizophrenia Bulletin*, 33 (1): 131–141.

Stanghellini, G. and A. Ballerini (2011), 'What is it like to be a person with schizophrenia in the social world? A first-person perspective study on schizophrenic dissociality – Part 2: Methodological issues and empirical findings', *Psychopathology*, 44 (3): 183–192.

Stanghellini, G. and T. Fuchs (2013), *One Century of Karl Jaspers' General Psychopathology*, Oxford: Oxford University Press.

Stein, M. (2021), 'Symbols and the transformation of the psyche'. Available online: http://www.murraystein.com/symbols.shtml (accessed 18 July 2021).

Steinman, I. (2019), 'The current state of psychodynamic treatment of psychosis', in R. Lombardi, L. Rinaldi and S. Thanopulos (eds), *Psychoanalysis of the Psychoses: Current Developments in Theory and Practice*, 247–258, Abingdon: Routledge.

Stephens, G. L. and G. Graham (1994), 'Self-consciousness, mental agency, and the clinical psychopathology of thought insertion', *Philosophy, Psychiatry, & Psychology*, 1 (1): 1–10.

Stephens, G. L. and G. Graham (2000), *When Self-Consciousness Breaks: Alien Voices and Inserted Thoughts*, Cambridge, MA: MIT Press.

Sterzer, P., A. L. Mishara, M. Voss and A. Heinz (2016), 'Thought insertion as a self-disturbance: An integration of predictive coding and phenomenological approaches', *Frontiers in Human Neuroscience*, 10: 502. Available online: https://doi.org/10.3389/fnhum.2016.00502.

Sterzer, P., R. A. Adams, P. Fletcher, C. Frith, S. M. Lawrie, L. Muckli, P. Petrovic, P. Uhlhaas, M. Voss and P. R. Corlett (2018), 'The predictive coding account of psychosis', *Biological Psychiatry*, 84 (9): 634–643.

Stokes, A. (2014), *Art and Analysis: An Adrian Stokes Reader*, ed. M. Harris Williams, London: Karnac.

Storch, A. (1924), *The Primitive Archaic Forms of Inner Experience and Thought in Schizophrenia*, New York: Nervous & Mental Diseases Publishing Company.

Storr, A. (1991), *Jung*, New York: Routledge.

Strauss, J. S. (1991), 'The meaning of schizophrenia: Compared to what?', in W. F. Flack, D. R. Miller and M. Wiener (eds), *What is Schizophrenia?*, 81–90, New York: Springer.

Sullivan, H. S. ([1956] 1973), *Clinical Studies in Psychiatry*, New York: Norton.

Sullivan, H. S. (1962), *Schizophrenia as a Human Process*, New York: Norton.

Szasz, T. (1987), *Insanity: The Idea and Its Consequences*, New York: Wiley.

Szasz, T. (1996), '"Audible thoughts" and "speech defect" in schizophrenia: A note on reading and translating Bleuler *Traduttori traditori*', *British Journal of Psychiatry*, 168 (5): 533–535.

Taine, H. ([1870] 1889), *De l'intelligence*, vols 1 and 2, trans. T. D. Haye, Paris: Librairie Hachette et Cie.

Tausk, V. ([1919] 1933), 'On the origin of the "influencing machine" in schizophrenia', *Psychoanalytic Quarterly*, 2 (3–4): 519–556.

Teichmann, R. (2015), *Wittgenstein on Thought and Will*, Abingdon: Routledge.

Teichmann, R. (2017), '"Not a something"', *Nordic Wittgenstein Review*, 6: 9–30.

Teichmann, R. (2021), 'Conceptual corruption', in M. Balaska (ed.), *Cora Diamond on Ethics*, 33–55, London: Palgrave Macmillan.

Thompson, M. (2008), *Life and Action*, Cambridge, MA: Harvard University Press.

Thornton, T. (1998), *Wittgenstein on Language and Thought*, Edinburgh: Edinburgh University Press.

Thornton, T. (2002), 'Thought insertion, cognitivism and inner space', *Cognitive Neuropsychiatry*, 7 (3): 237–249.

Thornton, T. (2004), 'Wittgenstein and the limits of empathic understanding in psychopathology', *International Review of Psychiatry*, 16 (3): 216–224.

Thornton, T. (2007), *Essential Philosophy of Psychiatry*, Oxford: Oxford University Press.

Thornton, T. (2008), 'Why the idea of framework propositions cannot contribute to an understanding of delusions', *Phenomenology and the Cognitive Sciences*, 7 (2): 157–175.

Trepper, T. and G. Shean (2013), *Understanding and Treating Schizophrenia*, London: Routledge.

Truly, Madly, Deeply (1990), [Film] Dir. A. Minghella, UK: BBC Films.

Turner, D. (1995), *The Darkness of God: Negativity in Christian Mysticism*, Cambridge: Cambridge University Press.

Urfer, A. (2001), 'Phenomenology and psychopathology of schizophrenia: The views of Eugene Minkowski', *Philosophy, Psychiatry, & Psychology*, 8 (4): 279–289.

van Duppen, Z. (2017), 'The intersubjective dimension of schizophrenia', *Philosophy, Psychiatry, & Psychology*, 24 (4): 399–418.

von Domarus, E. ([1944] 1964), 'The specific laws of logic in schizophrenia', in J. S. Kasanin (ed.), *Language and Thought in Schizophrenia*, 104–114, Berkeley, CA: University of California Press.

von Helmholtz, H. ([1860] 1962), *Treatise on Physiological Optics*, vol. III, New York: Dover.

von Herder, J. G. ([1772] 2002), *Treatise on the Origin of Language*, in J. G. von Herder, *Philosophical Writings*, trans. M. Forster, 65–166, Cambridge: Cambridge University Press.

Wahlberg K. E., L. C. Wynne, H. Oja, P. Keskitalo, L. Pykäläinen, I. Lahti, J. Moring, M. Naarala, A. Sorri, M. Seitamaa, K. Läksy, J. Kolassa and P. Tienari (1997), 'Gene-environment interaction in vulnerability to schizophrenia: Findings from the Finnish Adoptive Family Study of Schizophrenia', *American Journal of Psychiatry*, 154 (3): 355–362.

Wakefield, J. C. (1992), 'The concept of mental disorder: On the boundary between biological and social values', *American Psychologist*, 47 (3): 373–388.

Walker, C. (1991), 'Delusion: What did Jaspers really say?', *British Journal of Psychiatry*, 159 (suppl. 14): 94–103.

Ward, C. (2020), *Between Sickness and Health: The Landscape of Wellness and Illness*, Abingdon: Routledge.

Watson, G. D., P. C. Chandarana and H. Merskey (1981), 'Relationships between pain and schizophrenia', *British Journal of Psychiatry*, 138 (1): 33–36.

Watters, E. and R. Ofshe (1999), *Therapy's Delusions: The Myth of the Unconscious and the Exploitation of Today's Walking Worried*, New York: Scribner.

Weiskrantz, L. (1997), *Consciousness Lost and Found: A Neuropsychological Exploration*, Oxford: Oxford University Press.

West, J. (1983), 'Play therapy with Rosy', *British Journal of Social Work*, 13 (6): 645–661.

West, L. J. (1975), 'A clinical and theoretical overview of hallucinatory phenomena', in R. K. Siegel and L. J. West (eds), *Hallucinations: Behavior, Experience, and Theory*, 287–311, Chichester: Wiley.

Wiese, W. and T. Metzinger (2017), 'Vanilla PP for philosophers: A primer on predictive processing', in T. Metzinger and W. Wiese (eds), *Philosophy and Predictive Processing: 1*. Frankfurt am Main: MIND Group.

Wilber, K. (1982), 'The pre/trans fallacy', *Journal of Humanistic Psychology*, 22 (2): 5–43.

Williams, B. ([1976] 1981), 'Persons, character and morality', in B. Williams, *Moral Luck*, 1–19, Cambridge: Cambridge University Press.

Wittgenstein, L. (1958a), *Philosophical Investigations*, trans. G. E. M. Anscombe, Oxford: Blackwell.

Wittgenstein, L. (1958b), *The Blue & Brown Books*, Oxford: Blackwell

Wittgenstein, L. (1968), 'II: Notes for lectures on "Private Experience" and "Sense Data"', *Philosophical Review*, 77 (3): 275–320.

Wittgenstein, L. (1969), *On Certainty*, trans. G. E. M. Anscombe and G. H. von Wright, Oxford: Blackwell.

Wittgenstein, L. (1980a), *Remarks on the Philosophy of Psychology*, vol. I, trans. C. G. Luckhardt and M. A. E. Aue, Oxford: Blackwell.

Wittgenstein, L. (1980b), *Remarks on the Philosophy of Psychology*, vol. II, trans. C. G. Luckhardt and M. A. E. Aue, Oxford: Blackwell.

Wittgenstein, L. (1980c), *Culture and Value*, trans. P. Winch, Oxford: Blackwell.

Wittgenstein, L. (1981), *Zettel*, trans. G. E. M. Anscombe, Oxford: Blackwell.

Wittgenstein, L. (1993), *Last Writings on the Philosophy of Psychology*, vol.e 2, trans. C. G. Luckhardt and M. A. E. Aue, Oxford: Blackwell.

Wittgenstein, L. (2013), *Big Typescript*, Oxford: Blackwell.

Wollheim, R. (1980a), *Art and its Objects*, 2nd edn, Cambridge: Cambridge University Press.

Wollheim, R. (1980b), 'Seeing-as, seeing-in, and pictorial representation', in R. Wolheim, *Art and its Objects*, 205–226, 2nd edn, Cambridge: Cambridge University Press.

Wollheim, R. (1980c), 'Criticism as retrieval', in R. Wollheim, *Art and its Objects*, 2nd edn, 124–136, Cambridge: Cambridge University Press.

Woods, A. (2011), '"I suffer in an unknown manner that is hieroglyphical". Jung and Babette en route to Freud and Schreber', *History of the Present*, 1 (2): 244–258.

Woodward, J. F. (2008), 'Cause and explanation in psychiatry', in K. Kendler and J. Parnas (eds), *Philosophical Issues in Psychiatry: Explanation, Phenomenology and Nosology*, 132–195, Baltimore, MD: Johns Hopkins University Press.

Wundt, W. (1874), *Grundzüge der Physiologischen Psychologie*, Leipzig: Engelmann.

Yalom, I. (2002), *The Gift of Therapy*, New York: Harper Collins.

Yeats, W. B. (1889), *The Wanderings of Oisin, and Other Poems*, London: Kegan Paul.

Yeats, W. B. (1920), *Michael Robartes and the Dancer*, Dundrum: The Cuala Press.

Zahavi, D. (2000), 'Self and consciousness', in D. Zahavi (ed.), *Exploring the Self*, 55–74, Amsterdam: John Benjamins.

Index

splitting 95, 110, 116, 156, 157, 160,
218 n.4, 220 n.38, 221 n.48,
222 n.17
Stanghellini, Giovanni 207 n.27, 208 n.31,
220 n.27, 231 n.47, 231 n.49
Stephens, G. Lynn 219 n.8, 220 n.34–35
stigma 23–25
Straub, Babette 149–150, 154, 157,
161–164, 167, 232 n.6
Sullivan, Harry Stack 159, 229 n.25,
229 n.32, 231 n.47
suffering 20, 21–23, 143–147, 205 n.27
symbolization 10, 167–186, 231 n.2,
233 n.24, 234 n.37, 234 n.45
as substitution 181–182
Szasz, Thomas 205 n.14, 212 n.23

tacit reasoning 63–64
Taine, Hippolyte 224 n.6
Tausk, Victor 114, 221 n.3
Teichmann, Roger 211 n.6, 218 n.64,
223 n.34, 228 n.11, 229 n.22
Thompson, Michael 210 n.54
Thornton, Tim 206 n.42, 211 n.18,
211 n.19–22, 217–218 n.63–64,
220 n.28, 221 n.39, 222 n.26,
228 n.10, 236 n.12, 236 n.12
thought 153–155, 158–161, 165–166,
203 n.13, 228 n.11–13, 229 n.23
disorder *see* formal thought disorder
insertion 104, 109
totalizing 49
transitivism 115–117, 120, 121, 125,
222 n.9, 222 n.17

understandability/ununderstandability
psychological/motivational 37, 46–48,
166, 184, 185; *see also* motivation

rational/empathic 8, 23–24, 29, 31,
34–40, 46, 48–50, 55–56, 60, 66–67,
89, 105–106, 110–111, 120,
124–125, 155, 165–166, 183, 186,
187, 208 n.29, 208 n.31, 208 n.33,
208 n.36, 218 n.64, 235 n.4
understanding *see* thought
unreality 33, 52–53, 69, 70, 87, 108, 140,
221 n.43

violence 23, 199
von Domarus, Eilhard 191–192, 194, 195,
236 n.11

Wakefield, Jerome 206 n.42
Walker, Chris 207 n.7, 208 n.31
West, Janet 234 n.27–28
West, Louis Jolyon 142, 227 n.40
Williams, Bernard 213 n.42, 230 n.39
Wittgenstein, Ludwig 6, 11, 57–62, 89,
203 n.5, 203 n.12, 204 n.16,
204 n.20, 204 n.8, 205 n.13,
205 n.16, 205 n.17, 208 n.32,
211 n.14–16, 212 n.24–26, 212 n.30,
212 n.32–37, 212 n.41, 213 n.46–47,
214 n.18, 218 n.69, 220 n.22,
220 n.33, 220 n.36, 221 n.42–43,
228 n.11, 229 n.23, 236 n.22,
236 n.25, 237 n.27
Wollheim, Richard 203 n.6, 230 n.46,
233 n.24

Yalom, Irving 179, 234 n 35–36
Yeats, William Butler 76, 77, 78, 94, 95,
214 n.13, 218 n.1

Zahavi, Dan 214 n.8, 214 n.16, 216 n.36,
220 n.27